INTRODUCTION
TO
HEALTH PLANNING

Introduction to
HEALTH
PLANNING

THIRD EDITION

PHILIP N. REEVES
DAVID F. BERGWALL
NINA B. WOODSIDE

INFORMATION RESOURCES PRESS
Arlington, Virginia
1984

Available from
Information Resources Press
1700 North Moore Street
Suite 700
Arlington, Virginia 22209

Library of Congress Catalog Card Number 84-080535
ISBN 0-87815-050-1

CONTENTS

LIST OF FIGURES

LIST OF TABLES

ACRONYMS

ACIR	Advisory Commission on Intergovernmental Relations
ADC	Average daily census
AHA	American Hospital Association
AIP	Annual implementation plan
BLS	Bureau of Labor Statistics
CCU	Coronary care unit
CEO	Chief executive officer
CFF	Community funds flow
CHP	Comprehensive health planning
CON	Certificate of need
COO	Chief operating officer
CPI	Consumer price index
CRT	Cathode ray tube
DARE	Decision alternative rational evaluation
DHEW	Department of Health, Education, and Welfare
DHHS	Department of Health and Human Services
DRA	Actual death rate
DRE	Expected death rate
DRG	Diagnosis-related group
DSS	Decision support system
EMS	Emergency medical system
GIGO	Garbage in, garbage out
GNP	Gross national product
HAS	Hospital Administrative Services (of the AHA)
HMO	Health maintenance organization

HRSA	Health Resources and Services Administration
HSA	Health system agency
HSP	Health system plan
LRRA	Long-range recommended action
MIS	Management information system
MRI	Magnetic resonance imaging
M/S	Medical/surgical
NCHS	National Center for Health Statistics
NIMH	National Institute of Mental Health
OR	Operations research
PHS	Public Health Service
PMU	Program management unit
PPBS	Planning-Programming-Budgeting System
PPO	Preferred provider organization
PRO	Professional review organization
PSRO	Professional standards review organization
RFP	Request for proposal
RMP	Regional Medical Program
ROE	Return on equity
ROI	Return on investment
SBU	Strategic business unit
S.D.	Standard deviation
SHCC	Statewide Health Coordinating Council
SHPDA	State health planning and development agency
SMSA	Standard metropolitan statistical area
SRRA	Short-range recommended action
SWOT	Strengths, weaknesses, opportunities, threats
TIGER	Topologically Integrated Geographic Encoding and Referencing
UDI	Unnecessary death index
WOTS UP	Weaknesses, opportunities, threats, strengths underlying planning

PREFACE

The preface to the second edition of *Introduction to Health Planning* asserted our confidence in the usefulness and durability of the concepts of systems planning. We believe that confidence has been justified despite another set of dramatic changes in health services planning.

Some might characterize these changes as the shifting positions of opposing forces on a seesaw—shifts in the dominant focus between institutional planning and community planning. Others might see them as a movement along a circular path that is approaching the point of origin—in other words, where community influence on institutional development is exerted more through the actions of economically powerful groups and less through governmental or quasi-governmental agencies that purport to represent the interests of the general public.

In any event, although the scope of their work is more narrow than the work of community planners, institutional planners now generally recognize that they are designing for an entity composed of many diverse components rather than a homogeneous monolith. Furthermore, institutional planners pay special attention to the effects of the system's environment. Environmental forces include planning and regulatory agencies and, especially, consumers, who are taking a far more active role as informed purchasers of health services.

Because of these developments, we have prepared the third edition of *Introduction to Health Planning* with three objectives in mind:

1. To present an updated version of the generic elements relevant to health services planning wherever it is done

2. To expand the discussion of organizational planning to incorporate the latest innovations, particularly strategic planning

3. To describe the current status of community health services planning as a significant element of continuing importance in the health services system of the United States

Since it is our belief that health services administrators of the future will best be served by being taught the generic concepts and techniques that will remain relevant — regardless of shifts in focus or of social or technological change — we have emphasized in this edition those aspects that were stressed in the two previous editions.

In short, we are convinced that effective health services administrators must understand the rationale, theories, and methods of planning and their application in both organizational and community settings. It is our hope that the material presented here will serve them well in today's environment and, more important, provide the basis for continuing self-development throughout their professional careers.

The likelihood of achieving this goal has been considerably increased by the contributions of Tom Paivanas. His insightful comments have helped considerably to ensure that this book covers the major concerns of practitioners and to improve its usefulness for students. Because of the many advantages of word processing, the list of other acknowledgements has become somewhat shorter. Modern technology, however, has yet to devise a substitute for competent, dedicated editors. Consequently, we want to give special recognition to the major contributions to the style and quality of the book that were made by Gene Allen and Nancy Winchester, both of Information Resources Press.

1

OVERVIEW OF PLANNING

Planning, a widely used term, is perhaps almost as widely misunderstood and misused. This chapter discusses what planning is, why and where it occurs, by whom and how it is done, and, finally, how this book, with its limited scope, fits into the overall context of planning.

WHAT IS PLANNING?

Planning is making current decisions in the light of their future effects.

In the recent past, certain public organizations charged with regulation have been called *planning agencies.* Although it is true that some have based their regulatory activities on plans, it is nonetheless the case that planning and regulation are two separate and distinct functions. Unfortunately, many who feel that they have been disadvantaged by a regulatory decision have chosen to attribute their misfortunes to planning and thus to oppose planning as an unwarranted intervention into their individual affairs. Since this error is prevalent within the field of health services, it is important to understand that plans may be implemented by regulatory methods but that this connection is not certain. Conversely, it is essential to emphasize the positive effects that can be achieved through planning.

WHY SHOULD WE PLAN?

Ackoff[1] describes a style of planning that attempts to create the future. This is the true reason for planning. It is possible to anticipate what the future will be like if we allow events to follow their natural course (and, of course, if we assume that no external events will disrupt the pattern of development). Frequently, the predicted situation is not what we might prefer. Planning gives us the option of seeking interventions that will deflect events onto a path leading to circumstances that are better than the results of a laissez-faire approach and that conceivably could lead to the exact outcome we desire. There is no guarantee that our interventions will succeed, but the probability of success can be greatly increased if the interventions are developed through a systematic process based on a careful analysis of the information that is available. This is especially true because planning is done in a time frame that permits thorough, thoughtful decision making, in contrast to the hasty, perhaps frantic, actions that are typical responses to an unanticipated situation.

WHERE DOES PLANNING TAKE PLACE?

Planning activities relate to individuals and to organizations of all sizes. In this book, we focus on formal planning activities. Such activities require a relatively substantial base of resources to justify their existence (e.g., the average household would not be a candidate for establishment of a formal planning system). Therefore, planning activities are examined in two settings: large organizations and communities. The objectives of planning in these two settings may differ. Typically, planning in organizations seeks to maximize the results obtained by the activity of a single organization, whereas planning activities in communities strive to achieve an optimal balance among the efforts of many organizations within the limits imposed by the resources and values of the community. Nevertheless, the underlying principles and methods are relevant in both cases. Furthermore, because of the increasing interdependence of organizations and their environment, those who practice planning in one setting can succeed only to the extent that they are knowledgeable of and sensitive to the planning activities in the alternate setting.

Planning can be done by any organization and by any unit within an organization. The scope and time frame of a plan are determined by the

---

[1]Russell L. Ackoff. *Redesigning the Future.* New York, Wiley, 1974, pp. 26–31.

level of authority possessed by those doing the planning and the turbulence of the organization's environment. For instance, a department head in a traditional hospital would prepare plans of limited scope, usually for little more than a year into the future, because a department head has a very limited range of authority and a department's environment is the larger organization that tends to insulate it from the less-predictable events occurring in the outside world. On the other hand, an institution may use discretion in extending the scope of its activities to whatever range it deems feasible. It also has no buffer between it and the full impact of external events; consequently, it must use a planning horizon that extends far into the future. This will give an institution the time to anticipate events that are currently remote but that will eventually have a major impact on it.

When an institution is part of a larger organization (e.g., a hospital within a vertically integrated corporate structure), however, its planning role will be subject to additional constraints. Specifically, it must operate within the guidelines provided by corporate policies, and it must pay close attention to the effects of its decisions on other corporate members. In some institutions that have reorganized internally to create program management units (PMUs), the PMUs may have significant strategic planning responsibilities.

In the public sector, the scope of an organization's plan is usually determined by political jurisdictional boundaries and by a legislative charter. The effective planning horizon does not always reach far into the future because of the necessity to produce results in time for upcoming elections. Quasi-governmental agencies such as health system agencies (HSAs) and voluntary organizations like business coalitions tend to be insulated from these particular political considerations and are thus likely to have more extended planning horizons.

WHO PLANS?

Each of us plans to some extent in order to influence the course of our daily lives. For the purposes of this book, however, the question "Who plans?" will focus on the person(s) in an organization responsible for planning. There are both practical and theoretical reasons for assigning this responsibility to the organization's leader: The leader has the greatest amount of contact with the environment and thus is in the best position to know what the organization will face in the future. Furthermore, because the leader has the ultimate responsibility for the organization's performance and because planning is designed to enhance the outcome of the organization's efforts, it is reasonable that this individual must be the one to act toward this end. In other words, the leader may delegate the function, but responsibility for the result is not delegable. Consequently, the planning decisions remain the responsibility of the leader regardless of who actually makes them. The leadership role in community planning is typically assumed by a governing body. The members of this body are expected to make decisions based on the best interests of their constituents and of the community as a whole.

This formulation undoubtedly raises questions concerning the role of "planners." In simplest terms, the planner performs all the functions delegated by the leader, possibly including decision making if the leader attempts to abdicate his or her responsibilities. Ideally, the role of the planner is that of catalyst or facilitator of the planning process. In this role, the planner should be expected to provide and apply expertise in both the substantive and process aspects of planning.

HOW IS PLANNING DONE?

Decision making is frequently characterized as being one of two extremes: incremental or synoptic. Synoptic planning, which is the implementation of a rational model of planning, requires a complete analysis of each possible set of alternatives available to the organization during the foreseeable future. It emphasizes the avoidance of accepting current circumstances as limitations on what the organization seeks to accomplish in the future. Incremental decision making focuses on actions that are small deviations from the status quo. The advocates of this approach assert that it is preferable because the conditions required for synoptic planning can never be met. The advantages of incremental planning include the ability to operate from a strong base of information, since the changes are closely related to current experience, and the ability to reverse direction if the results are not satisfactory, since the modest changes implemented will not radically alter the situation that supported the status quo.

Clearly, the incremental approach has severe limitations, namely, that modest changes may be insufficient to deal with serious threats posed by the environment and that consideration of only small steps as sequential actions may not allow planners to respond in time to counteract threats or to take advantage of opportunities.

Of course, the synoptic approach is not without problems. These can be summarized by asserting that the decision maker does not have the scope and depth of knowledge that is assumed by the rational model of decision making (which, as its name implies, is based on a rational analysis of current and predicted situations). There is no doubt that this concern is justified, but it does not invalidate the synoptic approach, because the rational model can be approximated despite the lack of perfect information by using techniques such as mixed scanning,[2] simulation, and decision theory.

Use of the rational model for planning proceeds according to the following steps:

1. Identify the desired state (i.e., set goals and objectives).

2. Determine the discrepancy between the desired state and conditions that might occur if no action is taken (this involves forecasting).

3. Identify the resources that will probably be available to effect changes toward the desired state.

4. Develop feasible alternative methods for using these resources to make the necessary changes.

5. Evaluate these alternatives and select the ones that seem most likely to achieve the desired result within the limits imposed by resource availability.

6. Implement the chosen alternatives.

7. Appraise the performance of these alternatives, then make the necessary adjustments to bring them closer to achieving the desired objectives.

Clearly, these steps constitute a highly simplified model of the planning process. Planning is not and cannot be a straightforward, sequential process. Instead, it must be regarded as a cybernetic system with many iterative loops; that is, at each step along the way, the planners must be prepared to review what has occurred in all the preceding steps and to reevaluate these activities in the light of current developments. For example, it is entirely possible that, in the process of identifying available resources, the planners might discover that their initial objectives are either too high or too low. Should this occur, they must then go back and make the necessary adjustments to step one and proceed again through steps two and three. This iterative process will not be restated in this text but should be borne in mind in all considerations of planning.

---

[2]Etzioni's concept of mixed scanning as a planning strategy is described in George Chadwick, *A Systems View of Planning,* New York, Pergamon, 1971.

WHEN PLANNING OCCURS

Planning is an endless process. Since it is designed to help the organization cope with a turbulent environment, it follows that the successful planner must constantly seek information about new developments and incorporate these data into the plan. If this condition were met, there would never be a decision, because each analysis would be subject to revision based on the most recent information. Obviously, this situation is impossible, so a compromise must be made. The usual arrangement is to develop a plan with the intention of revising it on a periodic schedule with the expectation that the plan, although never truly current, will also never be seriously out-of-date. This, of course, assumes that the frequency of plan revision will be adequate for the rate of change in the environment.

A difficulty often encountered is that the resources required for complete revision of the plan are so great that the cost of frequent revisions is greater than the organization can afford. There is a related problem concerning the time required to prepare a revision of the entire plan. Charles Breindel[3] has proposed a solution that essentially leads to the continuous development of segments of the plan. This process allows the planners to allocate the available resources according to the relative importance of each segment and thus maximizes the benefit that can be obtained within a limited budget.

SUMMARY

This book emphasizes planning as a process that will allow leaders to maximize the performance of their organization within a turbulent environment. The approach described involves a simplified, rational model with some discussion of the values on which required choices are based.

A decision was made to avoid the issues of plan implementation and the more-or-less administrative aspects of the planning process (e.g., plan format, activity scheduling), which nevertheless are key ingredients in planning. These topics are absent because their omission does not detract from a discussion of the plan development process, but their inclusion would have expanded this book into a multivolume work.

This simplified approach should be useful in that it offers a basis for understanding the fundamentals of the planning process. Individuals can then adapt the process to meet the requirements of the various situations they will encounter during their professional careers.

---

[3]Charles L. Breindel. "Health Planning Processes and Process Documentation." *Hospital and Health Services Administration, 26*(Special II):5–18, 1981.

2

INTEGRATING POLICY, PLANNING, AND MARKETING

Policy, planning, and marketing, as they relate to health and health services, are inextricably intertwined. Considerable confusion arises because of different perceptions and uses of the terms in various settings. For instance, many governmental agencies are reluctant to use the term *marketing,* but these agencies are heavily engaged in functions that closely fit the standard definitions of marketing activities. Similarly, many people in the private sector regard policy as the exclusive province of government while performing policy functions under a different name. In this chapter, the relationships among these topics are demonstrated through a discussion focused primarily on planning.

PLANNING

Ackoff[1] provides a useful classification of approaches to planning: inactive, reactive, preactive, and interactive. Strategic planning, which is perceived as the sine qua non of health services administration,[2] is an interactive approach, defined by Ackoff as an effort to design a desirable

[1]Russell L. Ackoff. *Redesigning the Future.* New York, Wiley, 1974, pp. 22–31.
[2]Carl W. Thieme, Thomas E. Wilson, and Dane M. Long, "Strategic Planning for Hospitals Under Regulation," *Health Care Management Review, 6*(4):35–43, Spring 1981; Peter A. Nottonson, "Master Planning—Key to Survival," *Osteopathic Hospitals, 25*(16):8–11, June 1981; Kenneth M. Jones, Jr., "Long-Range Strategic Financial Planning," *Topics in Health Care Financing, 7*(4):23–29, Summer 1981.

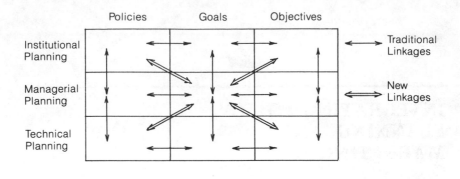

Figure 1   Modified Lorange-Vancil Model of the strategic planning process.

future. Jantsch[3] calls strategic planning "futures creative planning" and identifies its three essential characteristics as normative (value directed), integrative (system-wide), and adaptive (cybernetic). Ackoff points out that there will be occasions when some other approach to planning will be more appropriate. The skills and knowledge required for interactive planning, however, should be sufficiently adequate to allow the competent planner to meet the demands of any approach.

In this sense, it is important to note that Ackoff's four approaches do not represent types or levels of planning. Types of planning can be most usefully identified by using Parsons's[4] three levels of organizational structure: institutional/community, managerial, and technical. Each of these types should reflect the characteristics enumerated. This can be illustrated by an adaptation of a model originally developed by Lorange and Vancil[5] (Figure 1).

The model depicted in Figure 1 displays *normative* relationships, in that policies (values) have a direct influence on goals and objectives within each level and higher level policies affect those of a lower level. The model is *cybernetic,* in that each stage of the process receives and

[3]Erich Jantsch, *Technological Planning and Social Futures,* New York, Wiley, 1972, pp. 138-139; for a discussion of the necessity of adaptive systems in the modern environment, see Jay D. Starling, "The Use of System Constructs in Simplifying Organizational Complexity," in: *Organized Social Complexity,* edited by Todd R. LaPorte, Princeton, N.J., Princeton University Press, 1975, pp. 151-172.

[4]Talcott Parsons. *Structure and Process in Modern Societies.* Glencoe, Ill., Free Press, 1970, pp. 59-69.

[5]C. P. McLaughlin, C. M. C. Smythe, P. W. Butler, and A. B. Jones. *Strategic Planning and the Control Processes at Academic Medical Centers.* Washington, D.C., Association of American Medical Colleges, June 1979, p. 27.

adapts to information from adjacent stages. It is *integrative,* in that there are both vertical and horizontal flows of influence and feedback. These traditional linkages reflect the situation in a closely linked organization with a clear hierarchy of power. Vancil and Lorange[6] assert that in a decentralized organization with considerable autonomy at each level, the diagonal relationships more accurately describe the plan development process. For instance, the policies of a multihospital system (institutional level) will be strongly influenced by the goals of member hospitals (managerial level).

On several occasions, Jantsch[7] has described the three tiers in greater depth and applied different labels to each level. Figure 2 is an adaptation of Jantsch's models that incorporates Dror's[8] concepts of the components of policy. This figure is the basis for further discussion of each of the three levels of planning.

Note that the model in Figure 2 is actually a two-way matrix that reflects generic functions on the horizontal axis. Other authors suggest different functional sets, but there is general agreement that these generic functions are carried out at all levels of planning.

TYPES AND LEVELS OF PLANNING

Table 1 presents a complementary analysis of the three levels of planning. It links each of the purposes at the right-hand side of Figure 2 with a recapitulation of the appropriate approach, mode, level of detail, orientation, and supporting disciplines.

Policy Planning[9]

The purpose of policy (institutional) planning is to create the social institutions of the future. These new or revised institutions are reflec-

---

[6]This sort of arrangement is encouraged by Peters and Waterman. See "Simultaneous Loose-Tight Properties," in Thomas J. Peters and Robert H. Waterman, Jr., *In Search of Excellence,* New York, Harper & Row, 1982, chap. 12.

[7]Erich Jantsch, *Technological Planning and Social Futures,* p. 16; _____, "From Forecasting and Planning to Policy Sciences," *Policy Sciences,* 1(1):31–47, Spring 1970.

[8]Yehezkel Dror. *Design for Policy Sciences.* New York, American Elsevier, 1971.

[9]The term *institutional,* as used by Parsons and Jantsch, refers to social institutions (e.g., educational, religious). Since, however, in health services jargon, *institutional planning* is the term regularly used to denote facility or single organizational planning, the term *policy planning* is used in this book.

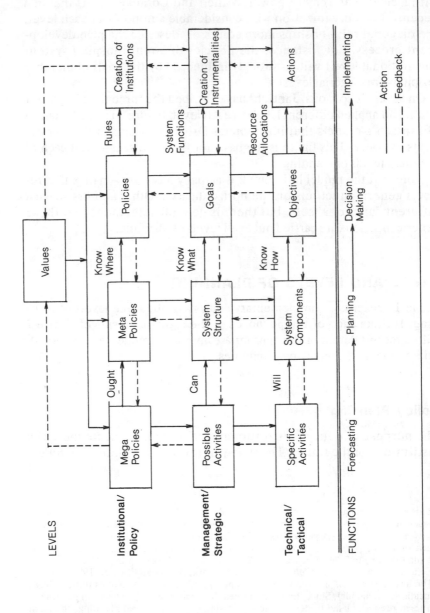

Figure 2   Planning levels and functions.

TABLE 1   Major Characteristics and Predominant Disciplines of
            Planning Levels

| | *Planning Levels* | | |
	Policy	*Managerial*	*Technical*
Purpose	Creation of institutions	Development of instrumental systems	Accomplishment of actions
Approach to Goal Attainment	Idealizing, Satisficing	Optimizing	Maximizing
Planning Mode	Normative	Allocative	Administrative
Nature of Content	General	Moderately specific	Detailed
Orientation of Decision Makers	General community interest	Health services generalist	Health services specialist
Predominant Disciplines*	Public administration, Political science, Ecology	Interorganizational behavior, Economics, Systems analysis, Epidemiology	Administrative theory, Behavioral science, Industrial engineering

*Does not include planning theory, marketing, and information systems, which are of
major significance at all three levels.

tions of society's values. To paraphrase Sir Geoffrey Vickers,[10] policy
regulates an institution over time in such a way as to optimize the realization of many conflicting values. Thus, policies are operational statements of society's values. According to Dror,[11] there are three types of
policy: *metapolicy,* which is policy on policymaking; *megapolicy,* which
expresses broad generic values; and *policy,* which is the focused application of megapolicy. (See Chapter 8 for further discussion of these concepts.) In the United States, for instance, there are

1. Metapolicies, which set out the rules for establishing megapolicy
and policy through legislative/regulatory/judicial processes
    2. Megapolicies, which espouse free-enterprise capitalism

---

[10] Sir Geoffrey Vickers. *Freedom in a Rocking Boat: Changing Values in an Unstable
Society.* London, Penguin, 1970.
[11] Yehezkel Dror. *Design for Policy Sciences.*

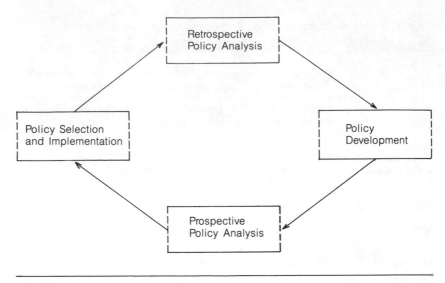

Figure 3   The policy cycle.

3. Policies, which govern our health services systems in a fashion that is more-or-less consistent with the free-enterprise model

The normative nature of planning at this level is obvious. Policy planning is integrative to the extent that it recognizes and attempts to deal with conflicting values between population groups and among policy dimensions (e.g., conflict between economic policy and social policy). The cybernetic aspect of policy planning is reflected in the phases of the policy cycle (Figure 3).

The policy cycle may begin at the point of retrospective policy analysis, an examination of the adequacy and completeness of existing policies. Such an analysis will stimulate policy development to fill identified gaps or correct perceived deficiencies. The proposed policies are then subjected to prospective policy analysis, which provides a basis for choice. Implementability is a crucial factor in choosing among competing policy proposals. Thus, a prospective policy analysis must incorporate the concepts of political science, as well as the cost-benefit analyses (economic, social, political, and the like) that are included in retrospective policy analyses.[12]

---

[12]The stages in the policy cycle were developed from ideas presented in Helen Abrams and Cyril Roseman, *State Health Policy Analysis,* Denver, Colo., PACT, 1978.

It is evident from the preceding description of the policy cycle that all the traditional policy concerns are encompassed within the scope of policy planning. The need to perform this level of planning is demonstrated by the relationship of policy planning and managerial or system planning. Policy planning establishes the nature of the institution, which, in turn, dictates the configuration of the system. For example, health services, as an institution in which the judgment of individual members of one profession is always paramount, cannot accommodate widespread development of systems similar to an institution such as public education, in which there is considerable standardization and centralization of decision making. In an organization, establishment of the mission is an example of policy planning.

Managerial Planning

Figure 2 indicates that the purpose of managerial (systems) planning is to create the instrumentalities that will perform the functions of the institution. Thus, managerial planning can be thought of as creating systems. Parsons's definition, however, also justifies the use of the term *systems* to indicate a broad perspective with a concern for multiple aspects of the institution's or organization's performance.

Managerial planning is *value-oriented,* in that it responds to the guidance of policy planning, as shown in Figure 2. It is *adaptive,* in that it relies heavily on assessment of the environment for direction within the constraints set forth by policy. It is *integrative,* in that it seeks to attain an optimum balance among the components of the system. It differs from policy planning, in that policy planning must generally seek to satisfice[13] because of the qualitative nature of many of its analyses, whereas managerial planning has the tools and data that make optimization at least a theoretical possibility. It differs from technical planning, which, because of its narrow focus, seeks to maximize the output of a single component of the system.

To illustrate, in community planning, megapolicy will determine the appropriate scope of health services as an institution. This might range from only medical care to the entire spectrum of health concerns implied by the World Health Organization's definition of health. Megapolicy will also determine the amount of resources available for the

---

[13]The term *satisfice* was coined by Herbert Simon to suggest that decision makers will not strive endlessly to reach an optimal position but, rather, will discontinue the search for better solutions after a threshold level of satisfaction has been achieved.

institution. On the other hand, technical planning tends to be the province of specialists, each of whom is motivated (for good, but sometimes self-serving, reasons) to provide the public with as much as possible of his particular service. Thus, technical planning seeks to acquire as many resources as possible. The managerial planners must bridge the gap between the other levels. They must distribute the allocated resources so as to maximize the system's total output, and they might seek, through the cybernetic process, to obtain a larger allocation of resources for their institutions. If they are not successful, the future instrumentalities that are created will be congenitally malformed. For instance, because of the historical lack of systems planning, health promotion is markedly underdeveloped, whereas medical care might be hypertrophic.

Technical Planning

Technical planning is where the action is. As Mao Tse Tung noted, there is no such thing as a "crossing-the-river" problem; there is a boat problem or a bridge problem. In other words, all of the abstraction of policy planning and managerial planning, no matter how sophisticated and elegant it may be, is of little value unless it leads to specific actions that will move the system, the organization, or the institution toward the realization of its purposes. Fortunately, we understand quite well how to plan in order to accomplish specific tasks. The processes (e.g., budgeting) and techniques (e.g., PERT) have been developed and refined over many years. Unfortunately, much of our technical planning as currently practiced does not meet Jantsch's three criteria: It is often done with little regard for institutional values (e.g., many facilities have established complex, expensive tertiary services in situations where there is little evidence of need and no indication of sufficient demand to ensure that the practitioners can develop and maintain clinical competence). It is seldom based on system-wide analyses (e.g., joint planning between independent acute care and long-term-care facilities). It is frequently not adaptive (e.g., continued maintenance of obstetric services in the face of declining usage and population projections that predict even fewer fertile females in the service area).

MARKETING

The evolution of health services institutional planning (described in Chapter 3) has led to the incorporation of a new discipline, marketing.

The recent decision to change the name of the Society for Hospital Planning to the Society for Hospital Planning and Marketing reflects this. The truth is, however, that formal recognition has only recently been given to this important element of both community and organizational planning activities. Indeed, many marketing techniques and concepts were introduced in health services planning long before their origins were recognized explicitly. This is probably attributable to a cultural bias that still exists.

As MacStravic and others[14] have pointed out, many people in the health services field have a distorted view of marketing as little more than hard-sell promotional techniques. Closer and more careful analysis of the marketing literature quickly dispels this misapprehension. For instance, any introductory marketing textbook describes a much broader range of activities than promotion and often identifies sets of generic functions that clearly relegate promotion and sales to a relatively minor role. One typical book, *Marketing Principles*,[15] lists six universal marketing functions and defines them in general terms to demonstrate their applicability to virtually any field of endeavor:

1. *Marketing Analysis:* learning about supply and demand for goods or services
2. *Marketing Communication:* conducting multidirectional exchanges of information between providers and consumers
3. *Product Differentiation:* adjusting product offers of both consumers and providers so that a mutually beneficial exchange can occur (includes product design)
4. *Market Segmentation:* identifying the likeliest consumers of products offered by providers
5. *Valuation:* making cost-benefit analyses of potential exchanges to determine if both consumers and providers will participate in the transfer of benefits between parties
6. *Exchange:* facilitating the transfer of benefits between parties in the marketing relationship

---

[14]R. E. MacStravic, "Marketing Curriculum for Health Services Administration," paper prepared for The George Washington University/Association of University Programs in Health Administration/Association of Schools of Public Health Conference on Curriculum in Policy, Planning, and Marketing, August 1981; Terrence J. Rynne, "The Third Stage of Hospital Long-Range Planning: The Marketing Approach," *Health Care Management Review,* 5(3):7–15, Summer 1980.
[15]William G. Nickels. *Marketing Principles.* Englewood Cliffs, N.J., Prentice-Hall, 1978, pp. 33–43.

TABLE 2   Examples of Planning Decisions that Relate to Marketing Functions

Marketing Functions	Planning Levels		
	Policy	Managerial	Technical
Product	Definition of health (e.g., Is gun control included?)	Assessment of aggregate need/demand for services (e.g., obstetrics)	Determination of types of service (e.g., midwifery)
Price	What proportion of resources should be allocated to health services (e.g., percent of gross national product)	Selection of methods of capital financing for health services	Determination of charges for individual services
Distribution	Level of trade-off between access and cost	Geographic locations for service delivery	Characteristics of health services facilities
Communication	Feedback from representatives of general community interest (e.g., elected officials or trustees)	Community health surveys	Utilization data

A shorter list, corresponding to MacStravic's "4 P's" (product, price, place, and promotion), can be used to show the relevance of marketing concepts at all three levels of planning. These functions, suggested by Lovelock,[16] are product, price, distribution (place), and communication (promotion).

Table 2 shows how each of these functions applies to each level of planning. Again, MacStravic[17] voices widespread concern about ethical issues in the use of marketing techniques. These issues reinforce

---

[16]Christopher H. Lovelock. "Concepts and Strategies for Health Marketers." *Hospital and Health Services Administration, 22*(4):50–62, Fall 1977.
[17]R. E. MacStravic. "Marketing Curriculum for Health Services Administration," pp. 8, 110–111.

Jantsch's assertion that effective planning must be normative, integrative, and adaptive. In other words, the values expressed by the megapolicies and policies within the policy plan must guide and constrain the use of marketing techniques throughout the entire system, and these megapolicies must reflect the changing expectations of the environment (i.e., the general public). For instance, if the general public accepts the notion that health services delivery should be regarded as a competitive industry, the prevalent social service ethos (which is a significant segment of current megapolicy) will have to be replaced by the economic imperatives of commercial enterprises.

Locations of Planning Levels

The preceding discussion has described planning in general terms and has shown that a complete planning system will encompass both policy and marketing. Now it is time to consider another division that often appears at the local level: community planning as contrasted to institutional planning.

Parsons made it clear that all three levels or types of activity existed for every organization but that the locus of a level would vary among organizational types. For instance, policy planning for a private corporation is typically carried out by the board of directors, and the social responsibility of such a firm is internally determined. A public entity, on the other hand, generally has the majority of its community responsibilities and its guiding principles mandated by the legislative and/or executive branches of government.

Within the health services industry, Stuehler's[18] model shows clearly that all levels must exist within institutional plans. Many authors,[19] however, have noted the rapid increase in multi-institutional systems. Zuckerman[20] specifically points out how the loci of many responsibilities (especially policymaking) shift from the individual institutional level to the corporate (system) headquarters.

The intense debate over the continuation of community health planning agencies (health system agencies [HSAs]) can be attributed largely

---

[18]George Stuehler, Jr. "A Model for Planning in Health Institutions." *Hospital and Health Services Administration, 23*(3):6–27, Summer 1978.
[19]For example, M. Orry Jacobs, "Cooperative Planning," *Hospital and Health Services Administration, 25*(4):23–35, Fall 1980.
[20]Howard S. Zuckerman. "Multi-Institutional Systems: Promise and Performance." *Inquiry, 16*(4):308–309, Winter 1979.

to disputes over the loci of various levels of planning. There appears to be continuing widespread agreement that system-wide planning is needed at the local level (witness the many proposals to form "voluntary" planning bodies sponsored by business coalitions to fill the vacuum that will occur if HSAs disappear). Health system agencies lost much local support because they were compelled to emphasize the federally imposed value of cost containment at the expense of the locally espoused values of system improvement. Furthermore, HSAs encountered extreme hostility from providers as it became evident that they were developing narrowly focused technical plans of great specificity to respond to the mandates of federal regulations that emphasized cost containment and to the regulatory requirements imposed by certificate-of-need laws.[21] Parsons's[22] predictions about such invasion of the technical planning turf by those responsible for managerial systems planning have proved, unhappily, to be all too true.

Nevertheless, despite the frequent misallocation of responsibility for various levels of planning, it is evident that all three levels are appropriate and necessary in both private and community planning. This confirms Breindel's[23] assessment that the distinctions between micro and macro planning are largely mythical. This is not to say, however, that planning functions are identical in all settings. Rather, it means that the competent planner will be acquainted with both organizational and public sector concerns and techniques (e.g., corporate funds flow analysis and measurement of community tax and debt capacity).

SUMMARY

Planning to create the future must be normative, integrative, and cybernetic. It is also a three-tiered process. The first tier is policy planning, which establishes the values that will guide actions in the other two tiers. Managerial planning, the second tier, creates the instrumentalities to perform the functions required by the policy decisions. Finally, technical planning encompasses the specific tasks needed to carry out the system's functions.

Marketing offers concepts, processes, and methods that contribute to successful planning at each of the three tiers. It establishes the

---

[21]Gordon D. Brown. "HSAs and Hospitals: Counter-Planning Strategies." *Hospital and Health Services Administration,* 23(4):65–74, Fall 1978.
[22]Talcott Parsons. *Structure and Process in Modern Societies,* p. 64.
[23]Charles L. Breindel. "The Myth of Micro and Macro Health Planning." *Hospital and Health Services Administration,* 25(Special I):38–47, 1980.

nature of products or services, how they will be made accessible to the consumer, how the consumers will be made aware of the ways the products fill perceived needs, and what the exchange relationship between provider and consumer will be; in other words, it determines the "marketing mix" of the organization. The three tiers of planning are required by all systems, but the responsibility for each of its aspects may be allocated to different elements within various systems, particularly if they have dissimilar organizations. This assignment of responsibilities is often a very controversial decision.

3

HISTORY OF HEALTH
SERVICES PLANNING

This chapter describes the evolution of health services planning in two segments: community planning and institutional planning. Although the two have interacted continuously, a separate discussion of each element will simplify and clarify the presentation.

COMMUNITY PLANNING

For many years, newspaper and magazine writers and authors of books and journal articles have written about the continuing health crisis in the United States. One such author was Lemuel Shattuck,[1] a Boston schoolteacher, writer, and publisher who became interested in vital statistics and active in community health and welfare activities. Shattuck has become known as the founder of public health in the United States. In 1849, he wrote,

The conditions of perfect health, either public or personal, are seldom or never attained, though attainable. Every year, thousands of lives are lost which might have been saved, tens of thousands of cases of sickness occur which might have been prevented. A vast amount of unnecessarily impaired health and physical debility exists among those not actually confined by a sickness, and means exist within our reach for the mitigation or removal of these evils.

---

[1]Lemuel Shattuck. *Report of the Sanitary Commission of Massachusetts, 1849.* Boston, Dutton and Wentworth, 1850.

21

Shattuck's report on health conditions in Massachusetts, which was buried by the Massachusetts legislature, included 50 recommendations of great importance.

A 1933 report[2] compared the conditions of the day to those of Shattuck's time and made several profound recommendations:

1. Medical service, both preventive and therapeutic, should be furnished largely by organized groups of physicians, dentists, nurses, pharmacists, and other associated personnel.

2. All basic public health services should be extended—whether by governmental or nongovernmental agencies—so that they will be available to the entire population according to its needs.

3. The costs of medical care should be placed on a group prepayment basis by means of insurance, taxation, or both.

4. The study, evaluation, and coordination of medical services should be considered important functions of every state and local community; state and local agencies should be formed to exercise these functions; and the coordination of rural and urban services should receive special attention.

5. Training for physicians should increasingly emphasize the teaching of health and prevention of disease; adequate training must be provided for nurse-midwives; and systematic training for hospital and clinic administrators should be available.

Today the United States is facing essentially the same health care challenge that it faced more than a century ago. Is this because we are not planning adequately to solve our health problems? Or are we not implementing the products of our planning process? Some insight into these issues can be gained from a review of the history of health services planning in the United States.

Public Sector Health Planning Levels

The planning process can be carried out at national, state, regional, and local levels and, at each level, can be accomplished through either

---

[2]Committee on the Costs of Medical Care. *Medical Care for the American People.* Chicago, University of Chicago, 1933. (Reprinted, Washington, D.C., U.S. Department of Health, Education, and Welfare, Health Services and Mental Health Administration, Community Health Service, 1970, pp. 103–144.)

voluntary efforts or governmental activities. Nationally, health planning is a fragmented operation, with its activities spread among various agencies within and outside the Federal Government. Therefore, planning generally has not been a well-focused, integrated effort, since there are no coordinated, long-range, national health goals of a general policy nature. Furthermore, although the delegation of many important federal decisions to the 10 regional offices of the Department of Health and Human Services (DHHS) might have made federal programs more sensitive to state and local concerns, it also has tended to create important differences in program implementation. These differences can become major problems for the many health organizations serving interstate metropolitan areas and areas that cross DHHS's regional boundaries, which are defined by state lines.

Each state government now has a health planning agency. If located within the governor's office, the agency can overcome fragmentation. If placed at a lower level in the state government hierarchy, such as the health department, it tends to become more parochial and limited in scope. This does not mean that the health department and other agencies and organizations in the health field should not maintain an internal organization for planning. The health planning agency, however, should be the overall coordinating agency for long-range planning.

Health planning at the regional level is complicated because, although the problems are local and the local point of view is the rationale behind planning, the solutions to today's health problems are, in fact, regional. But since regions involve more than one geopolitical entity, regional agencies generally lack the direct authority to implement planning at a regional level.

The "1400 governments syndrome," exemplified by a study of the New York City metropolitan area, is a description of fragmentation of local government. Although the average metropolitan area does not have 1,400 political subdivisions, the ratio of political entities to population and area is probably similar. Planning at the local level, then, can be as fragmented as actual health service at that level.[3]

Voluntary Efforts

Health planning in the United States has been accomplished through private efforts, as well as through the levels of government. Until very

---

[3] Robert C. Wood. *1400 Governments Syndrome*. Cambridge, Mass., Harvard University Press, 1961.

recently, in fact, these voluntary efforts have predominated in health planning. Usually, their efforts have been directed to the control of specific diseases. For example, at the turn of the century, organized groups of voluntary health workers recognized tuberculosis as a major national health problem. Their efforts resulted in the development of programs to prevent and treat tuberculosis in state and local public health agencies and in the formation of the National Tuberculosis Association. Later, the association extended its responsibilities and leadership and became the National Tuberculosis and Respiratory Disease Association; it is now the American Lung Association. The American Heart Association and the American Cancer Society are two more examples of large, well-known voluntary health agencies. All have numerous local affiliates and communicate and coordinate their activities through the National Health Council.[4]

Historically, planning for health manpower has also been done on a volunteer basis. Planning initially was stimulated by a study of medical education in the United States and Canada conducted by Abraham Flexner,[5] who reported his findings in 1910. The "Flexner Report" advocated that medical care be based on thorough knowledge of the biomedical sciences; that only high-quality medical schools receive accreditation; that these schools emphasize both laboratory work and intensive clinical experience; that many inadequate proprietary medical schools flourishing during that period close down; and that medical schools be affiliated with universities. Flexner's findings led to pronounced changes during the next 70 years in both medical education and the quality of medical care.

The Flexner, or research, model has two weaknesses in its plans for health manpower. First, it largely ignores health care delivery outside the medical school and teaching hospital. Second, it sets science in the medical school apart from science on the general campus, resulting in duplication of effort. To offset these weaknesses, two new models have been developed: the health care delivery model and the integrated science model.

Another voluntary effort was the Committee on the Costs of Medical Care. This group attempted to resolve the problems resulting from rising costs and unequal distribution of medical care before and during the depression years.

---

[4]Ernest L. Stebbins and Kathleen N. Williams. "History and Background of Health Planning in the United States." In: *Health Planning: Qualitative Aspects and Quantitative Techniques.* Edited by W. A. Reinke. Baltimore, Md., Waverly, 1972, pp. 3-4.

[5]Abraham Flexner. *Medical Education in the United States and Canada.* New York, Carnegie Foundation for the Advancement of Teaching, 1910.

Toward the end of World War II, the American Public Health Association, as a member of the National Health Council, conducted a study on the provision of full-time, local health services in the United States.[6] The study examined traditional public health services (environmental sanitation, communicable disease control, maternal and child health, vital statistics, health education, and public health laboratory services) and set minimum standards for these services based on a very limited scope of program activity. These standards became obsolete early on because the field of public health and its responsibilities expanded so rapidly.

The problems of the aged and the chronically ill came to the attention of the public through the Commission on Chronic Illness,[7] established under the auspices of the American Medical Association, the American Public Health Association, and the American Hospital Association. The commission's four-volume report, issued in the 1950s, contributed significantly to existing knowledge on the problems of finding and caring for the chronically ill. The impact of its recommendations, however, has not been fully realized.

In the 1960s, a voluntarily supported national planning effort, sponsored by the American Public Health Association and the National Health Council, was launched by the National Commission on Community Health Services.[8] The project was financed by foundation funds, as well as by the U.S. Public Health Service and the Vocational Rehabilitation Administration. The commission—representing health professionals, organized labor, industry, and the community at large—studied community health needs and existing services. Its goal was a plan for a system of preventive and curative medical and environmental health services for the next decade. The commission's report, published in 1967, was a compilation of monographs covering practically every phase of community health services; many of its recommendations have been implemented. Significantly, the commission recommended both greater federal participation in community health services and comprehensive health planning on a continuing basis. It was

---

[6]American Public Health Association, Committee on Administrative Practice, Subcommittee on Local Health Units. *Local Health Units for the Nation* (Emerson Report). New York, Commonwealth Fund, 1945.

[7]Commission on Chronic Illness. *Chronic Illness in the United States.* Vols. 1–4. Cambridge, Mass., Harvard University Press, 1956–1959.

[8]National Commission on Community Health Services. *Reports of the Task Forces on Environmental Health, Comprehensive Health Service, Health Manpower, Health Care Facilities, Financing of Health Services, Organization of Community Health Services.* Washington, D.C., Public Affairs Press, 1967.

through the research activities of this commission that certain fundamentals of the planning process evolved, including the concept of high-
quality health care and a healthy environment as civic rights, the definition of a "community of solution,"[9] and the recommendation of a
single system for health care delivery rather than a fragmented public
and private approach.[10,11]

Commissions

Several presidential commissions have influenced governmental health
planning. In 1951, President Harry Truman appointed the Commission
on Health Needs of the Nation, which represented professionals as well
as consumers, particularly in labor and industry. It studied the availability and adequacy of health services, facilities, and manpower and explored health needs and the extent to which they were being met. It
also examined consumer opinions on the adequacy of programs and services. The commission's report clearly identified deficiencies and
recommended major federal participation in financing more adequate
services and facilities. The report, however, had little impact on the
Eisenhower administration or on Congress.[12]

A more influential presidential commission was the Commission on
Heart Disease, Cancer, and Stroke, headed by Dr. Michael DeBakey.[13]
This group was appointed in 1964 to identify methods for reducing the
toll taken by these diseases, particularly through better and faster use
of existing medical knowledge. In less than a year, the commission explored the morbidity and mortality problems of heart disease, cancer,
and strokes and recommended, among other things, a nationwide net-
work of regional medical programs. The recommendation was enacted

---

[9]"Planning, organization, and delivery of community health services by both official
and voluntary agencies must be based on the concept of a community of solution—
that is, environmental problem sheds and health services marketing areas, rather than
primarily on political jurisdiction." National Commission on Community Health
Services. *Health is a Community Affair.* Cambridge, Mass., Harvard University Press,
1966, pp. 2–4.
[10]Ibid., pp. 129–131.
[11]National Commission on Community Health Services, Community Action Studies
Project. *A Self-Study Guide for Community Action Planning.* New York, American Public
Health Assn., 1967.
[12]Ernest L. Stebbins and Kathleen N. Williams. "History and Background of Health
Planning in the United States," pp. 6–7.
[13]President's Commission on Heart Disease, Cancer, and Stroke. *A National Program to
Conquer Heart Disease, Cancer, and Stroke.* Washington, D.C., U.S. Government Printing Office, 1964.

into law—although not exactly as the commission had intended—with almost unheard of dispatch, and the Regional Medical Program service began.

Major Government Initiatives

Increasing governmental action in the health care field during recent years stems from widespread dissatisfaction with health services in the United States. Historically, the medical care providers have insisted on a laissez-faire approach, which has made introduction of a planning process difficult. For example, planning cannot occur without the cooperation of physicians, and it has, on occasion, met with outright opposition from the American Medical Association. Even voluntary associations that operate as area-wide planning agencies on a private, nonprofit basis have encountered opposition in their efforts to allay consumer dissatisfaction.

Two alternatives appear to be available to the government: stimulation and coercion. At first, the government opted for stimulation via the grant-in-aid program; later, it moved toward coercion via legislation and regulation.

Grants-in-Aid

The federal grant-in-aid is a fiscal technique to assure that resources are allocated to dealing with major problems and to augment the revenues of less-affluent areas through the legal transfer of funds accumulated by wealthier areas. The funds are redistributed according to a formula based on population characteristics, health problems (morbidity and mortality), and financial needs. Also, the recipient area often must produce the required matching funds, which can range from one-third to two-thirds of the total budget for the project being supported by the grant.

The grant-in-aid mechanism is a potent tool for encouraging centralization and is consistent with the concept of federalism. Federal aid has been given to states since early in U.S. history and has focused on such areas as developing a militia (1808), land-grant colleges (beginning in the 1860s), and public health funds to control venereal disease (beginning in 1918).

During the depression years, the grant-in-aid mechanism was used more frequently when state and local governments either could not or would not fund programs that the Federal Government considered important. Since then, the number of federal grant programs has continually increased. Some attempts have been made to reverse this trend, notably during the Eisenhower administration, but these were unsuccessful. Many consider accepting funds from the government to be some sort of sinful dalliance, but few are practicing or supporting abstinence. There is always a constituency that protests vigorously against any threat to terminate an established grant program.

PURPOSE

The grant-in-aid programs serve a variety of purposes:

1. They equalize availability of programs. By redistributing revenues, grants-in-aid foster uniform availability of their programs throughout the nation by removing the financial reasons for not developing them.

2. They stimulate program development and continuation. The availability of categorical grant-in-aid funds specifically earmarked for disease control has made possible the development of programs to control tuberculosis, venereal disease, cancer, heart disease, and air pollution, as well as mental health programs, maternal and child health services, and radiological health programs. The broad spectrum covered by grants-in-aid even includes a general health category that can be used for such general programs as multiphasic screening.

3. Grants-in-aid support a program of specific interest to the grantor. In those instances where the grantor (namely, the Federal Government) has a specific interest and the locality may or may not share that interest, a grant-in-aid program can be developed with the intent that local support will be given as the need for the program is demonstrated. Service to the aged is an example of such a program.

4. They supervise and control. Requirements imposed on the use of federal grant funds provide indirect supervision and control over the scope and nature of local programs.

5. Grant-in-aid programs enforce minimum standards. For example, to use grant-in-aid funds, health personnel to be employed by the program are required to meet certain qualifications.

6. They distribute tax proceeds efficiently. Since local and state governments are not as adept as the Federal Government at tax collection, use of the federal collection agency for this purpose is more efficient.

MECHANISM

The grant-in-aid program is more than just a donation of funds to the states by the Federal Government. To receive these funds, states are required to meet several conditions:

1. The state or locality receiving the funds usually must produce its proportionate share of matching funds.
2. Formal acceptance is required at the state level; this sometimes necessitates legislative approval. Often, a state plan describing the purpose, objectives, methodology, and evaluation of a program must be developed and approved by the Federal Government.
3. The state must assure that it conforms to federal guidelines in such areas as record keeping, personnel qualifications, and program procedures.
4. The state must agree to report data in an acceptable format, provide regular progress reports, and submit to periodic fiscal auditing.

PROBLEMS

The federal grant-in-aid program has not been free of problems, some of which have been created by the program structure itself. For example, grant-in-aid programs generally are structured to observe scrupulously the rights and autonomy of state governments, but such a "hands-off" approach makes it more likely that states with less-effective governments will use the funds ineffectively or inappropriately. The program's categorical nature—that is, distribution of funds for specific programs—has resulted in fragmentation of health activities at state and local levels. Specific programs generally are planned and carried out independently, without effective coordination with other programs. Thus, the maternal and child health program usually is entirely separate from the tuberculosis control, venereal disease, or general health program.

Another problem is that federal priorities are foisted on states without considering state and local concerns. This means that the state occasionally is forced to forgo a program that it considers to have high priority in order to divert its funds to match a federal grant for a lower priority service. (Grant-in-aid funds cannot be used for any category except the one for which the funds are appropriated.)

States are uncertain as to whether specific grant-in-aid programs will continue to be funded. Funding is decided by the Federal Government on a year-to-year basis, with no guarantee that funds will extend beyond the current period, even though most grants are in fact renewed for many years. Although a grant program may continue, the funding levels may fluctuate from one year to another. Such uncertainty makes it extremely difficult to hire and retain qualified personnel. This problem becomes even more severe when the Federal Government fails to appropriate funds prior to the beginning of a fiscal year. In such cases, programs are authorized to spend funds at the level appropriated for the preceding year until an appropriation for the current fiscal year is enacted. (The legislative vehicle for accomplishing this is a "continuing resolution.") Since the new appropriation may be larger or smaller than the previous one, program administrators and staff exist in an environment of extreme uncertainty.

Frequently, a grant-in-aid program makes no provision for an increase in the yearly allocation. This means that annual increments for salary or cost-of-living raises must be met either from local funds or by reducing the program's scope to release funds to cover increased costs.

In summary, the most serious problems with the federal grant-in-aid program are fostering of fragmentation through development of categorical programs, lack of consideration for state and local priorities, and insufficient and uncertain funding.

The concept of general revenue sharing was developed to deal with the problem of insufficient and uncertain funding. In essence, revenue sharing implies that some of the Federal Government's revenues will be distributed to state and local governments for their unrestricted use. General revenue sharing has dealt effectively with concerns about local discretion. On the other hand, the exercise of local discretion has given rise to concerns about how the funds are used by various communities. Because funds are allocated without regard to the economic status of communities, there inevitably are cases in which an affluent community's highest priority projects seem frivolous in contrast to the needs in impoverished communities, even after the grant funds have been used.

Despite the problems with grants-in-aid, one should not forget that over the years, the program has resulted in developing and continuing efforts in all states to control tuberculosis and venereal disease, to provide maternal and infant care, and to perform additional services that otherwise might not have been uniformly available and might not have met acceptable standards.

The Reagan administration started with an intense commitment to drastically reduce the Federal Government's role in domestic affairs. Relevant keywords were "deregulation" and "New Federalism." Through the budgetary process, it effected dramatic changes in federal social programs. One of these changes was the concept of the block grant. (A block grant is a consolidation of a number of related categorical programs into a single grant.) The amounts of the block grants were substantially smaller (approximately 25 percent less) than the sum of the individual categorical grants they replaced. This reduction was rationalized by deregulating the affected programs (i.e., virtually eliminating federal oversight of the use of the money). In other words, it was assumed that one-fourth of program costs could be saved because of the reduced federal administrative requirements. Generally, the states accepted this with some reluctance, for although they badly wanted the increased latitude in the use of the funds, few had the resources to compensate for the obvious reduction in the available operating funds. After its overwhelming success during the first session of the 97th Congress, the Reagan administration began having difficulty in achieving the goals of the New Federalism. During its second session, Congress began to question the wisdom of many proposals, and state and local government officials became much more skeptical about the benefits they were supposedly being offered. The 98th Congress, elected in the middle of Mr. Reagan's term in office, included more members who opposed his fundamental philosophy. Thus, the New Federalism has been moving more slowly.

Specific health planning legislation at the federal level also began with a grant program, the Hospital Survey and Construction Act, described in the next subsection. During the several decades prior to passage of this and subsequent legislation, health program development followed two separate paths: The public sector of the health system dealt with the role of government in providing health services, and the private sector, including practitioners and hospitals, planned on an area-wide basis, principally to develop hospitals and other facilities.

Significant Federal Laws

HILL-BURTON ACT

The Hospital Survey and Construction Act, P.L. 79-725, was passed in August 1946. It comprised title VI of the Public Health Service Act and provided for the Hill-Burton program.

History

By 1946, there was a general shortage of hospital beds, and more than one-third of the nation's counties had no hospitals. Not only were these resources unevenly distributed geographically, but they were not coordinated with one another. The shortage resulted from a near cessation of new hospital construction during the depression of the 1930s and the years of restriction imposed by World War II and was further exacerbated by obsolescence of existing facilities. The problem was compounded by rapid population growth, migration from rural to urban areas, and rising construction costs. Also, the shortage of beds, especially in rural areas, was accompanied by a shortage of medical personnel.

A number of proposals were made calling for government action in the hospital field. Several years elapsed, however, before such legislation was enacted by Congress. In the aftermath of World War II, the Truman administration was preoccupied with foreign affairs rather than with domestic problems, and physicians and hospital associations were critical of proposed legislation and ignored the financial plight of the voluntary hospital. Once the Hill-Burton Act was passed, however, the program developed at an accelerating pace and, through the years, was expanded by amendments to the act.

Provisions

In its initial form, the Hill-Burton Act authorized grants to states for the following purposes:

1. To survey their health needs; to develop plans for the construction of facilities, including public and other nonprofit hospitals; and to establish adequate hospitals, clinics, and similar services
2. To help build and equip public and voluntary nonprofit hospitals (general, mental, tuberculosis, and chronic disease) and public health centers

The act authorized the appropriation of a minimum allocation to each state according to population; the states could draw on these allotments to meet up to one-third of their expenses in carrying out the new law. Each state was required to designate a single state agency and an advisory council to implement its program, and to establish a plan for conducting a survey of existing hospitals and related facilities to develop a program for needed construction.[14,15] The state agencies estab-

---

[14]U.S. Department of Health, Education, and Welfare, Public Health Service, Division of Hospital and Medical Facilities, Program Planning and Analysis Branch. *Facts About the Hill-Burton Program.* Washington, D.C., U.S. Government Printing Office, 1968.
[15]U.S. Department of Health, Education, and Welfare, Public Health Service, Division of Hospital and Medical Facilities, Program Planning and Analysis Branch. *Hill-Burton Is. . . .*Washington, D.C., U.S. Government Printing Office, 1968.

lished one or more regions within state boundaries for planning purposes. The Hill-Burton Act and its amendments, however, did nothing to encourage cooperation or regional coordination among health facilities, requiring only that there be a rational geographic distribution of hospital beds.

In 1949, amendments to the Hill-Burton Act authorized the U.S. Public Health Service to provide grants for and conduct research, experiments, and demonstrations on the development, effective use, and coordination of hospital services, facilities, and resources. It was 1956, however, before appropriations were made to carry out these amendments.

Additional amendments in 1954 broadened the Hill-Burton program to include specific grants for construction of public and voluntary nonprofit nursing homes, diagnostic or treatment centers, rehabilitation facilities, and chronic disease facilities.

The 1958 amendments to the Hill-Burton Act gave sponsors who met the standard eligibility and priority qualifications the option of taking long-term loans in lieu of grants. In 1961, under the Community Health Services and Facilities Act (P.L. 87-395), the annual appropriation authorized for construction of nursing homes and the annual research appropriation for experimental and demonstration construction and equipment projects were increased. This act also was used by the Federal Government to provide funds to planning agencies.

In 1964, amendments to the Hospital Survey and Construction Act extended that program through June 1969. The law's title subsequently was changed to the Health and Medical Facilities Survey and Construction Act (P.L. 88-443) and it became the Hill-Harris Act (P.L. 91-296). Its provisions included grants and loans not only for new construction but also for modernizing and replacing all types of facilities. In addition, project grants were authorized for development of comprehensive regional, metropolitan, or other local plans for health and related facilities (Section 318). Previously, demonstration grants supported area-wide planning efforts; however, in June 1967, funding for comprehensive health planning agencies was transferred to the new Comprehensive Health Planning (CHP) program. This program, authorized by the Partnership for Health Act (P.L. 89-749), repealed the Hill-Burton research and demonstration project grants and set up the National Center for Health Services Research and Development.

Problems

The Hill-Burton program, in addition to generating many small rural hospitals that were economically unsound, did not exert any influence on the delivery system itself, nor did it result in coordination among hospitals or between hospitals and other facilities beyond that which had developed sporadically as a result of the private practice of medicine. The act, of course, did not require such coordination, and there was no demand for it. Initially, the shortage of beds was so severe that the system under which the beds were provided was not important, and further coordination of health services was not recognized as a desirable goal.

By the late 1950s and the early 1960s, the need was apparent for a regional system with interrelationships and coordination among health facilities, but not necessarily with a medical center at its core. Thus evolved the concept of a partnership to link government and voluntary agencies. The Hill-Burton program would be one part of a total comprehensive health effort. This resulted in the Comprehensive Health Planning and Public Health Service Amendments Act of 1966, P.L. 89-749 (also known as the Partnership for Health Act).

More recently, the Federal Government decided that facilities assisted by the Hill-Burton program were not fulfilling their obligations to provide a reasonable volume of services to those unable to pay. Provision of such care was a major purpose of the original law and was retained through all subsequent years and then carried over into P.L. 93-641. For a long time, the regulations covering this aspect of the program were very general. Then, in 1972, the Department of Health, Education, and Welfare issued a revision that required state agencies to monitor compliance. Further study led to the conclusion that compliance was generally unsatisfactory. For instance, the state government of New York reported that of the state's 151 hospitals with Hill-Burton service obligations, only one was in full compliance and more than half failed to provide a reasonable volume of free or reduced-cost care.[16] Although this finding was disputed by the state hospital association, the proportion of hospitals involved was large enough to give credibility to the assertion that compliance was less than satisfactory. Moreover, there was no doubt that the level of expectations varied widely among the states. As a consequence, the Department of Health and Human Services published new regulations in 1979 that established uniform national standards based on specific dollar computations. These regulations also required full documentation of services rendered, in lieu of general assurances of compliance. The individual grant recipients and the American Hospital Association protested vigorously. Nevertheless,

---

[16]"State Accuses Most Hospitals of Hill-Burton Non-compliance." *Hospitals, 53*(18):17, September 16, 1979.

the revised regulations remain in effect and, as of 1984, 5,000 facilities are still required to provide uncompensated care as a result of having received Hill-Burton assistance. The total number of facilities that participated in the Hill-Burton program was 6,900.[17]

Accomplishments

The Hill-Burton program reduced the wide range of hospital bed-to-population ratios; increased the total number of beds so that few areas had shortages; helped modernize facilities; helped build new facilities; encouraged the states to adopt and improve licensure laws; reduced reliance on philanthropy as a source of funds; and, because public funds were involved, created a sense of community responsibility for health facilities. The program provided a good working example of cooperation among all levels of government while remaining attuned to local needs. The extension legislation for the Hill-Harris program (P.L. 91-296 [1970]) and for the Comprehensive Health Planning program (P.L. 91-515 [1970]) recognized the need to tie hospital and health facility construction planning more closely to the comprehensive health planning process.[18,19]

On the other hand, John W. Seavey's[20] recent analysis of data from the federal files of the Hill-Burton program reveals that, although the program did distribute funds to the states with the greatest needs, the allocation of funds within states was frequently inconsistent with federal aims (e.g., substantial amounts were awarded to tertiary and urban medical facilities, even though the law focused on aid to the community-level needs of small rural population groups). Seavey suggests that this might have reflected responsiveness to political power and possibly foreshadowed the distribution pattern of block grant funds provided to states under the New Federalism.

---

[17]American Hospital Association. *Washington Memo, 502*:7, May 25, 1984.
[18]U.S. Department of Health, Education, and Welfare, Public Health Service, Health Services and Mental Health Administration, Health Facility Planning and Construction Service, Office of Program Planning and Analysis. *Hill-Burton Program Progress Report, July 1, 1947–June 30, 1969.* Washington, D.C., U.S. Government Printing Office, revised 1969. (PHS 930-F-3)
[19]Philip N. Reeves. "Analysis of the Hill-Burton Program." Washington, D.C., The George Washington University, Department of Health Care Administration, 1967. Mimeographed.
[20]John W. Seavey. *State Allocative Health Politics: Hill-Burton Revisited.* Durham, University of New Hampshire, School of Health Studies, January 1983. Unpublished manuscript.

THE MENTAL RETARDATION FACILITIES AND COMMUNITY HEALTH CENTERS ACT OF 1963

This act was the cornerstone for improvements in mental health services. It was designed to combat the ravages of mental retardation and mental illness through provision of funds to construct research centers and service facilities. It also provided for the development of community mental health centers through construction, planning, and staffing grants. Amendments to the act provided for facilities to serve alcoholics and drug addicts.

Each state was required to designate a single state agency and an advisory council to develop a state plan providing for inpatient, outpatient, and emergency care; partial hospitalization; and consultation and education.

The overall intent of the Mental Retardation Facilities and Community Health Centers Act was to help prevent mental illness and to provide care for the mentally ill at the community level by offering a continuing series of coordinated programs within the community. This was an alternative to institutionalizing the mentally ill in large mental hospitals away from the community.[21,22]

Problems

In general, this legislation was successful in promoting community services, improved facilities, and increased knowledge about the care of the mentally ill and the mentally retarded. Nevertheless, the program was not without problems.

Many considered the target population required to establish a community mental health center (between 75,000 and 200,000 persons) too large for a community program. But the act offered little flexibility or local option relative to the size of a facility and its target population. For example, use of the "catchment area" concept was encouraged; this established the community mental health center as a reservoir, with patients and clients coming to it for services, rather than a decentralized program reaching out to the periphery of the catchment area. Some persons at the state level felt that the National Institute of

---

[21]Paul V. Lemkau and Wallace Mandell. "History and Special Features of Mental Health Planning." In: *Health Planning: Qualitative Aspects and Quantitative Techniques*. Edited by W. A. Reinke. Baltimore, Md., Waverly, 1972, pp. 279–288.

[22]U.S. Department of Health, Education, and Welfare, Public Health Service, Health Services and Mental Health Administration, National Institute of Mental Health. *The Comprehensive Community Mental Health Centers Program.* Washington, D.C., U.S. Government Printing Office, 1969.

Mental Health, which implements this act, superimposed its philosophy on state and local advisory boards and programs rather than pursuing joint and cooperative planning with states and localities. Furthermore, the program was structured to provide for a decrease in funds annually over a period of five years, at which time the states would take over funding. The states, however, found it difficult to provide funds for such a large and complex program within such a short period. In addition, the grants provided for the salaries of professional staff only, which meant that the local areas had to assume the responsibility for raising funds for nonprofessional and administrative staff salaries.

Finally, a longer range, programmatic problem faced the community; namely, community mental health centers were developed independently of physical health programs. Of course, the two should have been coordinated, since mental health is clearly part of total heath.

HEALTH REVENUE SHARING AND HEALTH SERVICES ACT, P.L. 94-63

Title III of P.L. 94-63, the Health Revenue Sharing and Health Services Act, was designed to deal with the problems of grants-in-aid, to fill service gaps by expanding the scope of the mental health program (e.g., by adding a requirement for activities to prevent rape and to aid its victims), and to force a recalcitrant administration to carry out congressional wishes by making requirements more specific than in the previous law (e.g., by providing a specific definition of a community mental health center and the services such a center must provide).[23] The Health Revenue Sharing and Health Services Act provides grants for planning and development; initial operation; consultation and education; assistance in cases of financial distress; and help in acquiring, building, and remodeling facilities.

Of particular interest is section 237, which sets forth requirements for a state plan for comprehensive mental health services. This plan must address the services to be offered by community mental health centers and the facilities required for such centers. It must parallel and be consistent with the state health plan and the state medical facilities plan required by the National Health Planning and Resources Development Act, P.L. 93-641 (discussed on pp. 46-56).

---

[23]For a description of congressional discontent with the administration's attitude toward community mental health centers, see U.S. Congress, House, Interstate and Foreign Commerce Committee, *Health Revenue Sharing and Health Services Act of 1975,* House Report 94-192, 94th Congress, 1st Session, May 7, 1975, pp. 48–52.

APPALACHIAN REGIONAL DEVELOPMENT ACT OF 1965

Although this legislation does not specifically require a health program, it has many provisions that affect health planning. Basically, it provides for public works and economic development programs in the Appalachian region of the United States, but two of these provisions are applicable to health planning.

First, the act provides for establishing the Appalachian Regional Commission. This joint state and federal commission is authorized to perform comprehensive planning and coordination, which can include the planning of health programs. (Some controversy has arisen over the power of the states versus that of the Federal Government in the functioning of this regional commission.) [24,25]

Second, the act provides for funding demonstration health facilities through grants for construction, equipment, and operation. Any agency or organization is eligible for these funds. [26,27]

HEART, CANCER, AND STROKE AMENDMENTS OF 1965, P.L. 89-239

This was the first significant attempt to organize health services along regional rather than geopolitical lines. It was a product of the President's Commission on Heart Disease, Cancer, and Stroke (the De-Bakey Commission), appointed in 1964 to study these three major causes of death in the United States.

A purpose of P.L. 89-239 was to encourage and help establish regional cooperative arrangements among medical schools, research institutions, and hospitals to enable them to conduct research, provide training and continuing education, and carry out demonstrations of patient care. The amendments also made available to patients the latest advances in the diagnosis and treatment of heart disease, cancer, and stroke (and later, under P.L. 91-515, kidney and related diseases).

P.L. 89-239 resulted in the creation of 56 regions (encompassing the 50 states and the territorial possessions of the United States), each with

---

[24]Edward Hearle. "The Regional Commissions: Approach to Economic Development." *Public Administration Review, 28*(1):17, January–February 1968.

[25]Randy Hamilton. "The Regional Commissions: A Restrained View." *Public Administration Review, 28*(1):20–21, January–February 1968.

[26]U.S. Department of Health, Education, and Welfare, Public Health Service, Health Services and Mental Health Administration, Office of Grants Management. *Profiles of Grant Programs.* Washington, D.C., U.S. Government Printing Office, 1971, pp. 3–8.

[27]Office of Economic Opportunity. *Catalog of Federal Domestic Assistance.* Compiled by the Office of Management and Budget. Washington, D.C., U.S. Government Printing Office, 1970.

its own Regional Medical Program (RMP). The RMP design for each region was determined locally, and the scope and nature of services were subject to decisions of the local planning body (known as the Regional Advisory Group). The initial general strategy for the various RMPs was to organize existing resources into cooperative arrangements for improving health care in the specific disease categories covered by the legislation (later coverage included kidney diseases).

Experience, legislation, and administrative interpretation produced substantial changes in the Regional Medical Program, and the basic disease-oriented thrust was eventually diminished. In its place, top-priority consideration was given to the availability and accessibility of quality health care. Furthermore, emphasis was placed on outpatient and ambulatory services rather than on institutional care at hospitals or medical centers, and disease prevention was stressed rather than treatment or curative services only.[28,29]

The RMP dealt not only with medical centers, hospitals, and related facilities but also with practicing physicians; therefore, it may be described as a direct link between the Federal Government and the private sector of medicine.

Problems and Issues

Many of the Regional Medical Programs successfully combined elements of the health care delivery system that previously were isolated and independent of each other. Others promoted the extension of new medical knowledge from the medical centers into the offices of private practitioners and community hospitals. But these many changes created confusion about the program's mission and means to achieve it. One particular issue of great concern was whether the role of the RMPs was to change the existing health care delivery system rather than simply to upgrade it. The threat of change seemed disturbing to health care providers.

Another problem involved the relationship of the Comprehensive Health Planning program with P.L. 89-239. There seemed to be insufficient justification for two separate programs, one dealing with providers

---

[28]F. R. Weinerman. " 'The Regional Concept,' from 'Regionalization of Medical Services.' " In: *Readings in Medical Care*. Edited by the Committee on Medical Care Teaching. Chapel Hill, University of North Carolina Press, 1958, pp. 350–356.
[29]Regional Medical Programs Service. *Progress Report*. Washington, D.C., U.S. Government Printing Office, 1970.

and heart disease, cancer, and stroke and the other primarily with consumers on a more comprehensive, but necessarily regional, basis.[30]

Concern also was expressed about the RMP responsibility for regionalization. Health providers opposed a highly structured regional system in which patient flow was from the periphery to the center and manpower and services were from the center to the periphery.

The major concern of the public was the accessibility and cost of health care; regionalization, although relevant, was not yet a public issue.

Furthermore, the Regional Medical Program did not have legislated authority for accomplishing regionalization. Yet its mission was to develop regional cooperative arrangements through voluntary efforts to bring together isolated elements of the health system.

RMP results must be considered in relation to program limitations, including funding restrictions, confusion in Washington over federal health policy and relationships between similar federal programs, and less-than-full cooperation from organized medicine. Despite these factors, RMPs took steps toward regionalization, brought increased attention to continuing medical education, and demonstrated the growing governmental belief of decentralizing authority in favor of local agencies. The program illustrated the move from categorical, institutionally based programs toward more comprehensive efforts to deliver health care services.[31,32,33]

COMPREHENSIVE HEALTH PLANNING AND PUBLIC HEALTH SERVICE AMENDMENTS ACT OF 1966 (PARTNERSHIP FOR HEALTH ACT)

P.L. 89-749 was enacted in 1966 to integrate the various activities that the health care delivery system had been developing on an ad hoc basis. Before passage of this legislation, planning agencies could rely only on persuasion and education to further their goals. By 1966, however, large increases had occurred in the number of health programs and activities, in the volume of funds spent within the health care industry,

---

[30]James E. Bryan. "View from the Hill." *American Family Physician,* 4(2):125–127, August 1971.

[31]Thomas S. Bodenheimer. "RMPs: No Road to Regionalization." *Medical Care Review,* 26(11):1125–1166, December 1969.

[32]Irvin H. Page. "Are Regional Medical Programs Worth It?" *Modern Medicine,* 39(13):61–66, August 9, 1971.

[33]Anthony L. Komaroff. "Regional Medical Programs in Search of a Mission." *The New England Journal of Medicine,* 284(14):758–764, April 8, 1972.

and in the number of official and unofficial groups involved in planning and service. Pressure had built up across the nation for legal authority and enforceable sanctions, control of financial resources, quality control through licensing, and even a federal agency to regulate the health care system as if it were a public utility.

The result of all this ferment was the "partnership for health" or "umbrella" concept embodied in the Comprehensive Health Planning and Public Health Service Amendments Act of 1966. It aimed to correct fragmentation; to link all planning and services — public, private, or voluntary — into a cooperative, coordinated system; and to include not only personal health services but also environmental health services, facilities, and manpower.

In passing these amendments, Congress declared that "The fulfillment of our national purpose depends upon promoting and assuring the highest level of health attainable for every person, in an environment which contributes positively to healthful, individual and family living." The legislative body then indicated that comprehensive planning for health services, manpower, and facilities was essential to carry out that purpose.[34]

Comprehensive health planning was intended as a process through which both providers and consumers could agree on health needs, goals, and priorities; resources and measures to achieve goals; and recommendations for action by public and private sectors to enhance existing resources and activities and to develop those needed for the future. Comprehensive planning, unlike functional or specialized health planning, focused on the total health needs of all, rather than only on a specific program (e.g., mental illness), a particular type of service (e.g., restaurant sanitation), or a specific population group (e.g., children). It did not, however, diminish the need for specialized health planning or for specific program planning by operating health agencies. Instead, it was intended to provide the framework within which planning for specialized functions and special programs could be related to state and community priorities and objectives.

Provisions

The most significant provisions of the Partnership for Health Act were in sections 314(a) through (e), described as follows:

---

[34]Public Law 89-749. *Comprehensive Health Planning and Public Health Service Amendments Act of 1966.* Washington, D.C., U.S. Government Printing Office, 1966.

Section 314(a)—Formula Grants to States for Comprehensive Health Planning. Each state was required to designate a single state agency that would administer the health planning function and develop a plan describing that function. The single state agency could be located in the office of the governor or in the state health department or it could be an interdepartmental agency or board. The state plan, which had to be approved by the Secretary of Health, Education, and Welfare, was to provide for the establishment of a state health planning council that would include representatives from state and local agencies, nongovernmental organizations, health practitioners, and other groups concerned with health. A majority of the council would represent consumers of health services.

Section 314(b)—Project Grants for Area-wide Comprehensive Health Planning. Public agencies and private nonprofit organizations could apply for grants to develop comprehensive regional or local health planning in coordination with existing and planned health services, manpower, and facilities. Approval of local applications by the state health planning agency was required to ensure coordination of local and state efforts. Most of the sponsoring agencies were local governments, and others were area-wide councils of government. If an area-wide planning agency was not part of the local government, it had to provide for representation of that government.

Geographically, project areas were not confined to a single county or state but ranged in size from single counties to several counties in two or more states. Grantees were required to establish health planning councils composed of persons representing providers and consumers of health services, with the latter predominating.

Section 314(c)—Project Grants for Training, Studies, and Demonstrations in Health Planning. Grants to improve health planning skills and knowledge were awarded to public agencies and private nonprofit institutions and organizations, including universities. Training to develop planning skills was emphasized. Grants supported graduate and continuing education and training of consumers to participate in comprehensive health planning.

Section 314(d)—Formula Grants to State Health Authorities and Mental Health Authorities for Public Health Services. Grants under this section were awarded to help establish and maintain a full range of public health services. Funds were intended primarily to provide the states with the opportunity to initiate new and different methods of health protection. The objective was to fund necessary innovations, particularly when important health services could not be supported with existing state or local funds. This section also authorized a single block grant that replaced 15 categorical formula grants.

A plan to provide public health and mental health services was required from each state. The plan was to be developed by the state health and mental health departments and was to be compatible with the comprehensive health plan of the state.

The amount of each grant was based on a state's population and its per capita income. States were required to allocate at least 15 percent of their block grant funds to the mental health authority and to provide at least 70 percent of their total grant funds for health services at the community level.

Section 314(e)—Project Grants for Health Services Development. Under this section, priority was given to projects (especially in disadvantaged communities) that were designed to deliver comprehensive primary health care services. Funding was allocated on a project grant basis to meet specific limited needs or to develop new methods of health care delivery. Innovation in the delivery of such services was encouraged, as well as new or improved health care systems to increase efficiency and reduce costs. Also, active consumer and provider participation was sought in developing and operating comprehensive health service projects.

Any public or private nonprofit agency could apply for a project grant to be used for health services development. In keeping with the intent of the legislation, health services supported by grants under this section were to be provided in accordance with the state comprehensive health plan.

Implementation and Functions

The Partnership for Health Program was amended by P.L. 90-174 and P.L. 91-515. These amendments strengthened the program by increasing and extending its funding authorizations and requiring a national advisory council on comprehensive health planning programs, with council membership to represent health consumers as well as providers.

This program represented an effort on the part of the Federal Government to consolidate many parallel programs operating at state and local levels, thereby eliminating duplication of services and improving efficiency. With its amendments, the program gave states greater flexibility to support comprehensive health services by allowing them to channel grant funds into programs having the greatest need.

The comprehensive health planning (CHP) agency sought to be an advocate of the public interest in health and to provide the mechanisms for consumer input into health planning. It further provided a setting and means for tripartite participation in rational decision making—that is, involvement by consumer, provider, and government.[35,36,37,38,39]

Issues and Problems

One issue of considerable importance was the relationship between the 314(a) state agencies and the 314(b) local or area agencies and, in turn, the relationship of these agencies to the Regional Medical Program.

The first of these relationships depended on similarities and differences in state and local functions and on the degree of authority available to carry out those functions. Comprehensive health planning at the area and state levels was similar in that it focused on all people and their needs. Its processes were similar in concept at both levels— although they varied in detail—and included such tasks as data gathering, goal setting, developing alternatives, and review or approval of government grants and government-supported programs.

The difference between the two levels lay chiefly in the subjects that were dealt with in planning recommendations and decisions. Initially, at the state level, these were chiefly matters of broad policy affecting the entire state or whole groups of institutions, activities, or resources. At the area level, these planning procedures and decisions were more often specific to particular institutions, activities, or resources. Later, as certificate-of-need processes were developed, the state agency retained decision authority over individual cases. As a result, state decisions often differed from the recommendations of local agencies, causing considerable controversy.

What authority did the comprehensive health planning agency have or what was its source of influence? Certainly, the legislation went far to encourage—indeed to provide—a mandate for comprehensive planning by supplying funds and establishing a structure for implementing the law. In effect, the influence of the comprehensive health planning agency depended to a considerable extent on its success in providing the means and setting for acceptable participation by all interested

[35]Cyril Roseman. "Problems and Prospects for CHP." *American Journal of Public Health,* *62*(1):16–19, January 1972.

[36]U.S. Department of Health, Education, and Welfare. *Comprehensive Health Planning, Comprehensive Health Services Fact Sheet.* Washington, D.C., U.S. Government Printing Office, 1971.

[37]Ibid.

[38]U.S. Department of Health, Education, and Welfare, Public Health Service, Health Services and Mental Health Administration, Community Health Service, Division of Comprehensive Health Planning. *1971-1972 Graduate Education in Comprehensive Health Planning.* Washington, D.C., U.S. Government Printing Office, 1971.(HSM 71-6103)

[39]Community Health, Inc. *Legislation—New Programs, New Philosophies.* Health Planning Issue Paper No. 1. New York, March 1970.

parties. Thus, the area-wide agency was given certain responsibilities for review and comment on applications for federally financed projects. As noted, however, the state has the final authority in applications related to a certificate of need.

The role of the consumer was still another issue in the Comprehensive Health Planning program and gave rise to additional questions. How was a truly representative consumer elected or selected? How could that consumer avoid being co-opted by the program when he became a functionary within it? Was the consumer's role controlling, advisory, or some combination of the two?

The formula or block grant under section 314(d) also posed problems. For instance, the total block allocation was very little more than the total funding formerly provided by the various categorical grants. If previous funding was obligated to existing programs that could not be reduced or eliminated, then, in effect, there was no advantage to combining all of these programs into a single block grant. Furthermore, special-interest groups complained about the block grant, because, by including their specific efforts with others, they felt they had lost the visibility associated with identification as categorical programs.

Health planners and workers also were discouraged because the comprehensive health planning program at state and local levels had developed at such a slow pace and, in most places, had not reached maturity more than seven years after passage of the law. At that time, most agencies were still performing essentially a review and comment function rather than actually practicing comprehensive health planning. In addition, there were some negative feelings about a relative underemphasis on environmental, as compared to personal, health services. Furthermore, the relationship of the CHP agencies to the Regional Medical Program, the area-wide council of governments, the Hill-Burton state agency, the model cities program, and other planning or coordinating groups was never firmly established.[40,41,42,43,44,45]

[40]Leonard Robins. "The Impact of Decategorizing Federal Programs—Before and After 314(d)." *American Journal of Public Health, 62*(1):24–29, January 1972.

[41]U.S. Department of Health, Education, and Welfare, Public Health Service, Health Services and Mental Health Administration, Community Health Service, Division of Comprehensive Health Planning. *An Advocate of the Public Interest.* Washington, D.C., U.S. Government Printing Office, 1971. (HSM 71-6108)

[42]U.S. Department of Health, Education, and Welfare, *1971–1972 Graduate Education in Comprehensive Health Planning.*

[43]Community Health, Inc. *Legislation—New Programs, New Philosophies.*

[44]Roger M. Batistella. "The Course of Regional Health Planning." *Medical Care, 4*:149–161, May–June 1967.

[45]Nancy N. Anderson. *Comprehensive Health Planning in the State: A Study and Critical Analysis.* Minneapolis, Minn., Institute for Interdisciplinary Studies, American Rehabilitation Foundation, 1968, pp. 30–38.

As experience was gained with programs enacted during the 1960s, particularly the Comprehensive Health Planning and Regional Medical programs, and because the Hill-Burton program followed a pattern established in earlier decades, the inadequacies of these efforts at health planning became apparent. One of the greatest was the CHP agencies' lack of authority or ability to use sanctions. Consequently, an attempt was made to give these organizations some control over investments made in the health services system with the enactment in 1972 of P.L. 92-603.

Section 1122 of P.L. 92-603 said, in effect, that providers of health care services would not be reimbursed for certain expenses related to capital investment unless those investments had received the prior approval of a state-designated planning agency. This requirement was the culmination of a process that began with local review by CHP agencies. In effect, that review gave CHP organizations an opportunity to comment formally and make recommendations on capital investment, with a clear implication that unless the CHP agencies viewed proposals favorably, reimbursement of certain expenses would be withheld for patients sponsored by federal programs (specifically medicare, medicaid, and maternal and child health programs, sometimes referred to as titles V, XVIII, and XIX).

Although this process did give CHP agencies some control over capital investment, planning and resources development still was fragmented, weak, and generally inadequate. Therefore, after much argument, debate, and negotiation, Congress enacted the National Health Planning and Resources Development Act of 1974 (P.L. 93-641).

P.L. 93-641

In essence, the new act sought to combine the planning function of the CHP agency with the medical resources development activities of the Regional Medical Program (RMP) and the Hill-Burton program. The law has two sections: title XV, on national health planning and development, which encompasses what were previously CHP and RMP functions, and title XVI, on health resources development, which is analogous to the Hill-Burton program because it relates only to medical facilities. The first section of P.L. 93-641 highlights the issues that led to its enactment. It states, for example, that achieving equal access to quality health care at reasonable cost is a priority of the Federal Government and that previous massive expenditures of federal funds have contributed to inflation without producing adequate changes in the supply of health resources and services. The law also points out that health providers are key participants in the health care delivery system; thus, it is essential that they participate actively in framing health policies at all levels of government.

In recognition of the extent and urgency of health problems, the new law was designed to ease the formulation of recommendations for a national health planning policy (note that this is national planning policy and not health policy) to enhance planning activities at state and local levels and to provide financial aid for the development of planning resources.

Details of the planning process are embodied in title XV. First, Congress announced a set of 10 health priorities; next, it established the National Council on Health Planning and Development. The purpose of this council is to make recommendations to the Secretary of the Department of Health and Human Services (DHHS) on the development of national health planning guidelines; implement the programs mandated by P.L. 93-641; and evaluate new medical technology in relation to the organization, delivery, and distribution of health care services.

Health System Agencies

The law also provided for the establishment of local planning bodies known as health system agencies (HSAs). The first step in this process was to divide the country into 205 areas. There was much debate on the configuration of these areas and the need to include entire standard metropolitan statistical areas (SMSAs) within any service area. Basically, each HSA would be responsible for what could be termed a *health trade area,* regardless of the political jurisdictions involved.

The law was implemented, but the realities of the American political scene clearly were impossible to ignore. For instance, governors often refused to allow the allocation of parts of their states (those within an SMSA) to the jurisdiction of an HSA located in another state serving the same SMSA. Also, HSA boundaries often did not coincide with those of organizations established under other laws administered by DHEW. A striking example was the discrepancy between HSA boundaries and those of the professional standards review organizations (PSROs) — groups of doctors who reviewed hospital utilization.

The law provided that an HSA could be organized either as a private nonprofit corporation or a government entity. The latter might be either a public regional planning body or a single unit of local government. In any event, the HSA was to be governed by a board composed of community representatives, local government, and the providers of health services. A majority of the board members, but not more than 60 percent, were to be area residents who were generally representative of the area's population and consumers, rather than providers, of health care. This mix of consumers was to represent the community's interest groups.

The remaining members of the governing body were to be area residents who were providers of health care. The law even divided these providers into five categories. Category 1 included physicians, dentists, nurses, and other health professionals; category 2 comprised representatives of health care institutions; category 3, health care insurers; category 4, professional schools; and category 5, allied health professionals.

To complicate the development of a governing body still further, the law also required that not less than one-third of the providers be in the direct provider category and that the membership of the governing body include publicly elected officials, a proportional percentage of individuals residing in nonmetropolitan areas, and representatives from Veterans Administration hospitals, if any were within the area.

One of the weaknesses of the earlier CHP agencies was inadequacy of funding and their heavy reliance on contributions from provider organizations. To alleviate this problem, the new law authorized annual grants of presumably sufficient size to enable HSAs to carry out all of their assigned functions without any additional financial support. The amount to be granted was generally based on population size, with the maximum set at $0.50 per capita, up to $3,750,000.

In contrast to the old law, the National Health Planning and Resources Development Act explicitly prohibited HSAs from accepting funds or contributions of any kind from any person or organization having a financial, fiduciary, or other direct interest in the health service system. Health system agencies *are* permitted to accept contributions from nonfederal organizations, and the law authorizes the Federal Government to provide—in addition to the initial funding—matching grants up to an amount equal to $0.25 per capita. It is important to note, however, that these funding levels are contingent on an agency achieving a status known as full designation, which is based on the ability to meet the law's organizational requirements and program mandates.

Until an agency reaches full designation status, it operates under a conditional designation for a period not to exceed 24 months. During that time, the agency performs a limited number of functions designated by the secretary of DHHS. The agency may not use area health service development funds until it has achieved full designation status. These funds supplement the planning grant intended to provide resources for accomplishing HSA functions. They are to be awarded to individuals or agencies within the HSA's area, to help them plan and develop efforts that the agency believes will achieve goals established in the health system plan.

The array of functions to be performed by a fully designated agency includes

1. Assembling and analyzing data on the health status of the population within the HSA's service area, the status of the health care delivery system and its use, the system's effect on residents' health, an inventory of the area's health resources and utilization patterns for those resources, and occupational and environmental exposure factors that may affect health status

2. Preparing a health system plan (HSP)

3. Establishing an annual implementation plan (AIP), which identifies objectives leading to the achievement of priority HSP goals, and developing specific plans and projects to achieve those AIP objectives

4. Implementing the HSP and AIP through various methods, including technical assistance to persons or organizations wishing to develop health services and, when available, allocation of development funds to such persons or organizations

5. Coordinating HSA activities with PSROs and other area organizations having an interest in health

6. Reviewing and approving (or disapproving) proposed allocations of federal funds to health programs within the HSA area

7. Reviewing and making recommendations to the state planning agency on proposals to develop new institutional health services within the area

8. Reviewing periodically the appropriateness of existing institutional health services

9. Recommending projects to the state to modernize, construct, and convert area facilities

It is particularly important to note that the ability to accomplish each function affecting the health system is contingent on the existence of a realistic, viable health plan.

State-Level Provisions

At the state level, the 1974 law authorizes the establishment of a state health planning and development agency (SHPDA), to be selected by the governor of each state. The functions of this agency include developing not only a state health plan but a state medical facilities plan that fulfills the title XVI functions of P.L. 93-641, the National Health Planning and Resources Development Act. In addition, the agency must implement those parts of the state health plan that relate strictly to the state government.

To be approved by the secretary of DHHS and thus receive federal support, each state agency must develop and administer a program that outlines in considerable detail how the agency will carry out its functions. One of its major activities will be preparing the preliminary state health plan, which initially will consist of a compilation of the health system plans developed by the HSAs within the state. (This preliminary plan will be submitted to another entity, the Statewide Health Coordinating Council [SHCC], described in this section.) In addition, the state health agency must serve the designated planning body under section 1122 of P.L. 92-603 and must administer a state certificate-of-need program. The latter is reinforced by a periodic review of institutional health services and recommendations.

The SHPDA will be advised by the Statewide Health Coordinating Council, composed of at least 16 members appointed by the governor from lists provided by the HSAs within the state. In addition, the governor may make other appointments, provided they do not exceed 40 percent of the total SHCC membership. In other respects, the composition of this coordinating council parallels that of the HSA governing bodies; for example, one-third of the providers on the council must be direct providers.

The SHCC has a number of important functions, one of which is to review annually the plans developed by the HSAs within the state. It must then prepare a state health plan based on the preliminary state health plan, which is partially derived from these HSA plans. Further, the SHCC will review HSA budgets and will advise the state planning agency on its performance.

The SHCC also will review applications for final approval by the state health planning agency of federal grants related to area health service development funds and categorical programs such as community mental health centers. To support the operation of the state program, the Federal Government may contribute up to 75 percent of the operating cost of each state health planning agency.

Title XVI describes in detail the process by which the Federal Government will provide grants, loans, loan guarantees, or interest subsidies for the modernization, construction, or conversion of medical facilities. The title also describes the state medical facility plan, which is closely related to the state health plan prescribed by title XV.

Implementation of the National Health Planning and Resources Development Act, P.L. 93-641

Despite some delays in the development of federal regulations and some significant controversy at state and local levels over the boundaries of planning regions and the choice of agencies to be designated as HSAs, the organizational mandates of P.L. 93-641 were implemented reasonably quickly. At one point, there were 57 state agencies and 204 local agencies blanketing the United States. It is estimated that these agencies involved almost 9,000 volunteer governing body members and another 40,000 volunteers who served on subarea councils and task forces.[46]

The law authorized substantial sums of money to be used to improve the technical quality of the planning process through education and technical assistance. These efforts were to be undertaken by the Department of Health, Education, and Welfare's central and regional offices and by centers for health planning. Political pressure from within and outside the Federal Government led to decisions that precluded any standardization of plan documents or the processes by which they were developed. This caused great anxiety and much confusion and recrimination when agencies sought federal approval of their plans as part of the process of becoming a designated health system agency. In addition, there was inefficient use of staff resources when the professional members of each agency sought a sound approach to the new concept of system planning. A few agencies made some truly creative contributions to the state of the art,[47] but most seldom created more than a complex of categorical resource plans placed between two covers.

While the Federal Government was in the process of implementing P.L. 93-641, the Carter administration arrived in Washington and, despite campaign promises to develop a national health insurance program, made "cost containment" the major initiative in the health field. To achieve this goal, it seized the health planning system as a potentially useful tool. Because it was believed that capital expenditures eventually led to increased operating expenses, emphasis shifted from planning as a system development concept to certificate of need (CON) as a means to restrict investment in health services and facilities. This was

---

[46]Draft of "Outline for Health Planning Portion of HRSA Background Book." Hyattsville, Md., Department of Health and Human Services, October 15, 1982, p. 3. Mimeographed.

[47]See, for example, *Community Health Analysis,* by G. E. Alan Dever, Germantown, Md., Aspen Systems Corp., 1979, especially chap. 10.

hardly a novel idea—CON-like activities had been introduced years earlier in many states—but this single-minded emphasis had two important effects.

First, it alienated many local constituents of the planning program. Some providers were hostile to the concept merely as a matter of principle, but most saw and supported the logic of controlled regional development of an integrated system. The nonprovider constituents were usually those who subscribed to the other priorities announced in the law (e.g., improvement of accessibility). As it became clear that the Federal Government's only concern was restriction of spending, both provider and nonprovider constituents withdrew their support of what they perceived to be a distorted program.

Second, by making the number or dollar value of disapproved applications for a certificate of need the only evaluative criterion, the executive branch made it impossible to defend the planning program to the legislative branch. Many members of Congress, particularly those not serving on health-related committees and thus not intimately acquainted with the details of health programs, were besieged by provider constituents who wanted the program abolished. When members of Congress inquired about the achievements of health planning, they were presented with numbers that indicated there had been little or no success in curbing new investment projects and with vague assurances that such positive things as consumer involvement were occurring at state and local levels. These assurances had little credibility in the eyes of many members of Congress, particularly those who relied on the reactions of their constituents to test the validity of the assertions in their district or state. Most constituents were either unaware of or indifferent to this program. Among constituents who were aware and involved, those who were disenchanted far outnumbered the program's supporters.

The degree of success of CON programs is still debatable. The studies usually cited suffer from serious methodological problems. For instance, most measurements of effectiveness were taken long before the impact of any of the programs had become evident. Also, there is no satisfactory method for identifying and evaluating the applications that were never submitted because of the CON program. Furthermore, there is dispute over measurement of the costs of the program, especially to the individual health organizations (these costs include the administrative/legal costs of processing and defending a proposal and the increased costs of carrying out the project because of the delay in starting).

Although many have concluded that the CON program was a failure, some recent information suggests otherwise. One study[48] showed that when CON was linked closely with other strong regulatory programs, such as rate review, the combined programs were likely to effectively slow the growth of hospital costs. Another study[49] concluded that CON's underlying concept is indeed valid. The analysis revealed that each dollar of capital investment led to an increase of $0.22 in annual operating costs. Furthermore, it pointed out that operating costs tend to build up over time and estimated that the present value of these operating costs for a 10-year period would be $1.84 per dollar of investment. Still another reviewer[50] concluded that "There is some evidence that certificate-of-need programs become more effective over time but the potential for these programs will remain highly dependent on the state's political commitment and support." Finally, several surveys[51] show that, despite the absence of positive formal evidence of CON's effectiveness, most states intend to continue their CON programs even if the Federal Government withdraws completely.

Because of the problems with CON, support for the planning program quickly began to wane. This was reflected in a decline in federal appropriations after an initial period of growth (from approximately $91 million in 1976 to $158 million in 1980, $116 million in 1981, and $58 million in 1982).[52] Also, the authorization levels for these years were never met (1976, $128 million; 1980, $191 million; 1981, $213 million; 1982, $140 million).[53] In short, the planning program was never funded at the levels intended by the original legislation and the gap widened over the years.

Congress made some modifications in agency responsibilities in P.L. 96-79, which was enacted in 1979. This law added six new goals; three

---

[48]Nicole Urban and Thomas W. Bice. "Measuring Regulation and Its Effects on Hospital Behavior." Seattle, University of Washington, September 1981 (unpublished). Cited in: Congressional Budget Office, *Health Planning: Issues for Reauthorization,* Washington, D.C., U.S. Government Printing Office, March 1982, p. 23.

[49]Arthur D. Little, Inc. *Development of an Evaluation Methodology for Use in Assessing Data Available to the Certificate of Need (CON) and Health Planning Programs.* Cambridge, Mass., Department of Health and Human Services, Contract No. 233-79-4003, April 1982. Cited in: *Health Planning: Lessons for the Future,* by Bonnie Lefkowitz, Rockville, Md., Aspen Systems Corp., 1982, p. 123.

[50]Jack Needleman. *Assessing Regulatory and Market Strategies.* Bethesda, Md., Alpha Center, June 1982, p. 3.

[51]Intergovernmental Health Policy Project, *State Health Notes,* Washington, D.C., The George Washington University, December 1981; *AlphaWaves,* Bethesda, Md., Alpha Center, October 1981.

[52]Congressional Budget Office. *Health Planning: Issues for Reauthorization.* Washington, D.C., U.S. Government Printing Office, March 1982, p. 3.

[53]Draft of "Outline for Health Planning Portion of HRSA Background Book," Appendix III.

focused on the accessibility of mental health services and three on cost containment. To restrain the relentless increase in health costs, agencies were required to foster competition. The exact nature of competition was not defined, but at least this law permitted a mix of market and regulatory efforts, recognizing that given the circumstances prevalent in the United States, a total regulatory system was politically unacceptable and pure competition without some reliance on regulation to ensure the maintenance of conditions required for competition could not succeed.[54]

This period of cautious adjustment ended abruptly in January 1981. The Reagan administration advocated total reliance on competition to control the escalation of health care costs,[55] a position strongly supported by certain policy analysis organizations.[56] The notion to immediately discontinue planning also found favor with members of Congress who strongly supported the administration's policies. They attempted to include in the budget provisions that would have terminated all funds for the health planning program at the end of fiscal year 1981. The administration's proposal was less drastic, providing a rapid phase-out over a three-year period. Nevertheless, many proponents of competition as the *primary* mechanism for reform of the health services system urged a more cautious approach.[57] Their concerns were shared by a wide range of individuals representing third-party payers, business executives, legislators, and financial experts; but other equally reputable thinkers tended to make light of these considerations. For instance, some members of the financial community asserted that it would be impossible to raise capital for projects that were not economically rewarding and that CON was therefore an unnecessary burden and expense.[58]

In 1982, the pendulum began to swing back toward support of some sort of planning program. The weaknesses of the program established

---

[54]Donald R. Cohodes. "Where You Stand Depends on Where You Sit: Musings on the Regulation/Competition Dialogue." *Journal of Health Politics, Policy and Law,* 7(1):54–79, Spring 1982.
[55]Linda E. Demkovich. "If the Health Planning Lid Is Removed, Will a Hospital Building Boom Erupt?" *National Journal, 13*(25):1110–1113, June 20, 1981.
[56]See, for example, *A New Approach to the Economics of Health Care,* edited by Mancur Olson, Washington, D.C., American Enterprise Institute, 1981; particularly good illustrations in Olson's book are "Health Care Competition: Are Tax Incentives Enough?" by Jack A. Meyer (pp. 424–449) and "Paying the Piper and Calling the Tune: The Relationship Between Public Financing and Public Regulation of Health Care," by Mark V. Pauly (pp. 67–86).
[57]See, for example, Clark C. Havighurst, *Deregulating the Health Care Industry,* Cambridge, Mass., Ballinger, 1982.
[58]Linda E. Demkovich. "If the Health Planning Lid Is Removed, Will a Hospital Building Boom Erupt?"

by P.L. 93-641 were identified, and proposals to overcome them were suggested. Among the deficiencies noted were

1. The program bypassed state government.
2. It required consumer participation but permitted providers to opt out, thus allowing the providers to put the onus of unpopular decisions on the consumers.
3. It was unable to implement many of its decisions (particularly decisions to make positive changes in the health services system) because the only significant power was the negative thrust of the CON program.[59]
4. The program required consumer participation (as a legacy from an earlier era), even though this effort to "open up the system" was regarded as inconsequential compared with the need to contain costs.
5. It was assigned regulatory responsibilities of such high priority that they consumed virtually all of the available resources, leaving little time or energy for the rational decision-making process that planning should be.
6. It was supported inadequately by both state and Federal Government, whereas the providers who opposed the planning decisions had ready access to those in power.[60]

Despite administration efforts to abolish the planning program by withholding funding in the budgetary process, and although the law was scheduled to expire in September 1982, Congress extended it by a continuing resolution that provided funds for an additional year. During that session of Congress, several legislators tried to secure passage of new legislation that would have corrected many of the program's problems (e.g., by increasing the thresholds of the CON program so that only projects of substantial import would have to be reviewed). But, during a lame duck session, a final compromise that had already been passed in the House was blocked by the Secretary of Health and Human Services, Richard Schweiker. Mr. Schweiker also authorized other actions that further reduced the size and effectiveness of the health planning program (e.g., termination of local agencies that, due to the reduction in federal funding, were unable to meet the staffing requirement established in the law). Once again, Congress intervened,

---

[59]John T. Tierney and William J. Waters. "The Evolution of Health Planning." *The New England Journal of Medicine, 308*(2):95–97, January 13, 1983.
[60]Symond R. Gottlieb, as reported in *Health Facilities Planning for the 1980's: Responses to a Changing Environment,* Bethesda, Md., Alpha Center, September 1982, pp. 2–4.

and the program was stabilized until new legislation could be developed and considered by the next Congress.[61]

Update on Community Health Planning Programs

After the 98th Congress convened in January 1983, numerous bills to renew the authorization of the federal health planning program were introduced in both the Senate and the House. There were many differences in the views of the bills' sponsors, however, and a final compromise measure had not been formulated by the end of the first session. Nevertheless, several significant events during the year suggested that continuation of the federal health planning program in some form was likely.

At the national level, Congress enacted prospectively priced reimbursement of the hospital portion of medicare. The prospective prices were to be based on typical costs incurred while treating patients with similar diagnoses. To accomplish this, diagnoses were placed into clusters called diagnosis-related groups (DRGs). This system was designed to revise the incentives in the reimbursement system to constrain the ever-increasing cost of hospital care.[62] But Congress temporarily postponed dealing with capital costs and permitted hospitals to continue to be reimbursed retrospectively for capital. It is now believed that until capital costs can be incorporated in the prospective pricing scheme, some mechanism to control hospital capital expenditures is essential. At this point, many people have come to realize that the only existing external check on hospital capital spending is the health planning program.[63] Consequently, language that would ensure temporary continuation of the federal health planning program in the absence of reauthorization was included in a law that appropriated funds for operation of the Federal Government.[64]

Also at the national level, the Director of the Office of Management and Budget, David Stockman, informed Congress that the administra-

---

[61]"Health Planning Odyssey Continues." *Washington Report on Health Legislation,* January 5, 1983, pp. 5–7.

[62]For a discussion of the implications of the recently enacted prospective payment legislation, see *Health Care Institutions in Flux: Changing Reimbursement Patterns in the 1980s,* edited by Warren Greenberg and Richard McK. F. Southby, Arlington, Va., Information Resources Press, 1984.

[63]Linda E. Demkovich. "When Medicare Tears Up the Blank Check, Who Will Lend Hospitals Capital?" *National Journal, 16*(3):113–116, January 21, 1984.

[64]*Today in Health Planning, 5*(19), October 3, 1983.

tion had abandoned its effort to eliminate the health planning program[65] but stressed that the administration preferred the least stringent bill among the various proposals.

Later in the year, the American Hospital Association, which had been a leading opponent of the federal health planning program, reached agreement with the American Health Planning Association and announced its support of a proposal to reauthorize the program. This proposal was based on a set of jointly developed principles.[66,67]

Various influential members of the health-related committees of Congress continued to press for the passage of legislation that would continue the national health planning program. For instance, in April 1984, Senator Lowell Weicker introduced a bill that would reauthorize the health planning program for three years. This bill includes provision for grants to both state and local agencies, grants for technical assistance from health planning centers, and continuation of the CON process.[68] The demands of campaigning in an election year and several other issues of greater urgency prevented Congress from taking any definitive action in 1984, so the future of the federal program remains uncertain.

During 1983 and 1984, there was also considerable interest in health planning at the state level. This often took the form of legislative activity in the states, but no widespread patterns were apparent. Some states revised their certificate-of-need statutes, others restructured their health planning organizations, and some provided state funding for local health planning agencies.[69] Also, some governors sought authority to reverse earlier decisions regarding the elimination of local health planning agencies in their states.[70]

Finally, there was considerable activity at the local level involving health planning agencies and business coalitions. Much of this work was supported with local funds, but resources also were made available through grants from prestigious national foundations and corporations.[71]

The business coalitions were often very similar to the voluntary local health planning agencies that disappeared for lack of a purpose after the implementation of the Comprehensive Health Planning Act. As government-sponsored local health planning agencies were disbanded

[65] *Washington Report on Medicine & Health, 37*(31), August 8, 1983.
[66] *Washington Report on Medicine & Health, 37*(45), November 14, 1983.
[67] *Today in Health Planning, 5*(22), November 14, 1983.
[68] *Today in Health Planning, 6*(7), April 2, 1984.
[69] *State Health Notes,* No. 39, October–November 1983.
[70] "Planning Revival." *National Journal, 15*(51–52):2642, December 17, 1983.
[71] *Business, Labor and Planning Notes, 1*(3), September 16, 1983.

or became less effective when federal support was drastically reduced, the coalitions emerged rapidly. In 1983, the number of extant coalitions was more than 150.[72] These coalitions were often influential at the state level because of the power of their members. For instance, the Hartford Business Coalition was instrumental in getting all-payer prospective payment system legislation enacted in Connecticut.[73] After a long and difficult struggle with the state hospital association, the Arizona Coalition for Cost Effective Quality Health Care obtained more than 109,000 signatures on a petition in support of a state constitutional amendment that would legalize public-utility-style regulation of health services.[74]

HISTORY OF INSTITUTIONAL PLANNING

The history of community planning can be described as a series of events that were more-or-less widely experienced at the same points in time. The history of institutional planning,[75] on the other hand, can be described as a series of levels of planning that have emerged over time and through which individual institutions are passing in an uneven evolutionary process. Indeed, some institutions have yet to take the first step toward planning; they are at Ackoff's inactive level of planning. At the opposite extreme are the innovators and early adopters who are now successfully engaged in strategic planning. The intermediate steps include basic financial planning, forecast-based program planning, and externally oriented market planning.

Basic financial planning focuses on the annual budget and strongly emphasizes operational control aimed at achieving very-short-run objectives. Forecast-based planning extends these efforts to include longer range goals based on estimates of the future state of the environment. Externally oriented planning seeks to improve forecast-based planning by taking into account a wider range of considerations, especially the anticipated reactions of consumers and competitors.

---

[72]"Hospital Research and Educational Trust." In: *Environmental Assessment: Overview 1984.* Chicago, American Hospital Assn., 1984. p. 11.
[73]"Connecticut Business/Planning Efforts Changing Reimbursement System." *Business, Labor and Planning Notes, 2*(4):3, May 14, 1984.
[74]"Arizona Coalition Gains Signatures Needed To Place Initiative on Ballot." *Hospital Week, 20*(21):2, May 25, 1984.
[75]The term *institutional* is used here to denote planning by organizations, whether they are individual institutions or, as is becoming more common, systems of institutions.

Strategic planning goes even further by adopting a proactive stance in which the planning organization attempts to create the future. Some of the notable differences between strategic planning and the other types of planning are that strategic planning

1. Stresses interaction analysis
2. Requires market research
3. Emphasizes social and economic aspects of medical care, as well as clinical considerations
4. Uses "futures" data, as well as historical data
5. Focuses on the wishes of the customer rather than on what the professional would like to offer the customer
6. Emphasizes long-run return on investment rather than short-run profit and budget balancing

The evolutionary process of institutional planning can be attributed to a number of factors. Among these are community planning activities, reimbursement patterns, stakeholder expectations, and technological change. The various government and private-sector community planning programs (e.g., the Hill-Burton program) rewarded planning behavior through the allocation of resources. This phenomenon was particularly evident in communities with strong "voluntary" planning programs that espoused a strategy of encouraging individual institutional planning as an alternative to mandated community-wide planning. Similarly, many institutions established a planning function as a means of coping with the regulatory requirements associated with CON programs. From the planners' point of view, this was doing the right thing for the wrong reason, but it did provide substantial impetus to the evolutionary process.

Prior to 1965, most health services organizations saw themselves as eleemosynary institutions. With the advent of medicare and medicaid, the government sought to ensure more widespread, more certain accessibility of health services by reimbursing providers who cared for persons who previously had relied on charity care. This changed the hospital's role and the orientation of its mission. Now, instead of providing as much care as possible within the limits of funds received from self-paying patients, privately insured patients, and philanthropy, the hospital sought to maximize reimbursements, particularly from government systems that agreed to pay hospitals for all "reasonable" charges attributed to government-sponsored patients. This reimbursement system not only provided sufficient funds for survival but also fostered expansion, since much of the cost of newly acquired facilities and technology could be included in the charges that government would pay. Furthermore, if the hospital managed its accounting and finances astutely, there would be surplus revenue that could be used for further expansion or transferred to stockholders as profit. Finally, even if the hospital had insufficient surplus revenue, expansion could usually be financed by borrowing.

Since the government programs virtually guaranteed the solvency of participating hospitals, hospital bonds became very attractive investments. The availability of capital financing and the opportunity to earn surplus revenues led to a rapid increase in both capacity and high-technology equipment. Institutional planning in this era concentrated on expansion of plant and equipment. As CON programs were implemented, some of the institutional planning effort was devoted to overcoming these constraints on organizational growth.

The 1122 program enacted in 1972 was the harbinger of federal concerns and responses to the rapid escalation of the annual federal expenditures for medical care. The later, more stringent CON requirements of P.L. 93-641 also proved inadequate to halt the continuing increase in federal expenditures, which was the natural consequence of the reimbursement system. They did, however, introduce competition into the system, in that different organizations vied for the implicit "franchise" to offer a particular service within their service area.

Competition, in the classic economic sense, was seen by many as the remedy for the excessive growth and utilization of health services. It was not a meaningful concept, however, until the reimbursement system was changed. This occurred when Congress included the prospective pricing system in the Social Security Amendments of 1983 (P.L. 98-21). Under this system, the hospital planning process must focus on surviving and prospering by providing services that cost the institution less than the level of reimbursement established by the government or other payer. (Many nongovernmental payers are seeking to prevent cost shifting and to minimize their own expenditures by entering into special arrangements with hospitals, such as preferred provider organizations, or PPOs.) This situation is similar to the circumstances faced by commercial enterprises; hence, hospitals have adopted the techniques of corporate strategic planning to meet the challenge.

The debate over ways to contain the costs of medical care has also influenced stakeholder expectations. Many of the most influential stakeholders have been convinced that hospitals are at least partly to blame for the cost problems because of inefficient operations. Since, in the culture of the United States, private-sector business is regarded as the epitome of managerial effectiveness, these stakeholders have begun to demand that hospitals demonstrate comparable competence in delivering health services and in producing an acceptable "bottom line." Other stakeholders—prospective patients—also have changed their perceptions of their roles, rights, and responsibilities. For instance, many now accept responsibility for maintaining their health with a minimum of medical intervention, and, when medical care is needed, they exercise their right to be active participants in the decision-making process. Such changes in stakeholder expectations have made it essential for hospitals to adopt a market-oriented approach to planning.

To prosper in this competitive environment, a hospital must position itself as a provider of high-quality care. High technology is often perceived as a manifestation of high quality. Consequently, the rapid appearance of new technologies (currently magnetic resonance imaging, monoclonal antibodies, genetic probes, and so on) compels the organization to develop strategic plans for its portfolio of service programs.

Finally, all the forgoing have contributed to radical changes in the organizational structure of health services institutions. Many have become parts of multi-institutional systems. Reorganization into diversified corporations is widespread. These structural changes require significant modification in management style, systems, and procedures. The approach of the traditional free-standing voluntary community hospital to governance and management is seen as inadequate for the current environment. Reactive, resource-oriented planning in particular is identified as an organizational weakness that cannot be tolerated.

The evolution of institutional planning has been uneven because of the substantial resistance it has encountered. Strategic planning requires new skills, additional knowledge, and different behavior; but people have learned that their present behavior produces rewards, and they are therefore unwilling to take the risk and commit the energy required to implement a process that is unfamiliar and/or untried. Nevertheless, it is clear that strategic planning is a key to institutional survival.

It is generally accepted that hospitals, as the largest organizations in the health services industry, have tended to be the leaders in the adoption of planning and other innovations that require a large economic support base. A sample survey conducted in 1980 by The Center for Health Services Research of the University of Southern California provides the most recent data available on the level of planning activity in hospitals. (A review of the professional literature suggests that these data are simply reflective of a point on an upward trend line.) Sixty-four percent of the planning departments identified in the survey had been in existence for less than three years. The results, as reported by the American Hospital Association, are as follows:

1. Thirty percent of all respondents reported having an in-house planner other than the chief executive officer (CEO). Teaching, urban, voluntary, and larger hospitals were more likely to employ planners.

2. Ninety-three percent of the responding planners indicated that they reported to the CEO.

3. The chief executive officers reported spending an average of 15 percent of their time in planning but felt that the allocation of effort should be increased to 19 percent. They also reported a strong commitment to the planning process by trustees and a low level of commitment by members of the medical staff.

4. In addition to in-house planners, 60 percent of all hospitals employed consultants for planning assignments. (The report does not say what proportion of the consulting effort took place in those hospitals with no planning staff, so it is not possible to estimate how many hospitals in the sample did no planning. Other responses, however, indicate that 69 percent of all hospitals claimed to have a written long-range plan.)

5. Finally, the respondents predicted a dramatic increase in the emphasis on market-based planning over the next five years, accompanied by a smaller, but still substantial, decline in the emphasis on planning for facilities.[76]

SUMMARY

This chapter describes the history of health services planning in the United States. It especially emphasizes community planning and hospital planning.

Community planning evolved from concerns with public health regarding availability, accessibility, quality, and cost of health services. Ultimately, cost became the dominant concern. Although this country's traditions favored a laissez-faire approach to medical care, serious, persistent problems led to government involvement. At first, the Federal Government sought to correct the identified problems by assisting state, local, and private-sector agencies with grants-in-aid. This

---

[76]American Hospital Association, Division of Hospital Planning. *Summary of Hospital Planning Survey: Final Report.* Chicago, American Hospital Assn., n.d.

led to individual successes but usually left many gaps in the system and sometimes created duplicate or overlapping services.

Next, the government attempted to foster comprehensive community-wide voluntary planning involving both providers and consumers. When it became evident that voluntarism was ineffective in dealing with the problems of the system across the nation, an elaborate national health planning program was mandated. Almost as soon as this program was established, the Carter administration chose to use it as its major tool for dealing with the problems of rapidly increasing federal expenditures for medical care. The technique emphasized was the certificate of need, a regulatory mechanism that had been attached to the planning process. Evaluation of CON effectiveness is difficult at best, and the evidence to date is inconclusive. The Reagan administration saw health planning as one of many regulatory programs that ran counter to its philosophy of government. Consequently, it sought, unsuccessfully, to terminate the program. The administration's efforts did, however, succeed in reducing support to the point that all agencies were incapable of fulfilling the mandate of P.L. 93-641 and many local agencies were forced out of existence. Despite the opposition of the executive branch, Congress has continued to support the national health planning program, and efforts to enact a revised program continue with the support of some organizations that had previously advocated abolition of a national health planning effort.

With the decline of vigorous federally supported local health planning, many voluntary organizations have emerged to fill the void. Most are business-sponsored coalitions with special concerns for the welfare of corporate employees and for the costs employers incur for health-related fringe benefits.

Hospital planning in a sense is a prototype of institutional planning. Until recently, few other health services organizations had the resources or the need to engage in formal planning. Hospital planning has evolved from limited intermittent responses to opportunities for expansion of medical services to strategic planning for diversified corporations. Intermediate phases in the evolutionary process included financial, program, and market planning. Although hospitals have progressed through this evolutionary process at a slow and uneven pace, current threats to organizational survival are providing greater impetus to the development of modern planning programs. These threats arise from factors such as a changed reimbursement system, technological advances, new stakeholder perspectives, and the effects of community health services planning.

4

PLANNING FOR HEALTH
SERVICES SYSTEMS

UNDERSTANDING SYSTEMS

To understand the idea of a health system plan, one must first have a good grasp of the concept of a system, which is well illustrated by a Zen proverb: "For the man who is ignorant, trees are trees, waters are waters, and mountains are mountains. When that man gains understanding, then trees are not trees, waters are not waters, and mountains are not mountains, and when at last the man attains wisdom then once again trees are trees, waters are waters, and mountains are mountains."

Sometimes, a person cannot see the forest for the trees. In other words, one must examine the big picture in order to make valid decisions. True understanding or wisdom occurs when those who grasp the picture also understand the symbiotic interaction of all its components. This is the essence of the systems approach.

It is useful to consider a system in terms of its purposes and methods, as shown in Figure 4. This simplified diagram illustrates the basic idea of a system, which can be defined as a set of elements linked together in a purposeful way to convert input into output. The part of the diagram labeled *Process* represents the actions and interactions of the elements of the system that transform inputs into outputs.

When using Figure 4 as a simplified representation of the health system, one must realize that the final output is different from what one might expect to find in, say, a manufacturing process. One could say that inputs, mainly health resources, are processed through the delivery system to create health services. These services, however, are

65

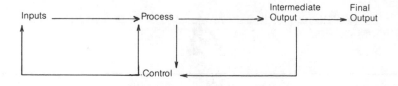

Figure 4   Simple schematic representation of a system.

not the end that is truly sought but simply a means to the ultimate end of health status, designated here as final output. A system, moreover, does not act in an uncontrolled fashion. Instead, it follows a cybernetic pattern in which those involved use information about what has occurred to adjust future actions so that they will be more likely to achieve the system's purposes. Specifically, information about the resources used, how they were processed, and the results is gathered into a control element. Through this element, it is decided whether the system should function differently in the future to better achieve the desired outcome. Starling[1] offers three descriptions of system performance that illustrate the importance of an effective control subsystem in today's environment:

1. *Equilibrium-seeking system.* It is assumed that the equilibrium state is efficient and, therefore, that disruptions cause inefficiencies. Consequently, the system seeks to prevent disruptions and, when they do occur, seeks to return to the equilibrium state as quickly as possible. Since the recovery of equilibrium is relatively slow, the system cannot tolerate many disruptions for any period of time because the cumulative impacts will become so great that the system will disintegrate. In view of this danger, leaders do their best to preserve equilibrium by resisting change and exerting more and more control. This tends to be self-defeating, however, because the system becomes ever more rigid and, thus, less able to cope with the disruptions that will inevitably occur.

2. *Homeostatic system.* Such a system attempts to maintain dynamic processes by responding to feedback messages. It focuses on maintaining an efficient ratio between inputs and outputs. These responses tend to alter the system's components so as to reduce the deviance

---

[1]Jay D. Starling. "The Use of System Constructs in Simplifying Organizational Complexity." In: *Organized Social Complexity.* Edited by Todd R. LaPorte. Princeton, N.J., Princeton University Press, 1975, pp. 151–172.

from preestablished goals. A homeostatic system does not attempt to adapt to the environment by altering its goals.

3. *Adaptive system*. This is an open system that is not disrupted by intrusive events in its environment. In fact, it needs these intrusions so that it can learn how to adapt to the environment. Consequently, some level of deviance among its members is valued as a resource of information and behavior that can be used in the future to make effective adaptations. Because of the high level of interaction with the environment, it is often difficult to determine the precise boundaries of an adaptive system. For instance, because of its involvement in emergency medical services, should a fire department be included in the definition of a medical system?

The systems approach suggested by the Zen proverb implies a holistic concept that considers all the alternatives and interactions among all parts of the system. Charles Lindblom[2] and others who subscribe to the incrementalist school correctly assert that it is impossible to achieve the ideal expressed in the systems approach. Their contention is that real-world decisions must be made incrementally; that it is not reasonable for human decision makers to cope with the vast amount of information required to make such comprehensive decisions; and, in fact, it is not even possible to generate all the data needed for these decisions. On the other hand, results of the incremental strategy would tend to be very small, marginal changes, possibly moving in a consistent direction but at a very slow pace.

An alternative to the incremental approach is suggested by Amitai Etzioni[3] in his model of mixed scanning. This model assumes that a system can be viewed in different levels of detail, so that a problem of immediate concern can be examined very closely and with a great deal of specificity. That problem, however, must also be considered within the context of a larger system, described at a much higher level of generality. Because more general descriptions can be synthesized from the specifics of a problem, one can reasonably deal with that problem in terms that are comparable to the general description of the remainder of the system.

This concept of mixed scanning is particularly important in developing a large and complex health system plan. It is surely beyond the

---

[2]Charles E. Lindblom. "The Science of Muddling Through." *Public Administration Review, 19*:79–88, Spring 1959.
[3]Etzioni's concept of mixed scanning as a planning strategy is described in George Chadwick, *A Systems View of Planning*, New York, Pergamon, 1971.

capacity of almost any organization to develop equally all elements of a health system plan in a short period of time, such as one year. Consequently, a feasible strategy for the organization is to describe the entire health services system in broad, general terms, to seek further definition of priority concerns in the community, and to provide sufficiently detailed descriptions that will enable decision makers to act in these priority areas. Gradually, the decision maker's attention can focus on other parts of the system, either by shifting priorities or through acting on proposals that require reviews and recommendations. Such parts will then be described as fully as those first addressed in the plan development process. Eventually, this evolutionary process will lead to the construction of a uniform health system plan for all elements of the system.

Definitions

Progression beyond this point will be difficult unless certain important terms are defined. The following definitions will be assumed throughout the remainder of this book:

1. *Environment.* Environment in this context does not relate to the physical or social milieu commonly associated with health planning. In other words, it does not mean clean air or pure water. In a systems context, environment refers to everything outside the system. The environment of the health system comprises the public education system, the public safety system, and the social welfare system, among others.

2. *Boundary.* The boundary of the system defines the system's scope in order to separate the system from its environment. To illustrate, the boundary of a health services system depends on what definition of health is adopted. A health planning body could, for example, adopt the very expansive definition of health proposed by the World Health Organization. Alternatively, it might decide to use a much more restricted definition, one that considers only medical care and services. The external boundary of an organization as a system is determined by its mission.

3. *Boundary Conditions.* This term can be used to describe how a system interacts with its environment. Usually, a system must make exchanges with outside elements. For instance, health planners may need to seek assistance from those in public education to ensure that a health promotional strategy is successfully implemented. On the other hand, those in the educational system might find it necessary to ask health

system planners to modify their activities in order to enhance the educational process (e.g., educators might ask health care providers to offer primary care services at various hours to minimize the number of school days lost when students obtain medical care). Longest[4] has developed an insightful analysis of how hospitals, as systems, must adapt their strategies to the demands and opportunities presented by their environments.

4. *Subsystems.* A system can be so complex that it often cannot be dealt with as a single entity. In such cases, the ability to manage the system effectively is much improved when one understands its components or subsystems.[5] In fact, one can imagine a hierarchy of systems. Each system is a component of a larger system and is itself composed of other smaller systems. For instance, one can envision a hierarchy extending from incredibly small subatomic particles to the expansiveness of the universe, with many intermediate levels. Within this range, each human being represents a system having a number of subsystems, such as the circulatory and respiratory systems. These, in turn, are composed of parts such as the heart and lungs. Moving in the opposite direction, we, as individuals, are part of larger systems: family, neighborhood, community, political jurisdiction, state, and nation. The question then becomes, how far should the planner explore in each direction when examining the expanses of the system. This is determined by the established boundary and by another concept, the *black box*.

5. *Element (Black Box).* This is the lowest level of subsystem that concerns decision makers. They are interested only in the performance, inputs, and outputs of a black box and have no concern with its internal workings. The hierarchy of subsystems ending in the black box can be illustrated by a familiar example. Each of us lives in a house or apartment, which is a shelter system. Within that system are various subsystems (e.g., for eating and recreation). The recreational subsystem has additional components, one of which could be a television set. For most of us, the television set is literally and figuratively a black box. In other words, we simply are not capable of or interested in critically examining the internal action of that device. Consequently, we concern ourselves only with the inputs (how much electricity does it consume?), the performance (does it begin to function as soon as we

---

[4]Beaufort B. Longest, Jr. "An External Dependence Perspective of Organizational Structure: The Community Hospital Case." *Hospital and Health Services Administration, 26*:50–69, Spring 1981.
[5]La Porte refers to this approach to dealing with complexity as the development of decomposable systems.

push the "on" switch?), and the outputs (does it provide clear pictures in realistic colors and a sound of reasonable fidelity?). Within health services organizations, the black box can be the program management unit (PMU). The PMU is a revenue center that provides closely related services (e.g., an oncology PMU or a cardiology PMU). In larger organizations, PMUs can be clustered into subsystems called strategic business units (SBUs).

6. *Attributes.* The characteristics of system performance that can be expressed operationally. Returning to our earlier example of the sound of a television set, we could ask for specifications of the audio output in terms of a frequency range, such as 20 hertz to 20 megahertz.

7. *Inputs.* Resources used by the system.

8. *Outputs.* Products or services the system creates by using its resources.

9. *Feedback.* Information on the system's performance that can be used to adjust its future operation. It is important to note that all the data in the feedback loop consist of historical information.

10. *Feedforward.* Information on expectations about future conditions in which the system will be operating. Feedback provides only historical information. The real concern is making changes in the system that will enable it to adapt to the circumstances in which it will be operating. This process is somewhat like leading the target in skeet shooting. Planners must anticipate where the system will be so they can make appropriate adjustments and achieve the desired performance.

11. *Closed System.* For all practical purposes, this system is independent of its environment. Analysis of such a system focuses only on what occurs within the system itself and ignores interactions between the system and its environment. This clearly is not a realistic representation of the usual social organization, but it has great merit as an analytic device because it allows planners to make a less-complex analysis of the system's operation as a preliminary step to considering the greater complexity of an open system.

12. *Open System.* The open system involves exchanges of resources, information, and outputs with the environment. Usually, the number of interactions is very large, and, thus, the complexities introduced are great.

13. *Control.* The control element makes decisions that will affect the system's operation. These decisions typically affect the quantity and nature of the inputs used, the structure or functioning of the system's components (process), or both inputs and process. They are based on analysis of feedback and feedforward in relation to values expressed as criteria and standards or as goal levels.

A Close Look at Systems

With these definitions in mind, one can take a somewhat more sophisticated look at a system diagram, as represented by Figure 5, which expands the simple system shown in Figure 4. The values, criteria, and standards that relate to the system's attributes are shown as important inputs to the control process. These inputs frequently derive from the environment rather than from the system itself. Similarly, it is evident that the final output—health status—is greatly affected by external forces, which reside primarily in the environment.

In the larger system, control is dependent on feedback from all components: external forces, final and intermediate outputs, process, and input. Without this array of information, an adequate assessment of the changes required is impossible. For instance, if the feedback indicates that the final output, health status, is unsatisfactory, one must know whether this represents a failure of the intermediate output (health services) or is the consequence of external forces over which we have no control. Similarly, one must be concerned with making the corrections that are most appropriate to the circumstances in which the system will be operating. Thus, one needs feedforward, which tells what to expect in the future in terms of external forces, processes (e.g., will there be a shift from solo to group practice in the provision of primary care?), and input (e.g., will medical education be changed to such an extent that future physicians will have different skills from today's doctors?).

A system has multiple purposes that can be described in terms of four specific functions. The first is goal attainment or achievement of the system's primary purpose. The second is self-maintenance. If the system cannot survive as an entity, its goals cannot be achieved. In other words, the system must devote a certain amount of its energy and resources to acquiring additional resources for future operation. Frequently, the latter function is regarded as bureaucratic overhead and spoken of in pejorative terms. Managers of clinical personnel frequently will be told, "I don't have time to prepare next year's budget; I'm too busy taking care of sick people." This attitude shows no comprehension of the reality that an approved budget is needed to provide the required resources if sick people are to be cared for next year. The third function is environmental adaptation. The system must maintain a satisfactory relationship with its environment or its efforts will be futile. This necessity implies a certain number of internal changes to accommodate the market for the system's output. It also implies that when some environmental factor is detrimental to system performance, those in the

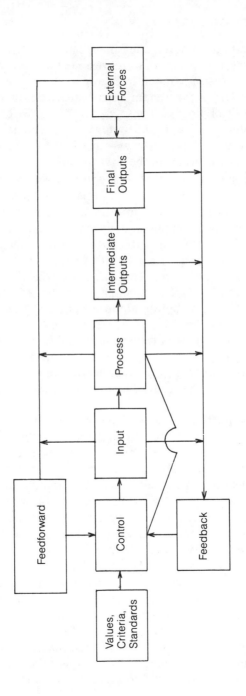

Figure 5 Schematic representation of a system.

system will try—through persuasion or other means—to effect a change that will accommodate the needs of the system. The fourth function is the integration of subsystem efforts. Each system must balance the activities of its parts so that one part does not maximize its performance at the expense of the others. This is a particularly pressing problem when dealing with professionals who are providing services. Because each professional is well aware of the importance of his work, he is strongly motivated to provide a maximum amount of that service to the beneficiaries. This attitude does not recognize that there is a point of diminishing returns, regardless of how excellent or important a service may be. For example, it is becoming clear that additional investments in high-technology medical care have far less impact on the health status of the population than do changes in environmental conditions or in individual behavior.

SYSTEM PLANNING

System planning can be contrasted with other types of planning commonly used in the past by examining two types that were prevalent in the days of comprehensive health planning agencies. The first of these is *problem-oriented planning*. As the name implies, this deals with specific, recognized problems. It tends to be short term rather than strategic and has a discrete focus, usually based on the assumption that a problem has a single cause and all will be well if this cause is eliminated. This single focus encourages a tendency to apply one solution to the maximum rather than seeking a suitable balance of resources within the system.

Earlier planning efforts using the problem-oriented approach experienced difficulties in keeping pace with the frequently changing focus of activity. Thus, a board of directors could meet monthly, using a "problem-of-the-month" planning process. Clearly, problems are far more persistent than this, and continually shifting the focus from one problem to another means that insufficient resources and time are allocated to deal effectively with any one issue.

At the other extreme are cases in which organizations or individuals are concerned with a single problem and persist in dealing with that issue long after it has ceased being major. This situation is typified by ad hoc groups that somehow become standing committees. Even though such committees make little or no contribution, unfortunately they still consume their original share of resources and thus prevent newer, more pressing needs from receiving deserved attention.

The second style of planning that has been replaced by system planning is resource oriented. This method also has a discrete focus, which is particularly damaging because it tends to overlook the fact that resources can be substituted for or can complement one another. This planning style assumes that maximizing resource availability is an end in itself. It does not consider that the demand for resources is in fact a derived demand. For example, people do not want hospitals as such; they want hospitals only because hospitals are a means of producing health services and they want the good health to which those services contribute.

The resource-oriented plan operates on the assumption that if the availability of some resources in a community can make a contribution to health status by providing services, then more of the same resources will lead to a linear increase in health status. This may be true up to a point, but it is clearly a simplistic assumption in that it ignores decreasing marginal returns.

In contrast to these outmoded approaches, the system-oriented planning process considers all system functions, not merely goal attainment. It also reflects the relationship between resources and output, in which health services are an intermediate output and health status is the final output. Finally, the health systems planning process permits analysis and understanding of interactions within and among subsystems. For instance, many hospitals have failed to achieve the results expected from an expansion of their patient-bed capacity because no consideration was given to the capacity of ancillary services. This can be illustrated at the community level by examining the effects of a decision to change the availability of nursing home beds in a community. If such a decision is made, the question then is what effects will occur within that subsystem and within related subsystems? If the number of nursing home beds is increased, it is probable that the geographic accessibility of these beds would also be increased, since it is unlikely that all the additional beds would be placed in the same location. This, of course, assumes that accessibility is defined in terms of geographic location. It also assumes that dispersing the beds throughout the community will mean that persons seeking to use these beds will be nearer to them. These clarifying statements illustrate the need to develop operational definitions for each of the system characteristics to be considered by the decision makers. Most people would agree that improved accessibility is desirable, but this apparent consensus might include the views of persons whose frames of reference are dramatically different. For example, it is apparent that the concept of accessibility easily could include spatial, temporal, financial, and cultural dimensions.

Another attribute of the subsystem to be considered here is the use of resources within the system. An increase in the number of nursing home beds would probably affect the level of bed usage, unless one began at a very high level of use and also had a very long waiting list. (In that case, unless the total number of beds were increased substantially, the number of persons on the waiting list might be large enough to maintain the high level of use that prevailed before the bed total was increased.) Furthermore, this probable change in bed use would likely have some effect on the cost of providing nursing home services. If the interactions between the long-term-care subsystem and related subsystems are then examined, one finds that there probably is no connection between the availability of nursing home beds and emergency services. On the other hand, in most communities, it is highly probable that some patients occupy acute care beds because there are no less-intensive-care beds available. If these persons could be moved into

SUBSYSTEM CHARACTERISTICS

	Availability	Accessibility	Utilization	Cost
Acute Inpatient Care	2		3	3
Emergency Service Facilities				
Long-term Inpatient Care	X	2	2	2
Mental Health Inpatient Care	2			

SUBSYSTEM OF MEDICAL CARE

X = Primary effect
2 = Possible secondary effects
3 = Possible tertiary effects

Figure 6 Interaction analysis related to increasing availability of beds in nursing homes.

nursing homes, more acute care beds would be available. The impact this would have on other attributes (e.g., utilization and cost) of the acute care hospital subsystem could then be studied.

The impact of additional nursing home beds on another component, the mental health facilities subsystem, depends on community policy regarding the location of mental patients. If elderly persons traditionally have been committed to state mental institutions in lieu of alternative care settings, the availability of nursing home beds may permit these individuals to move back into the community. On the other hand, if elderly persons have been served well by local community noninstitutional organizations, it is not likely that the decision will have any noticeable effect on the use of mental health facilities.

Figure 6 provides a conceptual framework for the analysis of these interactions. The matrix is limited to a small subset of all possible subsystems and to four general attributes. The primary effect of the decision to increase the number of nursing home beds is represented by the X in the cell describing the availability of long-term inpatient care services. Secondary or ripple effects of this action must also be considered by decision makers. These are most likely to occur in other attributes of the long-term-care subsystem or in the same attribute of other subsystems. Tertiary effects may be important in some cases. For instance, the secondary effect of increased availability of acute secondary care services is likely to cause changes in the utilization and cost of these services.

HEALTH SYSTEM PLANNING COMPONENTS

There are many advantages to the systems approach to health planning. The concepts of the systems approach can be incorporated in health system plans. The term *health system* includes the combinatio.is of health services and settings that are within the boundaries established by the decision maker. The matrix in Figure 7 portrays health services and settings that constitute a community health system. Policies and assumptions, community description, health status, health services, and health resources form the components of the health system plan. Figure 8, a flowchart of the process for developing such a system plan, shows the relationships among the plan's components.

Policies and Assumptions

The first, and perhaps most important, part of a health system plan embodies statements of health system policies and assumptions. This

HEALTH SYSTEM SETTING

HEALTH SYSTEM SERVICES		HOME	PUBLIC	AMBULATORY		SHORT STAY INPATIENT		LONG STAY INPATIENT		FREE STANDING SUPPORT	COMMUNITY
				HOSP.	OTHER	HOSP.	OTHER	HOSP.	OTHER		
PREVENTION AND DETECTION	COMMUNITY HEALTH PROMOTION AND PROTECTION — Health Education Services										
	Environmental Quality Management										
	Food Protection										
	Occupational Health and Safety										
	Radiation Safety										
	Biomedical and Consumer Product Safety										
	Individual Health Protection Services										
	Detection Services										
	DIAGNOSIS AND TREATMENT — Obstetric Services										
	Surgical Services										
	Diagnostic Radiology Services										
	Therapeutic Radiology Services										
	Clinical Laboratory Services										
	Emergency Medical Services										
	Dental Health Services										
	Mental Health Services										
	General Medical Services										
HABILITATION AND REHABILITATION	Medical Habilitation and Rehabilitation Services										
	Therapy Services										
MAINTENANCE											
PERSONAL HEALTH CARE SUPPORT	Direct Patient Care Support Services										
	Administrative Services										
	HEALTH SYSTEM ENABLING — Health Planning										
	Resource Development										
	Financing										
	Regulation										
	Research										

Figure 7 Health services and settings matrix.

section of the plan contains statements of the system's general goals, which provide the context and overall guidance for all other planning activities and make a major contribution toward the goal of an accountable planning process.

In addition to value statements, the system's governing body must clarify its assumptions about the health care system and its future. Some of the requirements here include an explicit definition of the

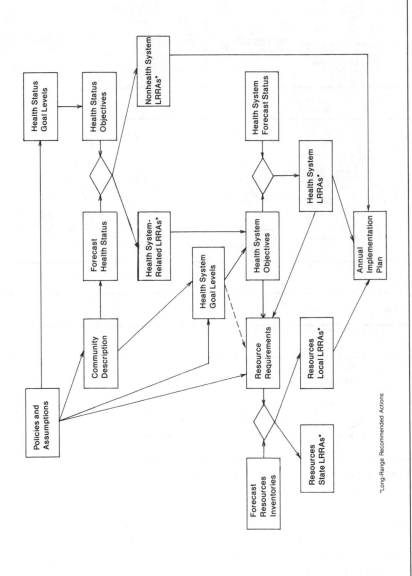

Figure 8   Health systems plan development process.

TABLE 3   Suggested Health Plan Policy Topics

1. Planning horizon
2. Emphasis on current or future program
3. Relationships with "peer" organizations
4. Board/committee/task force relationships
5. Board/staff relationships
6. Quality of information required by decision makers
7. Basic values and their relative priorities
8. Theory of health on which plan is based
9. Boundary of health system
10. Population groups to receive special attention
11. Subsystems to receive special attention
12. Goal levels uniform for entire health service area or variable
13. Assumptions about resource availability
14. Goal levels and objectives expressed at what level (minimum, national average, ideal)
15. Preference for investment or consumption activities

boundaries of that system and a determination of the planning horizon to be used in the decision-making process. (*Planning horizon* is simply the end of the time period for which planning has taken place. If a health system planning process establishes a five-year planning horizon, a plan developed in 1985 will have a planning horizon of 1990.)

The governing body must also state its expectations about the level of investment and operating costs that the community will approve for the health system during the planning period. Table 3 presents a list of topics that might be included in the policy section of a health system plan.

Community Description

The next major component of the health system plan is a community description. The concepts of marketing call for a population-based plan (i.e., a plan based on the needs of area residents as a whole rather than a process that deals with the proposals of individual institutions or providers as a basis for making planning decisions). In addition to describing the population to be served, the plan also should describe the conditions within which the plan will be implemented, including the social, economic, geographic, and political dimensions of the community. These factors are important from two perspectives. The social, economic, and political conditions will affect implementation of the plan. More important, they also will have great bearing on the health status of the population, if one assumes that an ecological model of health is to be used in the planning process.[6]

Because of these considerations, planners must incorporate the relevant data into this section of the plan. The word *relevant* is of particular significance; many plans have described communities in exquisite detail but have failed to indicate to the users of the plan the relationship between the community characteristics described and the health status of those to be served.

Health Status

Health status is the next component of the health system plan. Goal levels are established on the basis of the values expressed in the policy portion of the plan and are set for an indefinite time in the future. Consequently, the organization must move from the goal levels to a time-related set of objectives. In other words, planners must decide on reasonable health status levels at the planning horizon. These levels become the objectives that are compared with a forecast of community health status for the same time period. The forecast is developed from information provided in the community description.

The comparison of the health status forecast with objectives for the planning horizon will indicate the areas in which there are discrepancies—where problems exist. It must then be determined whether these discrepancies can be attributed to the health system or whether they are caused entirely or in part by factors outside the system. In the latter case, the organization might initiate appropriate actions vis-à-vis those who have power to make the necessary changes. This move is represented in Figure 8 by the box entitled "Nonhealth System LRRAS" (long-range recommended actions).

---

[6]An ecological model of health implies that health status is affected by many factors in addition to medical care. These often are grouped into three categories: biological (e.g., maturation and aging), environmental (e.g., housing conditions), and behavioral (e.g., leisure activities).

When some or all of the health status problems can be attributed to the health *system,* the organization must correct these internally. It cannot plan long-range recommended actions related to health *status;* there is no action, for instance, that will directly reduce infant mortality. Instead, the organization must design long-range actions that will somehow change the health system, the environment, or both, in such a way that the causes of infant mortality will be reduced. If the system for which the plan is developed is a health services organization rather than a community, the health status section of the plan will not contain goals. Instead it will be a major component of the environmental assessment used to identify market opportunities.

Health Services

The health system goal levels in Figure 8 are derived from the values expressed in the policy section and from the community's characteristics. The goal levels are translated into health system objectives that are appropriate for the planning horizon. These objectives can be compared with the LRRAs for health services that arose as a result of the examination of health status problems.

If the health system objectives are compatible with the LRRAs related to health, the planner can be confident that those objectives are appropriate. On the other hand, if they bear no relationship to each other, the planner can assume that the services objectives should be modified to encompass those actions needed to deal with a clearly defined health status problem. The health system objectives are contrasted with a health system forecast. This forecast is an inventory of the health system projected to the planning horizon so the planner can compare the two. This comparison is made along a number of dimensions represented by the attributes or characteristics specified within the planning law, plus any others that the governing body may have selected. The characteristics cited in the law are availability, accessibility, acceptability, quality, cost, and continuity.

In the event that the system's objectives differ from the forecast status of the system, the planner must then develop strategies and LRRAs that will bring the system's status into agreement with the objectives. At this point, it should be noted that a surplus may be as great a problem as a deficiency. As reimbursement shifts from a cost base to a prospectively set price, underused service capacity can become a serious drain on the financial resources of the system.

Health Resources

Whatever the case, the LRRAs for the health system generally will imply some adjustment in resource requirements, another important section of the health system plan. Ideally, one would hope that these requirements could be determined on the basis of the general values expressed in the policy portion of the plan, plus an aggregation of the more specific statements in the health system goal levels and objectives.

When such aggregate resource objectives are developed, they must be adjusted on the basis of the health system's LRRAs. During the interim, these LRRAs can be used to estimate changes in the projected supply of system resources. This supply is determined by taking an inventory of currently available resources and forecasting that inventory to the planning horizon. If the planners have succeeded in developing an aggregate system resource requirement, the forecast inventory and resource requirement can be compared to determine what action is necessary.

The adjustment that must be made in resources will become the basis for long-range recommended actions. In some cases, recommendations affecting the resource supply can be implemented at the local level, but many resource adjustments will require actions at the state or federal level. For instance, the state supposedly has control of facility development through the state medical facility plan. Similarly, a state might act to influence the output of the medical schools, but a community that is in complete control of the supply of physicians would be unusual. On the other hand, a community might influence the supply of inhalation therapy technicians through a community college that is the primary, if not the only, source of such technicians.

If the point of action is sufficiently remote, the system may have to set resource supply levels as budgetary constraints. If expenditures must be limited, the system can insist that no more than a certain amount of resources be allocated for the provision of specific health services. In such cases, LRRAs would be considered feasible only if their net resource requirements were less than the difference between quantities of resources required to provide existing health services and the resource ceilings derived from statements in the policy section of the health system plan.

IMPLEMENTATION PLAN

The data from the health system plan become part of an implementation plan, which describes what actions the organization intends to take to attain the objectives established for the planning horizon. Figure 9 is a flowchart of the process for developing an implementation plan. The decisions concerning which of the long-range recommended actions are to be implemented during the coming year are dependent on knowledge of organization resources and other data that may be relevant to priority determination (e.g., availability of community resources) and on the policies and assumptions contained in the health system plan. When all these factors have been taken into account, the organization can establish annual objectives related to changes in the health system, health resources, and those aspects of the environment that have an adverse effect on health status.

For each of these objectives, planners will develop both short-range recommended actions (SRRAs) and project plans to implement them. If the system is an organization, the actions must be preceded by strategies (e.g., marketing strategy, finance strategy) that will guide the choice of actions.

Table 4 presents a list summarizing plan development activities. This list should not be regarded as a sequential set of actions, since many of these activities can be accomplished concurrently. For example, once the indicators for health status and the health system have been

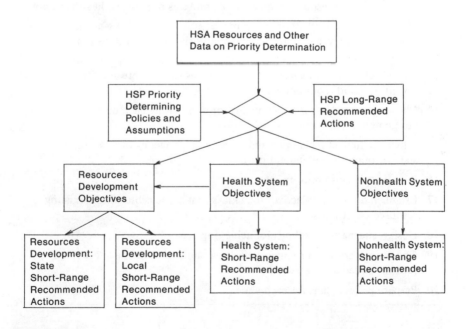

Figure 9   Annual implementation plan development process.

TABLE 4   Plan Development Activities

1. Establish planning policies and assumptions
2. Prepare community description
3. Determine indicators and goal levels for health status and health systems; optimize goal levels
4. Set objectives on basis of goal levels
5. Prepare forecasts of community health status, status of health system, and inventories of health resources
6. Compare health status and health system forecasts with objectives
7. Arrange observed disparities in priority sequence
8. Design alternative means for eliminating disparities that have the highest priority
9. Choose preferred means for eliminating each priority disparity and designate it as a long-range recommended action (LRRA)
10. Examine health system objectives to ensure consistency with health-system-related LRRAs designed to achieve health status objectives; modify health system objectives as necessary
11. Establish health resource requirements on basis of policies, health system objectives, and health system LRRAs
12. Compare forecast health resources inventories with health resources requirements
13. Design alternative means for eliminating disparities between forecast inventories and requirements
14. Choose preferred alternative means for eliminating each disparity and designate it as an LRRA
15. Inform state health planning and development agency of LRRA related to state resources development plans
16. Put all LRRAs into priority sequence
17. Establish one-year objectives for LRRAs that are feasible within existing resource constraints
18. Design alternative methods for achieving each objective
19. Choose preferred alternatives and designate each one as a short-range recommended action (SRRA)
20. Prepare project plans for each SRRA

determined, planners can begin to prepare the forecast of community health status, the status of the health system, and the inventory of health resources, because the indicators represent the decision variables, that is, the measurable characteristics of the system that are used in making decisions. Collection of other data would be unnecessary, since these additional factors would not be used in actions affecting the system. The process of preparing a forecast is not affected by determining goal levels, and, consequently, the latter can occur concurrently with the preparation of the inventory. Obviously, however, both of these forecasts must be completed before they can be compared, as required in step 6 of Table 4.

Table 4 also shows items not fully addressed in the description of the health system planning flowchart (Figure 8). For example, step 3 calls for optimizing system goal levels. This step recognizes the need for trade-offs between certain attributes of the system—one would not expect the highest level of quality at the lowest possible cost. Experience has shown that in the initial process of setting goal levels, health care decision makers tend to establish a maximum as the desirable level. Unfortunately, maximization of all attributes is seldom possible, and it is particularly unlikely that the ultimate in other attributes (e.g., accessibility, quality) will be attained for a minimum cost. Therefore, after goal levels are initially stated, they must be reexamined to ensure that they are internally consistent. If they are not, then decision makers must seek to achieve a reasonable balance among the desired levels for each of the many attributes.

Several steps in Table 4 imply a choice among different options. For example, step 7 indicates that disparities or problems must be placed in priority sequence. This implies insufficient resources to deal with all the trouble spots or opportunities, so one must address the most important to the extent allowed by available resources. Similarly, step 9 requires decision makers to choose among a number of means of dealing with a problem to determine which is preferred in terms of cost and benefit. This is a constant challenge to planners and, in fact, can be seen as the real reason for planning. Because resources are insufficient to accomplish all possible aims, planners must help decision makers choose the most desirable achievements and determine how to attain them with the scarce resources available. The system plan and the process by which it is developed are the means by which planners can accomplish this task.

The system planning process is not dependent on the assignment of all planning functions to a single agency. The allocation of responsibilities is more of a political or administrative matter than a requirement of the process. It would be easy from a technical standpoint to separate the three levels of planning (policy, strategic, and operational) that are incorporated in the process. The shift of responsibility for policymaking from the planning organization to some other body would result in the establishment of two easily delineated sets of tasks. The line of demarcation between strategic and operational planning is less obvious, but it is significant because the strategic planning organization must understand clearly the implications of being involved in operational planning. Specifically, if the role of the planning organization were limited to strategic planning or to strategic and policy planning, its plan development responsibilities would end with the establishment of objectives for each attribute of each component of the health services system, in keeping with resource budget limits. The operational planning phase could then be carried out by the operating organizations. The decision makers would hold the operators responsible for developing health services in accordance with the objectives and budgetary constraints. The organizations responsible for operational planning must have the high level of expertise needed to select the best means of achieving an objective (long-range recommended action) and the best combination of resources to carry out the chosen action. Furthermore, the effort involved in this kind of detailed analysis and planning is so great that the strategic planning group must either avoid the task or resort to mixed scanning. For this reason, planners must be concerned with two things: First, they must be especially meticulous in setting priorities, because they will be able to develop operational level plans for only a few concerns. Second, they must not succumb to pressures to develop operational plans at the expense of completing the strategic plan. It is essential that performance standards (objectives) for the entire system be known when LRRAs are chosen, because the selection process must consider the likely effects of choices on the performance of other parts of the health services system.

SUMMARY

General systems theory provides a useful framework for planning the organization and delivery of health services. The integrative systems approach overcomes many of the deficiencies of earlier styles of planning, which focused on the acquisition of resources as the purpose of planning or on individual problems as discrete and isolated issues. A health system plan contains sets of elements, each of which evolves in a logical progression from the preceding elements. Policies and assumptions set the overall guidance for the plan. Within that guidance, a community description characterizes the environment and population that the health system is intended to serve. Health status data, as a subset of the environmental information, reflect the community's needs that are to be met by the system. The health services section describes the organizations and services required to satisfy those needs in a way consistent with the community's policies. The next element of the plan identifies the resources required to maintain and operate the desired system. Finally, there is a specific action plan that describes what will be done to achieve the most immediate objectives of the health system plan. This chapter has discussed systems planning from the perspective of community-wide health services planning. The systems concepts are also directly relevant to organizational planning because each organization is, in fact, a system. Organizational planning is discussed in Chapter 5. Although systems concepts will seldom be mentioned explicitly, the reader should keep them in mind while reading that chapter.

5

ORGANIZATIONAL PLANNING

ANOTHER LOOK AT SYSTEMS

Although the concepts of systems planning are appropriate for institutions,[1] there are some important differences between institutional and community-wide planning. The individual institution can be designated as the black box of a community-wide health system plan. The principles of systems hierarchy, however, show that the black box itself is a system with numerous subsystems. For example, within an individual health institution or black box such as the community hospital, there are subsystems for patient care, medical education, research, management, and logistics. Each of these can be subdivided further— the management subsystem into administration, finance, public relations, personnel, and planning; the patient care subsystem into medical and surgical care, pharmacy, radiology, and laboratory; and so on. Depending on the size of the organization, these are designated as strategic business units (SBUs) or program management units (PMUs). Performance standards and criteria can be designed for each of these subsystems. For instance, data from the American Hospital Association's (AHA's) Hospital Administrative Services (HAS) might be used as the norm for setting performance standards for certain management and logistical functions.

---

[1]The words *institutional* and *organizational* will be used interchangeably in this chapter. The concepts and methods discussed are relevant to the traditional free-standing institution, the corporation that includes one or more health institutions, and the noninstitutional health services provider organizations.

Each institution must be concerned with four system functions: attaining its goals, acquiring resources, adapting to its environment, and balancing the activities of its own subsystems. Undoubtedly, the major focus of every institution is to attain its goals, and this function often obscures the importance of other functions. The function of acquiring resources usually depends on the availability of funds, without which the system or institution cannot maintain itself. This particular function, then, is frequently an overriding factor in decisions about changing the scope or methods of operation in an institution.

Tucker[2] highlights the two major environmental adaptations made by institutional managers. For any institution to survive, it must first maintain effective exchange relationships with both the patients and the medical staff. According to Tucker, patients demand certain amenities but also are influenced by the caliber or prestige of the medical staff. A good medical staff, in turn, will demand the best of everything for its patients. Institutional management can refuse these demands, however, when the requested equipment or services will pose an economic threat to the institution's survival. Historically, most institutions have been reimbursed on a full-cost basis, so there was usually no reason for management to deny requests for more or better equipment and services. With the advent of reimbursement based on prospectively determined prices, management clearly has a major task in balancing the activity and use of resources among the various parts of an institution. Without that balance, inefficiency would soon result; those parts of the institution favored with resources would be producing large volumes of high-quality output that could not be fully used, and there would be inadequate output from those parts that were deprived of resources. Consequently, the hospital will lose the revenue that could have been generated by the less-favored units and will receive insufficient revenue from the favored services to cover their full costs.

A significant difference between institutional and community planning lies in the task of balancing activities and resources; namely, institutional decision makers have much greater influence over the activities they supervise. Thus, the institutional system as a whole is much likelier to respond quickly to its own planning initiatives than is the general community health system.

---

[2]Stephen L. Tucker. "Introducing Marketing as a Planning and Management Tool." *Hospital and Health Services Administration, 22*(1):37–44, Winter 1977.

THE RELATIONSHIP BETWEEN INSTITUTIONAL
AND COMMUNITY PLANNING

The similarities between institutional and community planning have been noted. We have emphasized the great need for cooperation and collaboration between institutions and community health service planners if the planning process is to be effective and efficient. These relationships and the potential for collaboration between the two groups are illustrated in Figure 10.

In this diagram, steps 1 through 5 at the institutional level represent the development of a strategic plan as a direct analog to the community's health system plan. The figure further illustrates ways that the institution can benefit from a cooperative relationship with regional planners through such activities as data exchange and technical assistance. The data exchange and technical assistance that public agencies provide to institutions would solve many institutional needs for what are essentially marketing data. In the past, data have frequently been collected for individual institutions by consulting firms as part of a role study. These studies are expensive and generally focus on the institution and its potential for expanding its "market share," without regard to the rest of the community's health service system. Furthermore, the role study and subsequent recommendations often are based on analyses using methods and data that are inconsistent with those of other institutions in the community, including the community planning agencies.

This is not to say that the data and methods used by the majority of institutions in a community are necessarily correct or better than those of an individual institution; however, to avoid counterproductive conflict and to raise the quality of the planning process throughout the community, negotiation should occur among all planning entities so that the planning process is raised to its highest possible level of accomplishment. Furthermore, the data exchange and technical assistance activities of the public agency could clarify community expectations for the individual institution. This information could be used to ensure that both planning efforts and ongoing activities are appropriately focused in terms of the community's needs and wishes.

If these tasks are successfully carried out, the review processes (e.g., review of proposals to offer new services), which must necessarily be conducted on an arm's length basis, are quite likely to result in favorable recommendations after a rigorous analysis by local and state planning agencies. If such results can be achieved, the institutional planning process will have made a worthwhile contribution to the

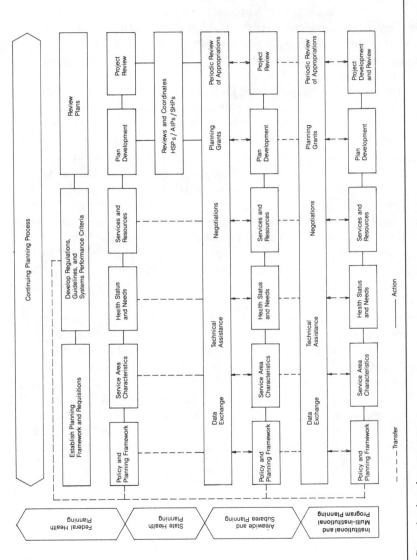

Figure 10 Generic planning process.

organization it serves, and the organization itself will be better able to serve its community.

ORGANIZATIONAL PARTICIPATION IN COMMUNITY PLANNING

The benefits of planning apply to institutions, as well as to larger systems. Indeed, the lack of planning would surely jeopardize an institution's survival. An institution's motivation to survive is sometimes a major point of conflict in the relations between institutions and community health planners and sometimes is seen by the latter as taking priority over the general community welfare. This attitude leads to planning by confrontation rather than cooperation—certainly an undesirable development and one that should be avoided. Community planners must recognize that the survival of existing institutions will ensure a stable base to provide needed health services. In turn, institutional planners must make every reasonable effort to see that institutional survival is compatible with community well-being. This goal can best be achieved by ensuring that institutional decision makers have an opportunity to understand and participate in the development of community health system plans that ensure their organizations of meaningful roles that contribute significantly to the community's health. Unfortunately, the assumption that all institutions are prepared to participate in this type of planning is naive. Too many have failed to establish planning processes. As a result, they react only to internal pressures (Tucker[3]) rather than engage in a long-run developmental process that will be mutually beneficial to the institution and the community it purports to serve.

There is currently much external pressure on institutions to initiate internal planning efforts. For example, during the days of the voluntary planning movement, the health facilities planning agency of Pittsburgh (under the direction of Robert Sigmond and later Steven Sieverts) emphasized the development of individual institutional plans. More recently, requirements for planning have been imposed by federal and state law. Section 234 of P.L. 92-603, the Social Security Amendments of 1972, requires each hospital participating in medicare or medicaid to have an annual operating budget and a capital expenditure plan covering at least a three-year period. These documents are to be reviewed and updated at least annually, and their preparation must be

---

[3]Ibid.

supervised by a committee comprised of representatives from the institution's board, administration, and medical staff. In 1974, Section 1532 of P.L. 93-641 established a requirement that reviews of certificate-of-need requests must consider the relationship of the proposed project to the long-range plan, if any, of the provider proposing the service. Although this law did not insist that every provider have a long-range plan, it implied that reviewing agencies would look more favorably on providers who did. The state of New Jersey has enacted a law requiring each hospital to develop a long-range plan that includes a five-year forecast of health care needs, services, and institutional capacity. The plan must include a community profile, a patient origin study, goals, and alternative courses of action.[4]

A study of community hospitals in Missouri showed that many institutions had no planning process because of either resistance to external pressure or lack of concern for the potential benefits involved. It was found that in a representative sample of hospitals throughout the state, none of the administrators interviewed had any staff person with primary responsibility for planning and only a few of the larger institutions had any formal planning process. Moreover, the study concluded that very few of the institutions examined had given adequate consideration to the needs of the community, as well as to the aspirations of the institutions.[5]

Some attribute the lack of participation in the planning process to the negative attitude of many state and national professional organizations and individual providers who view community-wide planning as a threat to their legitimate decision-making role in the delivery of health services.[6] This is in spite of the language in planning laws, such as P.L. 93-641, which explicitly recognizes that provider concerns must be incorporated into the community plan development process. Others point out that since some 40 percent of health service expenditures are public funds, "those who object to regulation qua regulation, as many still do, probably should not accept assignment as hospital trustees except in institutions that have no public patients. Elsewhere, hospital governance is in part a public responsibility and not less because the hospital may be an unwilling partner to the public contract." This is because "responsibility goes where the money comes from, so public

---

[4]"New Jersey Requires Hospitals To Do Long-Range Planning." *Hospitals, 49* (18):94, September 16, 1975.

[5]Douglas C. Mankin and William F. Glueck. "Strategic Planning." *Hospital and Health Services Administration, 22*(2):6-22, Spring 1977.

[6]Charles A. Frankenhoff. "The Planning Environment of Health Systems Agencies: A Strategy for Intervention." *Inquiry, XIV*(3):217-228, September 1977.

policy requires that there should be some public effort to safeguard against unnecessary expense."[7]

ORGANIZATIONAL PLANS

Organizations are involved in several types of planning, including contingency planning, program planning, project planning, and strategic planning. Contingency planning involves the establishment of a course of action to be followed if certain unusual or unanticipated events should occur. Disaster planning falls within this category. Contingency planning also should include plans for holding the line when a strategic plan fails because it was based on incorrect assumptions or because of dramatic, unexpected shifts in the environment (e.g., rapid introduction of a statewide, all-payer system of reimbursement). Since contingency plans are designed for short-term administrative responses to crises, they fall outside the scope of this book. Similarly, other administrative implementation plans are excluded, such as project plans and program plans. Their purpose is the implementation of the organization's strategic plan.

STRATEGIC PLANNING[8]

Strategic planning is essential to the survival and growth[9] of organizations. Until recently, it was generally assumed that health services institutions (especially hospitals) were providers of essential and highly valued services and, thus, were virtually assured of survival so long as day-by-day management was competent and honest. The expansion of services fostered by this assumption has meant the allocation of ever-increasing portions of our national resources to the health industry, and now the value of health services relative to other uses of our nation's wealth is increasingly under question. More

---

[7]Robert M. Cunningham, Jr. "Who's Minding the Store?" *Hospitals,* 52(6):115-120, March 16, 1978.

[8]Much of the material in this section was developed with the support of the American College of Hospital Administrators. It originally appeared in *Case Studies in Health Administration Volume Three: Strategic Planning for Hospitals,* Chicago, Foundation of the American College of Hospital Administrators, 1983. It is used here with their permission.

[9]Growth is not the expansion of physical facilities only; it may mean maturation and transition into a new style or type of service that is more responsive to the demands of an evolving market.

recently, shifts in federal policy away from widely accepted commitments to ensure access to needed health services with little regard for ability to pay have made it even clearer that there are definite limits to the amount of resources available for medical care and other health-related services. Thus, expectations about the future size and nature of the health services market have been altered significantly.

The proportion of gross national product committed to health expenditures has reached an upper limit. In fact, it may be declining because of the priority assigned to competing uses (e.g., national defense). This limitation has become more severe with slower growth of the national economy, which has meant that both the absolute and relative amounts of money available for health services are virtually certain to remain constant or decrease. So, to survive, health services organizations must now compete vigorously for their share of fixed or shrinking resources.

This competition becomes more complex with the shift in payment policies. Most likely, there will be a shift in the demand for health services as certain economic groups become less able to avail themselves of needed services. This shift will be reinforced and perhaps amplified by the need for providers to maximize reimbursement to avoid bankruptcy. Strategic planning was originally developed to help commercial enterprises survive and prosper in such an environment. Leaders in the health services field anticipated a need for it years ago. Now this innovation is widely diffused throughout the industry, but it still is too new to be thoroughly familiar to most of those participating in it.

Definition of Strategic Planning

Every organization has a mission or purpose. *Strategy* is an integrated approach to move the organization toward accomplishing its mission. *Mission* is a high-level, abstract statement of what the organization should become. Strategy offers rules for making the trade-offs necessary to carry out the mission in a changing environment characterized by scarce resources. *Planning* is the process of making current decisions on the basis of their future effects. Ackoff[10] calls this "creating the future." In summary, *strategic planning* is making current decisions on the basis of rules designed to aid the development and maintenance of an ideal organization during a period in which that

---

[10]Russell L. Ackoff. *Redesigning the Future.* New York, Wiley, 1974, pp. 3-4, 26-31.

organization's environment is constantly changing and frequently hostile.

Clearly, strategic planning is different from operational planning, which is simply the development of schemes to accomplish specific, limited objectives (e.g., building a facility or setting up a new program). Furthermore, strategic planning is not necessarily long-range planning. Operational planning may have a very long time span; strategic planning may entail an immediate response to a sudden shift in the organization's circumstances (e.g., a change in the method for reimbursement of hospitals).

Since strategic planning deals with a constantly changing environment, the process must be continuous. This is not to say that all steps of the process will be carried out concurrently and with equal intensity. It does mean that the organization must be continually scanning its internal and external circumstances and must be prepared to modify earlier decisions in the light of new intelligence. Strategic planning should be regarded as a continuous, cyclical process in which the plan completed during one phase becomes the input for the first phase of the next cycle. Strategic planning is not done by planners. The planner's role is to design a planning process and to facilitate the use of that process. When strategic decisions are to be made, the actual planning must be done by an organization's leadership. Because of interaction between planners and leaders and the broad scope of strategic planning, however, serving as an organization's principal planner can be key in preparing for the responsibilities of a chief executive officer (CEO). In fact, because of the CEO's concern with external affairs, the planning position provides invaluable experience that is seldom available to persons serving as chief operating officer.

Strategic planning is a continuous cycle of activities, referred to here as steps. Although it is possible and desirable to accomplish some of these steps concurrently, they are linked in a logical developmental sequence, as shown in Figure 11. Each of these activities is described in detail in the following section.

The Strategic-Planning Process

Step 1: Establish the Planning Process

There are at least three general approaches to strategic planning: gap analysis, problem solution, and SWOT (strengths, weaknesses, opportunities, threats). In gap analysis, an ideal future situation is defined

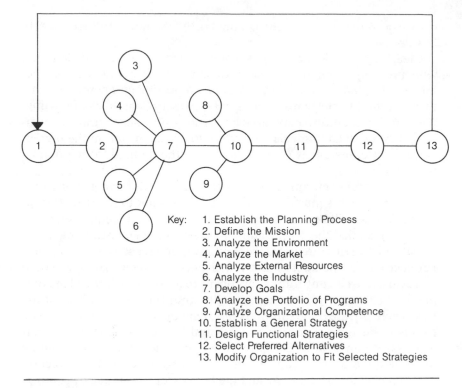

Figure 11   The strategic planning process.

and contrasted to a reference projection[11] of current activities. The differences between this projection and the ideal are the gaps that strategic planning must address. The aim in problem solution is to focus the strategic plan on significant problems expected to exist at the planning horizon. These problems may be entirely new results of environmental shifts, exacerbations of current minor issues, or the persistence of currently serious deficiencies. The SWOT approach focuses on both the opportunities and threats likely to exist at the planning horizon. It also explicitly forecasts the strengths and weaknesses of the organization as factors that must be considered while developing strategies.

Regardless of the approach selected, the direction of the planning process within the organization—top-down or bottom-up—must be

---

[11]A reference projection is simply an extrapolation of current activities to the planning horizon on the basis of historical trends. It must be remembered that strategic planning is not necessarily long-range planning.

decided. Because of the widely accepted notion that a system is more than the sum of its parts, the bottom-up approach, which tends to be little more than an aggregation of plans prepared by lower echelons, is generally discredited as an initial approach to strategic planning. Instead, an organization's leadership must establish a mission that reflects both the contributions of individual organizational components and the effects of synergistic interactions among them.

The degree of involvement of others in the organization after this first step varies, but it is generally accepted that there should be some input from each organizational level. This could be done by organizing a planning team on which all levels are represented; or a sequential, cyclical process could be set up in which the output from one level's planning effort becomes the input for the next planning step by an adjacent level. For example, the mission developed by the top level in the first cycle becomes the basis for the intermediate level's goal development. These goals become the purposes for which the operating level designs functional programs. After validation by the intermediate level, these programs, in turn, become the basis of the top level's second-cycle activity—resource allocation. Ackoff[12] combines these two ideas by recommending that the higher level should have a representative involved in the planning process of the lower level.

Figure 11 does not reflect this cyclical approach, but it does assume that many levels in the organization will help to create the final product for each stage in the process. This is related to Breindel's[13] recommendation that, rather than seeking to develop a total master plan, the organization should prepare a series of related documents. He believes this will enhance the process by making it more flexible. To some extent, this proposal addresses Quinn's[14] assertion that a formal planning process may become an impediment to true strategic planning. More important is Quinn's message that the process is incremental and iterative—incremental in that major, far-reaching decisions are avoided for as long as possible so that leaders can have the best possible information before making a commitment and iterative in that prior decisions frequently must be modified as a result of new

---

[12]Russell L. Ackoff. *Redesigning the Future*, pp. 49–53.
[13]Charles L. Breindel. "Health Planning Processes and Process Documentation." *Hospital and Health Services Administration*, *26*(Special II):10–17, 1981.
[14]James B. Quinn. "Formulating Strategy One Step at a Time." *Journal of Business Strategy*, *1*:42–63, Winter 1981. (Those familiar with the writings of C. E. Lindblom will recognize that he too does not equate incrementalism with "muddling" as that word is usually understood.)

knowledge gained through current activities; such modification usually leads to repetition of all intervening steps to ensure agreement with the modified decision. Even more important are Quinn's concepts that the formal planning process, if properly developed and used, is an essential complement to the related power-behavioral processes that affect implementation, and that incrementalism is a clearly conceived, carefully managed strategy of effective executives.

The planning process and its support structure must accommodate the characteristics of the organization, including size, management style, environmental complexity, and the nature of the production process (e.g., medical staff arrangements for hospitals clearly require a structure different from that of a hierarchical commercial enterprise). Despite these varying features, there are three roles (planner, chief executive officer, and chief operating officer) about which important generalizations can be made:

1. The planner should not do the planning. That is a responsibility management cannot delegate. The roles of the planner or planning office are to design the planning process, serve as a catalyst to carry it out, and provide continuing staff support. These responsibilities could be located elsewhere within the organization, but the required skills and knowledge have become so specialized that it is quite unlikely a generalist manager could function as effectively as someone with special preparation for these tasks.

2. A related issue is the priority assigned to planning. Typically, if a person has both planning and operating responsibilities, the pressures of current situations will crowd out the seemingly postponable planning activities. This presents a dilemma for the chief executive officer, especially in a smaller organization. If the CEO's chief responsibility is the future survival and growth of the organization, then that person should delegate internal operating responsibilities to a chief operating officer (COO) and concentrate on strategic and external concerns. In a small organization, however, there may be no COO-type position. In this case, the CEO would have to remain the focal point for operations and, to assure that strategic concerns were not ignored, would assign some other member of the top management team as the organization's strategist.[15] Needless to say, there must be a concomitant reduction in the strategist's other duties.

---

[15]William W. Wommack. "The Board's Most Important Function." *Harvard Business Review, 57*:48–54, September–October 1979.

OPTIONS FOR A PLANNING UNIT

Various options are available to chief decision makers who decide to delegate responsibility for planning functions. This section describes four of those options.

Governing Board and Committee of the Board

If the organization's governing body is to perform the planning function, then the plans can deal only with the most complex, comprehensive, and significant problems. This type of planning usually is done in very broad terms unless subcommittees are formed and adequate staff is provided. One advantage of subcommittees is that they are an excellent means of obtaining the advice and consent of the external interest groups (stakeholders) invited to participate in the planning process. This benefit can be realized by expanding the membership of subcommittees to include persons who are not members of the organization's governing board. Thus, there can be many subcommittees, each having at least one member from the formal governing board of the organization, with other members being the representatives of affected groups and/or professional experts.

Perlin[16] describes a board planning committee that receives inputs from community advisory, management planning, and medical staff planning committees. Presumably, this gives all key sectors a stake in the process, making them more receptive to the final planning results. Such a structure indicates that each section of the triad of hospital governance has its own separate planning committee, with the community advisory committee acting as the counterpart of the trustee, who represents community interest in the process of institutional governance. This arrangement also has the virtue of involving the medical staff. As Stevens[17] noted in his article on hospital costs, the traditional governing arrangement tends to separate professional responsibility and fiscal responsibility, with physicians having little or none of the latter. Other authors have noted that although the board works harder in the kind of committee arrangement envisioned by Perlin, it is better informed than a board that works as a committee of the whole or one that only reacts to proposals by the chief executive officer. These same

---

[16]Martin S. Perlin. *Managing Institutional Planning.* Germantown, Md., Aspen Systems Corp., 1976, pp. 46–47.
[17]Carl M. Stevens. "Hospital Costs: On Rationalizing the Physician-Hospital Relationship." *Inquiry, XIV*(3):303–305, September 1977.

authors, however, state that the nonmanagement members of the triad can function effectively only when they have been adequately educated to assume the added responsibilities that are involved.[18]

The American Hospital Association's *Guide to Institutional Planning* describes the following roles for the board and the committees of the board: The board establishes the general policy. Then, a planning-policy committee reports to the governing board and generally reviews all proposed planning activities. A third component, a building committee that does not plan, carries out plans for adding or modernizing physical facilities.[19] (This division of responsibility between planning and building committees is often not recognized in practice, where planning and facility development frequently are regarded as synonymous.) The AHA's *Guide* further notes that the responsibility for executing any part of the plan does not lie with these committees—it is the province of the chief executive officer.

Committees of Chief Operating Officials

If a committee of this scope does the planning itself, the plans will tend not to be very specific. Chief operating officials generally are very busy individuals, with neither the time nor the inclination to concern themselves with the minute details of final plan implementation. Additionally, if the members of this committee are not part of the decision-making echelon but rather subordinates, then the committee may lack the authority to make the commitments necessary to carry out the plan.

The primary advantage of the style of planning where chief operating officials act as decision makers is that it allows the persons who will be directly affected by the plan and who probably have the greatest expertise in the functions involved to participate in the planning. Furthermore, their participation increases the likelihood that they will accept the plans that eventually evolve. One way to offset the tendency of such a committee to avoid detail is to organize a committee of key decision makers and to provide that group with a project organization that will perform all the specific detailed planning that is needed—subject, of course, to the approval of the committee itself.

---

[18]L. E. Weeks and R. A. Devries. "The Status of Hospital Trustee Education." *Hospital and Health Services Administration, 23*(1):72–96, Winter 1978.

[19]American Hospital Association. *The Practice of Planning in Health Care Institutions.* Chicago, 1973, p. 14.

Planning by Committee

Another option for a planning unit is to have the planning function executed by a specific planning committee, with membership other than governing boards or operating officials. Since committees play such a vital role in the planning process, it is worthwhile to examine some of the considerations involved in creating them.

Committees may be of several types. A control committee acts as a pluralistic decision maker, whereas an advisory committee merely evaluates the proposals of others. An investigative and advisory committee initiates actions and develops recommendations for solutions. This group, however, does not have the authority to carry out the recommendations it makes. To be effective, a committee must have authority commensurate with its role. It must be staffed with capable members and supported by adequate technical assistance. Also, it must have a clear charter, or it will spend all of its time deciding what to do.

The committee approach to planning has a number of important advantages. First, it has the ability to achieve informal but effective coordination among members who represent the diverse interests affected by the plan; as we noted, people tend to accept solutions made by groups of which they are members. Second, this diversity of membership brings a wider range of knowledge to the problem at hand. Third, and significantly, a skilled executive can use the committee as a delaying device when it is necessary to prevent a person or group from launching an ill-conceived or premature project. An opportunity for delay, of course, represents one of the most significant disadvantages of the committee approach. Committees tend to be very expensive and quite slow, and time is a critical factor in the planning process. For example, given the problems of inflation, postponing decisions often involves a substantial increase in the cost of a project. Another disadvantage is that committees tend to develop compromise decisions, and consensus does not necessarily represent the best choice. Finally, responsibility for committee activities cannot effectively be placed on any one individual. Even the head of the group can easily rationalize delaying tactics and indecisiveness by attributing problems to other members.

Staff Planning Groups

This option offers an alternative to the committee approach when an executive wishes to delegate some of the work involved in the planning process. The advantages and disadvantages are essentially the opposite of those described for planning by committees.

The major drawback to planning by staff groups is the potential for noninvolvement of those most directly affected by the plan. The greatest advantage is that a specific person is assigned primary responsibility for carrying out the planning process. This person can be regarded as an "integrator" of organizational functions.[20] Consider the following description of the job of assistant administrator for planning at Mount Carmel Mercy Hospital in Detroit:[21] "These objectives and functions cannot be performed by one person without a great deal of cooperation from within the hospital and from outside it. The most dominant and time-consuming task of the assistant administrator for planning is cultivating effective planning relationships within hospital, among hospitals, and between the hospital and many agencies that inspect it."

The integrator task requires a staff of specially talented people, who are hard to find. Further, integrators must contribute to decisions on the basis of their expertise rather than on the authority of their positions. They must have a balanced orientation between operation and development, between service and cost, and between specialty concerns and the total plan. They must also be acceptable as arbitrators of intraorganizational disputes, which inevitably will arise while planning is being done. They must not ignore disputes, hide conflicts, or use arbitrary measures, because such tactics, although sometimes initially successful, eventually will destroy the effectiveness of the planning process.

SUPPLEMENTARY RESOURCES

On occasion, decision makers may require assistance beyond that provided by their own internal resources. Where special expertise is needed, they may turn to supplementary resources, that is, the use of outside consultants. Consultants are persons who have special knowledge, usually derived from a high level of education and intensive experience within a limited scope of activities. The use of consultants is fairly common within the health industry for two reasons. First, health agencies have historically lacked specialized managerial and administrative expertise. Even in a well-staffed organization, consultants can offer skills that are not available within the organization

---

[20]Paul R. Lawrence and Jay W. Lorsch. "New Management Job: The Integrator." *Harvard Business Review, 45*(6):142–151, November–December 1967.
[21]Sister Mary Leila, R.S.M., T. R. O'Donovan, and L. T. Schwartz. "Planning: A Full-Time Responsibility." *Hospital Progress, 57*(9):95, September 1976.

because those skills are not required on a day-to-day basis. Second, very few health agencies have adequate staffing to perform more than their regular operations. The consultant is another source of manpower that the chief decision maker can use when a planning project unit or task force would divert too many resources from ongoing work.

Consultants can do anything from creating an entire plan to carrying out a very specific assignment related to one small segment of the plan. For example, a general consultant might produce an entire plan, whereas an architect would convert the functional plan into a construction plan and supervise its implementation. Some of the most common consultant tasks include identifying the need for a plan, that is, establishing organizational objectives, gathering and analyzing data for a plan, developing and evaluating alternatives, and simply evaluating plans developed by others. These tasks are essentially a recapitulation of the planning process.

Consultants can make some very important contributions to planning, one of which is their ability to sell a plan. They can serve as the outside, "unbiased" expert that proposal authors often deem necessary to gain acceptance of ideas from the people most affected. They also can provide the special knowledge and experience that plan implementation often requires. For example, architects are skilled at supervising construction because they have gained experience on past similar projects, but an individual hospital, which has construction projects under way only at infrequent intervals, most likely lacks personnel with this expertise.

Selection of Consultants

The use of consultants creates special problems for the chief decision maker, all of which revolve around selecting persons who are competent, ethical, and not inclined toward self-interest. A limited amount of free consultation might be obtained by dealing with manufacturers' representatives. Because these agents have something to sell, however, they clearly do not meet the criterion of being disinterested. Nevertheless, they are competent and, for the most part, ethical, so the decision maker can get a certain amount of free input into the planning process if he carefully observes the dictum of caveat emptor.

Once the decision maker determines that he may have to go beyond the free contributions of manufacturers' representatives, he must then consider the conditions within his institution that necessitate engaging outside consultants. The most important of these include

1. The available staff lacks well-rounded experience.
2. The needed specialists are not available internally.
3. Additional staff and training time are not available.
4. The project involves a total organization survey.
5. The project is a broad study that extends beyond the organization.
6. The project requires advanced, special techniques.
7. Outside appraisal, "sales" assistance, or experience from other businesses is desired.[22]

For efficiency, the decision maker should devise a step-by-step procedure for selecting a consultant that includes a preliminary investigation, the release of a request for proposal (RFP), and an evaluation of the RFP responses and of the references of the consultants.

PRELIMINARY INVESTIGATION   There are many types of consultants; some have highly specialized staffs and function only in very limited areas, whereas others have broad skills and can offer a wide range of talents. Thus, at the outset, the decision maker should clearly and precisely define the exact nature of the project he wants to undertake; this will determine to a large extent the persons or firms to be approached. He should then identify and conduct informal but specific interviews with persons or firms who are qualified to participate and who might be interested in the proposed project.

Professional associations and other health agencies that have recently conducted similar projects are good sources of information for the preliminary investigation. Once the initial list of contenders is compiled, the decision maker should determine for each

1. The history of the company
2. The background of its personnel
3. Its financial status
4. How easy it has been to work with in the past
5. Its inventiveness (Does the company come up with new ideas or give the impression that it has predetermined solutions for problems that might develop?)
6. The number and type of satisfied clients and the amount of repeat business the company receives from its former clients
7. The pertinence of the consulting company's specific experience to the project at hand (Most consultants have broad expertise and can

---

[22]J. W. Haslett. "Decision Table for Engaging a Consultant." *Journal of Systems Management,* 22(7):12–14, July 1971.

legitimately claim to have the relevant knowledge and skills; however, in terms of the kind of experience the decision maker is seeking, this might not be so.)

8. Fee arrangements (Is compensation based on a fixed price, a time-and-materials cost basis, a retainer fee, or some other kind of arrangement?)

Any consulting company that fails to meet or just barely meets these preliminary screening criteria should be eliminated immediately.

REQUEST FOR PROPOSAL   Once the field of contenders has been determined, the qualified firms should be invited to discuss the project in more detail. The project specifications should be given to all contenders so that each can submit a formal proposal for the service to be performed; specifications should be provided in a formal document (RFP) to avoid ambiguity concerning project requirements. The RFP must clearly identify the nature of the problem and the objectives of the project. It also should state the mandatory requirements and desired capabilities that will be used to judge the competing companies and their proposed approaches. In other words, the RFP must require that each bidder's proposal cover the following points:

1. A statement of the bidder's understanding of specific project objectives

2. The bidder's technical approach

3. Staff that will be allocated to the project (important, because many persons have hired consultants on the basis of the principal's qualifications only to discover that the principal seldom, if ever, contributed to the study of the problem)

4. A specific time schedule

5. Cost factors, including the method of billing

6. The consulting firm's methods of project control and status reporting

7. Specific areas of responsibilities that the consultant will assume, as well as those areas of the project for which the consultant disclaims all responsibility

8. Assistance needed from the hiring agency

9. The contractual terms and conditions under which the proposal is offered

10. References from satisfied clients

EVALUATION OF RFP RESPONSES   Four areas are of special importance to the decision maker in evaluating RFPs:

1. Adequacy of the proposal's technical features
2. The consulting organization's fee
3. The consultant's qualifications
4. The adequacy of the consultant's references

A major step in the evaluation process is to determine each consultant's performance history, particularly among organizations having experience with similar projects. This is a difficult undertaking because organizations obviously are reluctant to admit having made serious errors. Thus, the reference checker must be prepared to do some probing by asking questions such as, What kind of work did the firm do? Was it done completely and on time? Were the solutions practical and economical? Did the assigned personnel perform competently and objectively? How did the assigned personnel work with the client staff? Did the firm's supervisory personnel spend adequate time controlling and supervising the project? Would the reference hire the same consulting firm for similar work or for a different kind of technical endeavor?

Decision makers should not be reluctant to shop around. Consulting services represent a substantial investment, and organizations naturally want to get the most for their money. This can best be accomplished by a careful analysis of the capabilities of each person or firm competing for the contract.

In fairness to the consultants, the fundamental issue in determining the success or failure of a consulting project is how well the client agency has specified its goals and objectives. Without a clear picture of what its client wants, the consulting firm will succeed only by accident or by luck, or by investing a large amount of time in trying to determine the client's objectives. Furthermore, a client organization will be unable to evaluate proposals unless it knows exactly what it wants.

Step 2: Define the Mission

An organization's mission statement is a broad, abstract description of its purpose and, implicitly, its philosophy and values. It is an essential element of the organization's policy planning, for it is a statement of direction, analogous to the architect's conceptual model (versus schematic drawings or blueprints). Finally, it is an operational definition of the organization's driving force.[23] The mission statement should be

---

[23]Benjamin B. Tregoe and John W. Zimmerman. "Strategic Thinking: Key to Corporate Survival." *Management Review, 68*:9–14, February 1979.

fairly general, but Peters[24] suggests that these specific points be included: major functions, philosophy, levels of care, services or specialties, populations or geographic areas served, and relationships with other health care providers.

The mission statement sets the boundaries of organizational endeavor, within which more concrete goals and objectives will be specified. Its purpose is to put the organization in a distinctive position that will give it a competitive advantage. It is a response to three questions: What do we want to do? What should we do? What can we do?

Frequently, the initial mission statement is simply an answer to the first question. It is modified as the planning process produces information that makes it possible to consider the second and third questions. Some practitioners assert that mission definition should not be undertaken until there are enough data to deal with all three issues. Such a course of action seems dangerous, since the absence of an explicit and broad mission statement could lead to data collection and analysis that would be incomplete, partially irrelevant, or both.

It is clear that the values of the CEO and, perhaps, those of an organization's board will be the basis of the initial mission statement. This is one responsibility that no true leader can abdicate. In today's society, however, such an autocratic, self-serving approach, if sustained over a long period, would become counterproductive. Thus, even though the first iteration of the mission may be unilateral, later versions must be based on a thorough analysis of the interests of all major stakeholders in the organization (e.g., physicians, patients, staff, and community residents).[25]

After the *what* has been established, it is important to define *how*. In other words, the policies that will guide the selection of means for accomplishing the mission must be made explicit.

Step 3: Analyze the Environment

The term *environmental analysis* is often used to represent an analysis of all factors outside the organization that could affect its activities to a significant degree during the period covered by the plan. In this book, the term implies consideration of factors in the broad environment

---

[24]Joseph P. Peters. *A Guide to Strategic Planning for Hospitals.* Chicago, American Hospital Assn., 1979, p. 70.
[25]Russell L. Ackoff, *Creating the Corporate Future,* New York, Wiley, 1981, pp. 30–34; William R. King and David I. Cleland, *Strategic Planning and Policy,* New York, Van Nostrand Reinhold, 1978, pp. 152–156.

only. It includes economic, demographic, technological, sociocultural, and political/legal issues. Furthermore, it focuses only on factors external to the industry. Thus, market, resource, and industry analyses are separate later steps, and the integration of all the information is the culmination of step 6, industry analysis.

Step 3 has in common with steps 4–6 a requirement for forecasts as well as current facts. Because the effects of current decisions will be felt now and in the future, planning is likely to fail unless the changes between now and the planning horizon are anticipated. As Utterback[26] has pointed out, however, the requirements of the forecasting process and, consequently, its costs will vary with the nature of the situation. In simple and static circumstances, no formal methods are required, and, at most, expert opinion will suffice. If the situation is complex but still static, trend monitoring and extrapolation might be useful. Finally, if the situation is both complex and dynamic, quantitative models, simulations, and other sophisticated methods are probably appropriate.

Although most of the data gathered in the categories listed here will be objective, there is a qualitative data set that deserves explicit recognition: the expectations of stakeholders in the organization.[27] The level of effort needed to identify stakeholder interests is an indication of the organization's sense of social responsibility. In fact, the attention given by an organization to the environmental analysis reflects the degree of that organization's understanding of the reality that it is an open system that depends heavily on and is influenced by its environment. Except for government regulation, most of this influence tends to be indirect, subtle, and, consequently, easily overlooked, whereas the short-run, bottom-line results are overemphasized.

Step 4: Analyze the Market

Market analysis is a critical step in strategic planning. It symbolizes a major difference between strategic planning and the facility or program approaches that, until recently, characterized planning by health organizations. In these, the underlying assumption is either that the service is so inherently good that the patient will demand it without any stimulus

---

[26]James M. Utterback. "Environmental Analysis and Forecasting." In: *Strategic Management.* Edited by Dan E. Schendel and Charles W. Hofer. Boston, Little, Brown, 1979, p. 139.

[27]Ackoff defines stakeholders as those persons inside and outside the organization who are directly affected by its actions. For a hospital, the stakeholders would include such groups as employees, medical staff, patients, and community residents. See Russell L. Ackoff, *Creating the Corporate Future,* p. 30.

or that the demand can be created by educating the consumer (selling). The marketing approach reverses this paternalistic orientation and seeks to discover and satisfy the needs of the consumer. To do this requires knowledge of who the consumers are and how they obtain health services. This raises a particularly thorny issue in regard to many medical services: The analyst must decide whether physicians and other prescribing professionals are the consumers or the channels of distribution. This book will proceed on the premise that patients are the direct consumers of health services. Consequently, the analysis will discuss physicians as resources or channels of distribution. (The analysis could easily take the other point of view, however. In such a case, the analysis of physician characteristics would become part of the marketing study.)

The first step is to identify the consumers. This is typically determined by a patient-origin study. These locational data can be refined by computing relevance and commitment indexes.[28] Spatial identification gives access to census data, the main source of information on the demographic characteristics of consumers. These data then become the basis for market segmentation, a critical step in formulating strategy. Market segmentation permits the organization to focus on subgroups based on use rates, types of service used, tastes, and the like. Many of these factors affect technical decisions on the amount and kinds of services needed, but need does not equate with use. Ordinarily, ability to pay is recognized as an important factor in differentiating between need and demand. The key intervening variable that is frequently overlooked is consumer tastes.

Consumer tastes include preferences for different methods of service delivery, perceptions of service quality, and the image of the organization. The significance of this information is reflected by a recommendation in *Marketing Your Hospital*[29] that 0.5 percent of a hospital's annual budget be allocated to consumer research. Market research, per se, represents only a small portion of the analytic effort, however. The use of readily available operational data will usually be the principal basis of market analysis.[30]

---

[28]Philip N. Reeves, David F. Bergwall, and Nina B. Woodside. *Introduction to Health Planning.* 2nd Edition. Washington, D.C., Information Resources Press, 1979, pp. 125–127.

[29]Norman H. McMillan. *Marketing Your Hospital.* Chicago, American Hospital Assn., 1981, p. 20.

[30]Roberta N. Clarke and Linda Shayvitz. "Marketing Information and Marketing Research—Valuable Tools for Managers." *Health Care Management Review,* 6:1, 73–77, Winter 1981.

Step 5: Analyze External Resources

Current and future supplies of key resources are critical elements in assessing opportunities and threats to which an organization might respond. In some cases, the characteristics of the suppliers are as important as the available quantity of the resource. For instance, if nurses, the suppliers of essential skills, are unionized, that fact may affect the use of nursing services. This section discusses four types of resources: finances, personnel, technology, and facilities.

Usually, the availability of capital is regarded as the key factor in analyzing resources. But given the expectation that some organizations will provide urgently needed health services to the indigent, the ability and willingness of the community to reimburse providers for services received is another financial factor that may significantly affect an institution's survival. Consequently, the analysis should include both insurance coverage and, as a proxy for ability to pay direct out-of-pocket costs, income levels in the various market segments.

Capital financing is a necessary, although not sufficient, condition for attaining most goals. It represents the value that must be exchanged for the productive resources required to carry out the plan. Capital can be acquired through borrowing, by retaining surplus revenue (profits), or by sale of equity. In any case, the analysis must examine the availability of capital through the means chosen and the cost of capital.

Supply of personnel has exhibited some interesting trends in recent years (e.g., a shift from an apparent shortage of physicians to a projected surplus). Once again, quantity alone is an inadequate descriptor. Forecasts of supply also must consider types or subcategories, productivity, and personal characteristics. For example, what is the age distribution of physicians within each specialty? How will physicians behave when they embark on their careers with the burden of a huge debt incurred to complete their education?

New technology must not be accepted uncritically. Several questions should be asked. First, how rapidly will the technology be diffused throughout the professional community? Second, what effect will it have on costs? Will adopting the technology raise or lower unit and aggregate expenditures for health services? The third question is the matter of consumer tastes. Will the new technology be acceptable, or will it be regarded as dehumanizing or depersonalizing?

The supply of facilities may be particularly vexing because of their inflexibility and high cost, and both of these factors are significant barriers to leaving the health industry. Who wants to buy a hospital building that is underused because it is in the wrong location for its intended purpose? Who would buy or rent such a facility for another purpose when conversion costs are so high? Furthermore, the existence of underused facilities, no matter how inconvenient or inappropriate they have become, might result in disapproval of proposals to establish new facilities within an "overbedded" community.

Step 6: Analyze the Industry

The mission statement developed in step 2 set broad parameters that delimited the collection of data on the environment, markets, and resources. It is now necessary to define more precisely what business the organization is carrying out, that is, what is its industry? For instance, does the organization offer general acute inpatient care, general and specialty acute inpatient care, or health services? This industry identification will become the basis for translating the broad mission statement into more specific goals. The development of goal statements, however, must be guided by an analysis of the industry's situation now and at the planning horizon.

Porter[31] asserts that an industry analysis should focus on five factors: rival firms, potential entrants, buyers, suppliers, and substitute products or services (all but rival firms, including those offering substitute services, were mentioned in steps 3–5). Industry analysis entails the development of information with an industry profile based on data collected in steps 3–5. The end result should be a macro description of the industry and a micro description of an institution's potential rivals.

The macro description should highlight emerging trends to facilitate identification of threats and opportunities. Areas of particular concern are growth rate,[32] costs of resources, and development and diffusion of technology. In addition to these industry-specific issues, market shifts (e.g., demographic changes), changes in government policies, and general economic trends should receive special attention.

The micro description of rival organizations should include data on marketing (e.g., charge structure), production and products (e.g., costs of providing services), finances, and organization (e.g., philosophy and assumptions of trustees).[33] The philosophies and assumptions of trustees are crucial to an effective assessment of a rival's probable strategic moves and future goals. Particular heed must be paid to rivals seeking

---

[31]Michael E. Porter. *Competitive Strategy.* New York, Free Press, 1980, p. 4.
[32]Analysis of growth rate should examine both aggregate growth of health services and growth of individual institutions and services.
[33]William R. King and David I. Cleland. *Strategic Planning and Policy,* p. 248.

to enter the industry or to introduce substitute services. Frequently, these will be firms outside the boundaries of the industry as defined by the organization doing the analysis. Thus, it is easy to overlook them and be taken by surprise. A good intelligence system is necessary to provide early warning of these threats.

The term *intelligence* usually evokes images of spies, secret meetings, and other clandestine activities. This is, in fact, a grave misperception. Intelligence is merely data that are analyzed and focused on a critical issue; the data are readily available to anyone who will maintain a consistent, systematic intelligence-gathering system. First, much of the data is distributed widely by organizations (e.g., annual reports, speeches by trustees or the CEO). Second, some data come into the public domain as a result of government requirements (e.g., licensure applications, certificate-of-need applications). Finally, data become available as a by-product of business transactions (e.g., requests for proposals, documents developed in support of bond issues). In fact, there is danger of drowning in data. To avoid being overwhelmed, the intelligence system must be built on a conceptual framework that will identify which data are relevant and suggest how they should be analyzed to contribute to the strategic planning process. Porter's *Competitive Strategy* is an excellent guide to developing such a framework.

Step 7: Develop Goals

Goals are restatements of the organization's mission—more specific assertions of what the organization seeks to achieve. Specificity is attained by establishing measurable objectives to accomplish. These accomplishments are "what must actually be done to enable the institution to achieve its mission."[34] Thus, goals are ends, and strategies are means.

Note the transition from the singular, *mission,* to the plural, *goals.* The mission encompasses the interests of all stakeholders; a goal often relates to only one or a few of these constituencies. Because of the broadness of the single mission statement, it is important to have these explicit and specific goals as the linkage between mission and strategies. But goals, because of their specificity, also serve as standards to control progress and evaluate performance while the plan is being carried out. These uses imply that goals should be developed in a more

---

[34]Joseph P. Peters. *A Guide to Strategic Planning for Hospitals,* p. 72.

participatory process than the mission statement. If those whose performance is to be measured participate in the goal-setting process, they will find the goals more credible and thus will be more committed to achieving them. Furthermore, the greater specificity of goal statements often requires more detailed knowledge than the CEO is likely to have.

Goals are derived from the situational analysis completed in step 6. They are designed to satisfy stakeholder claims to the maximum extent feasible, given the environmental context, threats, and opportunities. Since some stakeholder interests are likely to be competing, it is imperative that the final set of goals be carefully analyzed to ensure that they are internally consistent. Goal development is a critical juncture at which the mission statement must be revalidated. The mission was created as a broad abstraction of an idealized purpose with little basis for estimating its feasibility. Now it must be tested and, if necessary, modified in the light of detailed information on environmental constraints and operational definitions of what it commits the organization to accomplish.

Step 8: Analyze the Portfolio of Programs

Portfolio analysis is a device to assess how significantly current activities are contributing to attainment of the organization's aims and to suggest appropriate ways to enhance the organization's performance. In business literature, portfolio analysis is characterized as a system that provides visibility of performance in both strategic and financial terms, selectivity in resource allocation, and differentiation in administrative attention given to different organizational components.[35,36] We suggest a fourth purpose: display of information on how programs contribute to each of the organizational goals.

The first step in portfolio analysis is to divide the organization's activities into SBUs or PMUs. Two theoretical principles are important. First, the elements within each unit should be as similar as possible.

---

[35]Philippe Haspeslagh. "Portfolio Planning: Uses and Limits." *Harvard Business Review, 60*:61, January–February 1982.

[36]Visibility of performance is provided by the two axes of a typical diagram such as Figure 12. Resource allocations are suggested by the notion that surplus revenues generated by the profitable but strategically less important SBUs (lower left of figure) should be directed toward expansion of strategically more important SBUs (upper left or upper right). Similarly, administrative attention should not be allocated equally among stable SBUs, SBUs of decreasing significance, and SBUs whose growth is strategically important.

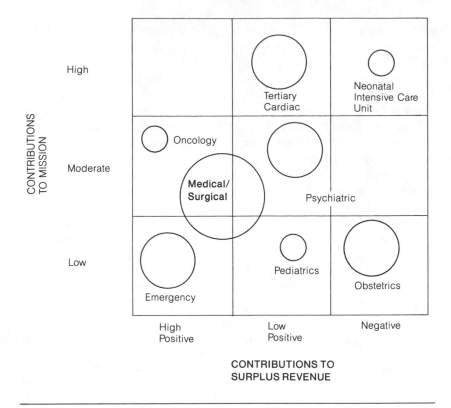

Figure 12   General portfolio analysis matrix.

Second, the units should be as different from each other as possible. Units should be established to facilitate delegation of responsibility, authority, and accountability for performance. The next step is to construct a two-dimensional matrix. The designations of the axes differ, but, typically, one relates to profitability (sometimes called *competitive position*) and the other, often called *industry attractiveness,* reflects major organizational purposes, such as growth. The scales for each axis usually result in a matrix of four or nine cells.

Figure 12 illustrates a nine-cell matrix. The horizontal axis represents contributions to surplus revenue, a measure of financial success and survivability. The vertical axis measures support of the organization's mission. SBUs or PMUs can be located on each axis on the basis of ratings assigned by the organization's decision makers.[37] The SBUs are placed

---

[37]The ratings may be assigned by any one of several methods. Often the goals developed by the organization are used as a set of factors reflecting contribution to the mission.

within the matrix on the basis of their ratings on the two scales. More information can be provided by depicting SBUs or PMUs as circles, with diameters that are proportional to their gross revenue or to some other significant performance measure.

Some business analysts categorize the cells of the matrix in terms of the strategic actions that should be taken in regard to the SBUs or PMUs that fall into them. For instance, an organization would want to discontinue an SBU or a PMU that made only a small contribution to the mission and also was losing money.

As noted earlier, the mission statement is broad and general and must be clarified by operational definitions in the form of goals. Consequently, an aggregate rating based on contribution to the overall mission tells little about how an SBU or PMU achieves the organization's purposes. Factor or weighted-factor ratings make explicit assessments of the contribution of each SBU or PMU to each goal (see Chapter 10). This information is lost in the visual display, however, since only the sum of the ratings is used. Furthermore, there is no effort to show the relative support provided for each goal. It is easy to remedy this deficiency and thus provide critical information to decision makers by preparing an additional matrix for each goal. The horizontal axis would remain unchanged, but the vertical axis would measure contribution to that specific goal.

Step 9: Analyze Organizational Competence

The preceding portfolio analysis showed how the organization's programs contributed to its two generic goals: survival and achievement of its mission. Graphic displays often will suggest the need to add programs, modify existing ones (e.g., increase the market share of a profitable high-level contributor), or both. The organizational competence analysis is designed to determine what the organization can realistically expect to accomplish.

Many texts on strategic planning advocate WOTS UP (weaknesses, opportunities, threats, strengths underlying planning) analysis as a combined process. In this book, that process has been divided. It is assumed here that most, if not all, opportunities and threats are the result of environmental factors; therefore, they were considered in the environmental analysis. It is possible, however, that opportunities or threats could arise as a result of some special combination of internal factors (organizational characteristics and portfolio composition). If such a situation is discovered during the analysis, the results of step 7 (goal development) must be reexamined in the light of the new information.

The goals developed in step 7 are designed to exploit opportunities and to counter threats. Weaknesses or strengths can now be determined in the light of those goals; this would not have been possible at an earlier stage, since the classification of an organizational characteristic as a strength or weakness depends on the purposes of the organization. For instance, a large number of trained specialists on a clinical staff would probably be assessed as a weakness in an organization that offered only primary medical care. In other cases, determining whether a factor is a strength or a weakness will be based on ability to meet the organization's internal needs rather than ability to respond to external circumstances. For instance, how does the organization's financial status look according to generally accepted standards (e.g., the acid-test ratio)? Weakness and strength analysis is a key input in formulating strategy. Weaknesses obviously are constraints; strengths must be further categorized. Does the strength represent a distinctive competence? If it does, can it be used as a competitive advantage?

In general, the identified competences and weaknesses must not only be listed, but the strategic implications of each must be explicitly stated. Characterization of strengths and weaknesses should consider resource, organization, and program or service aspects. This could quickly become an overwhelming task, but it would be easier if the analysis was limited to a set of factors identified as critical determinants of success. For medical staff, for example, age, specialty distribution, and level of admitting activity may be the critical factors. For technology, position of the organization on the learning curve in contrast to other organizations may be key. (This assumes that productivity and, thus, profitability increase with advances along the learning curve.) For programs, their distribution in the portfolio in terms of their cash demands might be the determinant.

Step 10: Establish a General Strategy

Strategy can be defined as the organization's approach to achieving its goals. There must be a general overall strategy to serve as a guide for later development of more specific functional strategies. This master strategy lays down the central concepts on which the organization's actions are based. It must be consistent with the internal capabilities of the organization and flexible, so that the organization can adapt readily to environmental changes. Flexibility can be gained by focusing not on products (services) and markets but rather on the useful benefits of the products.[38] For example, railroads would have more flexibility if they defined their business as transportation of people and cargo rather than as operation of trains.

Hofer and Schendel[39] assert that a good strategy statement will be expressed in functional rather than physical terms. They also suggest that a good statement (1) be as precise as possible; (2) describe each of the four components of the strategy: scope of activity, resource deployments to develop competencies, competitive advantages to be exploited, and intended synergy from joint effects or scope and resource-deployment decisions; and (3) indicate how the strategy will lead to accomplishing the organization's goals.

Quinn[40] states that the strategy should have a clear pattern or thrust, which can be based on principles such as concentration of resources to ensure sufficient strength to overcome the likely obstacles to achievement of the chosen goals. In a similar vein, Porter[41] suggests that there are three generic strategies: cost leadership, differentiation, and focus.

Whatever their nature, these general strategy statements emerge as the products of steps 1–9. In particular, they bring into focus opportunities and threats; organizational strengths and weaknesses; and management values as exhibited in the stakeholder analysis and expressed in the goal statements, in an effort to fill the gaps that exist between the organization's goals and the performance of its portfolio of programs.

Porter[42] has suggested another classification scheme that identifies the organization's strategic posture as reactive, active, or proactive. Reactive strategies seek to position the organization based on its strengths and weaknesses with respect to the existing environment. Active strategies attempt to change existing factors. Proactive strategies search for ways to create new circumstances.

Abell's[43] analysis is a reminder that it is not necessary to use an identical approach to all aspects of a strategy. He notes that a strategy may be focused, differentiated, or unfocused along each of three dimensions: technology mix, customer segments, and customer needs, yielding 27 possible outcomes. One outcome could be to focus on a

---

[38]Max D. Richards. *Organizational Goal Structures.* New York, West Publishing Co., 1978, p. 32.
[39]Charles W. Hofer and Dan E. Schendel. *Strategy Formulation: Analytical Concepts.* New York, West Publishing Co., 1978, pp. 25, 42.
[40]James B. Quinn. "Formulating Strategy One Step at a Time."
[41]Michael E. Porter. *Competitive Strategy,* p. 35.
[42]_____ . "How Competitive Forces Shape Strategy." *Harvard Business Review, 57*: 143–144, March–April 1979.
[43]Derek F. Abell. *Defining the Business: The Starting Point of Strategic Planning.* Englewood Cliffs, N.J., Prentice-Hall, 1980, pp. 174–175, 187.

single technology mix, differentiate several customer segments, and ignore the various ways in which customers use the service. This might be an effective strategy for hospital emergency services. The service would always be the same (single technology mix), charges might be scaled on the basis of ability to pay (differentiation of market segments), and the organization would be indifferent as to whether the service was used as a substitute for a personal physician (no attempt to focus on different needs being met by the service).

Most of the literature on strategy emphasizes growth, but this must be critically examined. There are unique aspects of service businesses that require approaches different from those appropriate for product-based businesses.[44] The type of growth must be suitable for the extant state of organizational/environmental relations.[45] Historically valid assumptions on economies of scale are no longer certainties.[46] Changes in general economic conditions may have affected the market such that previously successful strategies are now inappropriate.[47]

Despite their diversity, the processes for developing strategies will not highlight these hazards. Higgins[48] identifies six of these processes: WOTS UP, strategy profile, product/market matrix, product portfolio, directional policy matrix, and life-cycle analysis. Steiner's[49] list also adds gap analysis and a search for synergy. These processes should result in several distinct alternatives for each major strategic thrust. For example, if the general strategy calls for growth through addition of a new service, the alternatives might be to establish a new business in a separate organization, to develop the new service within the existing organization, or to conduct a demonstration project.

These options seem mutually exclusive, but the choice need not be. In this case, the options could become sequential steps in a developmental strategy. In other instances, the final strategy should be some combination of the alternatives.

---

[44]Dan R. E. Thomas. "Strategy Is Different in Service Businesses." *Harvard Business Review, 56*:158–165, July–August 1978.

[45]Beaufort B. Longest, Jr. "An External Dependence Perspective of Organizational Structure: The Community Hospital Case." *Hospital and Health Services Administration, 26*:50–69, Spring 1981.

[46]Robert A. Leone and John R. Meyer. "Capacity Strategies for the 1980s." *Harvard Business Review, 58*:133–140, November–December 1980.

[47]Alan J. Resnik, Peter B. B. Turney, and J. Barry Mason. "Marketers Turn to 'Countersegmentation.' " *Harvard Business Review, 57*:100–106, September–October 1979.

[48]J. C. Higgins. *Strategic and Operational Planning Systems.* Englewood Cliffs, N.J., Prentice-Hall, 1980, pp. 22–27.

[49]George A. Steiner. *Strategic Planning.* New York, Free Press, 1979, pp. 144–145.

Step 11: Design Functional Strategies

Once again, there is a need to translate a broad, guiding statement into operational terms that will help in making specific decisions. The developmental process is essentially the same as that for the master strategy, but now the aim is to develop options in a number of relatively narrow areas. This specificity can be described in terms of categories and types.

The master strategy addresses growth, price, focus, timing, and investment.[50] There should be specific strategies to support each of these major thrusts; hence, there will be strategy statements addressing capacity, price, service line, markets, and investment. An additional category, organizational structure and process, is also required, for reasons that will be discussed in step 13.

These categorical designations focus on outcomes; strategy types are distinguished on the basis of means or processes to attain the outcomes. (Some authors refer to specific strategies as functional strategies.[51] Thus, they equate type with function.) Rothschild describes in detail strategic options for marketing, producing services (manufacturing), financing, and innovating. These are rather broad definitions that can be further refined—for example, "marketing" includes the well-known four P's (product, price, place, and promotion).

Strategy types can be combined with categories in a two-dimensional matrix that will give considerable information to the astute analyst (Figure 13). At the very least, the matrix will indicate whether all significant outcomes have been addressed and whether the opportunities offered by all strategy types have been exploited.[52]

Hofer and Schendel[53] outline a decision-tree approach that is likely to lead to a comprehensive, integrated set of strategies. Functional marketing strategies are first developed to determine the nature of the organization's products and services and the processes by which they are

---

[50]In this context, growth is a strategy, not a goal. For example, growth is a strategy for reducing the organization's vulnerability to environmental influence by increasing its strength and self-sufficiency. Focus strategies relate to the scope of the product/service line, the structure of the markets, or both.

[51]William E. Rothschild. *Strategic Alternatives.* New York, AMACOM, 1979, pp. 75–164.

[52]For example, if the organization has chosen growth as a general strategy, the analyst should explore the possibility of developing a specific strategy in each of the subtypes identified on the vertical axis of Figure 13. Then, after the full set of feasible strategies has been identified, it must be carefully examined to assure internal consistency. For instance, a marketing strategy emphasizing service tailored to the wishes of individual clients will run counter to a production strategy that seeks to achieve efficiency and to contain costs by using standard materials and procedures. For a service such as health care, scheduling of services is a likely point of conflict between marketing and production strategies.

[53]Charles W. Hofer and Dan E. Schendel. *Strategy Formulation,* p. 37.

Strategy Types		Strategic Categories				
		Growth	Price	Focus	Timing	Investment
Marketing						
Producing	1 2 • • n					
Financing	1 • • • n					
Innovating	1 • • • n					

Figure 13   Strategic category/strategy type matrix.

made available to the customers. Next, strategies are developed for producing these goods and services. Finally, strategies are established for acquiring necessary resources to support the production and marketing functions.

Since these more detailed options usually will be developed below the top management level by committees, task forces, or operating units, the leadership of the organization must have a means to review these products, select the preferred ones, and then balance them.

Step 12: Select Preferred Alternatives

The first phase of this step is to screen each proposed alternative for consistency with the mission, goals, and general strategy of the organization. Special emphasis must be placed on supporting the organization's basic thrusts or principles.

Proposals that survive this initial screening should then be evaluated on the basis of four general tests:

1. *Frame test:* Does the strategy focus on the critical issues in this area?

2. *Competence test:* Does the strategy pose subproblems within the range of those solvable by organizational skills and competences?

3. *Workability test:* Does the strategy require only resources that are available to the organization? Will it produce the results sought?

4. *Asymmetry test:* Does the strategy create or exploit an asymmetry, or difference, constituting an advantage over rival organizations?[54]

The proposals passing these tests should be assessed on the basis of additional, more specific criteria. Various authors have proposed comparable sets of criteria; the following list was developed by Steiner:[55]

1. Is the strategy consistent with the environment?

2. Is the strategy consistent with internal policies, management styles, philosophy, and operating procedures?

3. Is the strategy appropriate in the light of resources? (This is analogous to the workability test previously described.)

4. Are the risks in pursuing the strategy acceptable?

5. Does the strategy fit the product life cycle and market strength-market attractiveness situation?

6. Is the timing of the proposed implementation correct?

Steiner provides 34 questions that make these criteria operational. Another factor that also deserves consideration is the degree to which the proposal will create or contribute to synergistic interaction with other strategies.

The four tests previously described yield "yes" or "no" decisions. Thus, a proposal either survives or is rejected. The criteria, however, can be met to varying degrees, so the issue to be decided is which set of proposals is best. The answers are ultimately judgmental, but rating schemes such as those mentioned in Chapter 10 can be very helpful to the decision maker.

Step 13: Modify Organization to Fit Selected Strategies

The organization is the vehicle for implementing the strategic plan; therefore, it must be suitable for the task. Some would argue that strate-

---

[54]Richard P. Rumelt. "Evaluation of Strategy: Theories and Models." In: *Strategic Management.* Edited by Dan E. Schendel and Charles W. Hofer. Boston, Little, Brown, 1979, pp. 199–203.

[55]George A. Steiner. *Strategic Planning,* pp. 144–145.

gies are selected on the basis of compatibility with an organization as it exists; this may be true in some cases. In those instances, this step would be limited to verification of the fit. When organizational congruence is not used as a constraint on strategy development, however, the implementers must act to assure the suitability of three facets of the organization: structure, process, and behavior. It has been widely accepted that structure should follow strategy. The dissenters seem to feel that a better explanation is provided by a hypothesis focused on the fit between people and structure.[56] But there are also strong beliefs about the fit between people and strategy types. Consequently, the argument may be circular. In any case, several authors have prepared useful tables showing organizational characteristics in relation to types of strategy. Following are a few items from a table presented by Schendel and Hofer:[57]

Strategy Characteristics	Managerial Type	Organizational Characteristics
Growth	Entrepreneur	Must enable future growth
Earnings maximization	Solid businessman	Must provide flexibility at moderate cost
Divestiture	"Hard-nosed" operator	Must be low cost and no frills

Apparently, there is no controversy about the need to adapt processes to accommodate the strategies selected. For instance, it is clear that the evaluation-and-reward system for a strategy emphasizing current profit would be ill-suited for a strategy focused on research or long-range development. Bower[58] singles out two processes—specialization and integration—as particularly critical for successful implementation. Similarly, there seems to be agreement on the requirement that behavior support the chosen strategies. This implies that style and shared values must be compatible with organizational aims and the means chosen to attain them. The essence, then, of this step is the concept of achieving a strategic fit among the well-known *Seven S's*. The Seven S framework was developed by the McKinsey Corporation and has been widely used by successful firms.[59] In short, the decision makers must

---

[56]Dan E. Schendel and Charles W. Hofer (eds.). *Strategic Management.* Boston, Little, Brown, 1979, pp. 222–225.

[57]Ibid., p. 132.

[58]Joseph L. Bower. "Solving the Problems of Business Planning." *Journal of Business Strategy,* 2:38–41, Winter 1982.

[59]Robert H. Waterman, Jr. "The Seven Elements of Strategic Fit." *Journal of Business Strategy,* 2:69–73, Winter 1982.

assure a match between the strategy selected (the first S) and the organizational factors identified by the other six S's (see the following).

The S's

Factors Affecting Strategy	The Six S's Affecting Strategy
Structure	Structure, Staff
Process	Systems, Skills
Behavior	Style, Shared Values

SUMMARY

The systems planning concepts usually associated with community planning must also be applied to the process of organizational planning. Further, to achieve maximum value from the effort expended, organizational planning should be integrated within the community health system planning process. Organizational planning includes contingency planning, program planning, and project planning. Each of these are subsidiary to and guided by the organization's strategic plan. Strategic planning is a 13-step activity beginning with the establishment of a planning process and culminating in modification of the organization to facilitate achievement of the strategic mission. Intermediate steps encompass identification of opportunities and threats within the environment, analysis of the organization's strengths and weaknesses in relation to the goals derived from the environmental assessment, and selection of a feasible strategy for achievement of the goals.

REFERENCES

Abell, Derek F. *Defining the Business: The Starting Point of Strategic Planning.* Englewood Cliffs, N.J., Prentice-Hall, 1980.

Ackoff, Russell L. *Creating the Corporate Future.* New York, Wiley, 1981.

American Hospital Association. *The Practice of Planning in Health Care Institutions.* Chicago, 1973.

———. *Redesigning the Future.* New York, Wiley, 1974.

Bower, Joseph L. "Solving the Problems of Business Planning." *Journal of Business Strategy, 2*:32–44, Winter 1982.

Branch, Melville. *Planning Aspects and Applications.* New York, Wiley, 1966.

Breindel, Charles L. "Health Planning Processes and Process Documentation." *Hospital and Health Services Administration, 26*(Special II):5–18, 1981.

Carithers, R. W. "What to Expect from an Outside Consultant and How to Get It." *Health Care Management Review, 2*(3):43–46, Summer 1977.

Chi Systems, Inc. *Health Facility Planning and Development: A Position Paper.* Ann Arbor, Mich., October 1977.

Chi Systems, Inc., and Stone, Marraccini, and Patterson. *Health Facility Planning and Development, Generic Planning Process: State of the Art.* Ann Arbor, Mich., Chi Systems, Inc., February 1976.

Cunningham, Robert M., Jr. "Who's Minding the Store?" *Hospitals, 52*(6):115–120, March 16, 1978.

Domanico, Lee. "Strategic Planning: Vital for Hospital Long-Range Development." *Hospital and Health Services Administration, 26*:25–50, Summer 1981.

Frankenhoff, Charles A. "The Planning Environment of Health Systems Agencies: A Strategy for Intervention." *Inquiry, XIV*(3):217–228, September 1977.

Frankenhuis, Jean Pierre. "How to Get a Good Consultant." *Harvard Business Review, 55*(6):133–139, November–December 1977.

Galbraith, Jay R., and Daniel A. Nathanson. *Strategy Implementation: The Role of Structure and Process.* New York, West Publishing Co., 1978.

Hardy, O. B., and L. P. Lammers. *Hospitals: The Planning and Design Process.* Germantown, Md., Aspen Systems Corp., 1977.

Haspeslagh, Philippe. "Portfolio Planning: Uses and Limits." *Harvard Business Review, 60*:58–73, January–February 1982.

Hayes, Robert H., and Steven G. Wheelwright. "The Dynamics of Process-Product Life Cycles." *Harvard Business Review, 57*:127–136, March–April 1979.

Higgins, J. C. *Strategic and Operational Planning Systems.* Englewood Cliffs, N.J., Prentice-Hall, 1980.

Hillestad, Steven G., and Richard Berry. "Applying Strategic Marketing." *Hospital and Health Services Administration, 25*(Special II):7–16, 1980.

Hofer, Charles W., and Dan E. Schendel. *Strategy Formulation: Analytical Concepts.* New York, West Publishing Co., 1978.

Jaeger, B. Jon (ed.). *Hospital Corporate Planning.* Durham, N.C., Duke University, 1981.

Jay, Antony. "Rate Yourself as a Client." *Harvard Business Review, 55*(4):84–89, July–August 1977.

Kantrow, Alan M. "The Strategy-Technology Connection." *Harvard Business Review, 58*:6ff, July–August 1980.

King, William R., and David I. Cleland. *Strategic Planning and Policy.* New York, Van Nostrand Reinhold, 1978.

Leone, Robert A., and John R. Meyer. "Capacity Strategies for the 1980s." *Harvard Business Review, 58*:133–140, November–December 1980.

Longest, Beaufort B., Jr. "An External Dependence Perspective of Organizational Structure: The Community Hospital Case." *Hospital and Health Services Administration, 26*:50–69, Spring 1981.

Lorange, Peter, and Richard F. Vancil. "How to Design a Strategic Planning System." *Harvard Business Review, 54*:75–81, September–October 1976.

Mankin, Douglas C., and William F. Glueck. "Strategic Planning." *Hospital and Health Services Administration, 22*(2):6–22, Spring 1977.

Mason, R. Hal. "Developing a Planning Organization." *Business Horizons, 12*(4):61–69, August 1969.

McMillan, Norman H. *Marketing Your Hospital.* Chicago, American Hospital Assn., 1981.

"New Jersey Requires Hospitals To Do Long-Range Planning." *Hospitals, 49*(18):94, September 16, 1975.

Parston, Gregory; Hila Richardson; and Barbara A. Hill. *Multi-Future Strategic Planning.* San Francisco, Western Center for Health Planning, July 24, 1981. (Technical Assistance Memo 75)

Perlin, Martin S. *Managing Institutional Planning.* Germantown, Md., Aspen Systems Corp., 1976.

Peters, Joseph P. *A Guide to Strategic Planning for Hospitals.* Chicago, American Hospital Assn., 1979.

Pierce, Charles F., Jr. "Partnerships in Planning: Getting Everyone into the Act." *Hospitals, 50*(12):113–116, June 16, 1976.

Porter, David. *Health Design Administration.* Washington, D.C., 1973.

Porter, Michael E. *Competitive Strategy.* New York, Free Press, 1980.

———. "How Competitive Forces Shape Strategy." *Harvard Business Review, 57*:137–145, March–April 1979.

Quinn, James B. "Formulating Strategy One Step at a Time." *Journal of Business Strategy, 1*:42–63, Winter 1981.

Resnik, Alan J.; Peter B. B. Turney; and J. Barry Mason. "Marketers Turn to 'Countersegmentation.' " *Harvard Business Review, 57*:100–106, September–October 1979.

Richards, Max D. *Organizational Goal Structures.* New York, West Publishing Co., 1978.

Rijvnis, Arie J., and Graham J. Sharman. "New Life for Formal Planning Systems." *Journal of Business Strategy, 2*:100–105, Spring 1982.

Rothschild, William E. *Strategic Alternatives.* New York, AMACOM, 1979.

Schendel, Dan E., and Charles W. Hofer (eds.). *Strategic Management.* Boston, Little, Brown, 1979.

Schlenger, Mary Jane. "Marketing Audits for Health Organizations." *Hospital and Health Services Administration, 26*(Special II):32–51, 1981.

Steiner, George A. *Strategic Planning.* New York, Free Press, 1979.

Stevens, Carl M. "Hospital Costs: On Rationalizing the Physician-Hospital Relationship." *Inquiry, XIV*(3):303–305, September 1977.

Stuehler, George, Jr. "The Hospital-Based Planner 'In His Time Plays Many Parts.' " *Hospitals, 50*(12):75–79, June 16, 1976.

———. "A Model for Planning in Health Institutions." *Hospital and Health Services Administration, 23*(3):6–27, Summer 1978.

Thomas, Dan R. E. "Strategy Is Different in Service Businesses." *Harvard Business Review, 56*:158–165, July–August 1978.

Tregoe, Benjamin B., and John W. Zimmerman. "Strategic Thinking: Key to Corporate Survival." *Management Review, 68*:9–14, February 1979.

Tucker, Stephen L. "Introducing Marketing as a Planning and Management Tool." *Hospital and Health Services Administration, 22*(1):37–44, Winter 1977.

Unterman, Israel, and Richard H. Davis. "The Strategy Gap in Not-for-Profits." *Harvard Business Review, 60*:30ff, May–June 1982.

Vancil, Richard F., and Peter Lorange. "Strategic Planning in Diversified Companies." *Harvard Business Review, 53*:81–90, January–February 1975.

Waterman, Robert H., Jr. "The Seven Elements of Strategic Fit." *Journal of Business Strategy, 2*:69–73, Winter 1982.

Weeks, L. E., and R. A. Devries. "The Status of Hospital Trustee Education." *Hospital and Health Services Administration, 23*(1):72–96, Winter 1978.

Wommack, William W. "The Board's Most Important Function." *Harvard Business Review, 57*:48–62, September–October 1979.

Wrapp, H. Edward. "Organization for Long-Range Planning." *Harvard Business Review, 35*(1):27–47, January–February 1957.

6

INFORMATION SYSTEMS FOR HEALTH SERVICES PLANNING

Data are essential ingredients in the planning process, and implementation of various planning methods depends almost totally on the availability of data. The purpose of this chapter is to acquaint planners with fundamental principles related to information systems and to provide them with a basis for evaluating, either prospectively or retrospectively, the information systems designed to support the health planning process.

THE NEED FOR DATA

Planning theory illustrates very clearly the need for data. For example, theorists Davidoff and Reiner[1] cite three types of planning choices: choosing goals, choosing methods for attaining goals, and choosing revisions based on evaluation. Davidoff and Reiner recognize that all choices ultimately are based on good judgment (which, in turn, depends on a rigorous analysis of *information*) that makes the purpose and the impacts of the choices very clear.

Hauser[2] aptly describes the need for data in a decision-making process in *Social Statistics in Use*. He writes that "Statistics are quantitative

---

[1]Paul Davidoff and T. A. Reiner. "A Choice Theory of Planning." *Journal of the American Institute of Planners, 28*(3):103–115, May 1962.
[2]Philip M. Hauser. *Social Statistics in Use*. New York, Sage, 1975, p. 1.

facts collected, aggregated, and analyzed to provide intelligence to facilitate understanding and to serve as a foundation for the formulation of policy, development and administration of programs." What Hauser describes as the application of statistics is in fact the total planning process.

Congress also has recognized the need for data in developing federal health planning laws. House Report 93-1382,[3] for example, states that the functions of health system agencies are to "gather data about a specific health system; then based upon the problems and deficiencies which these data reveal, develop and specify goals, objectives, priorities, and specific plans which will correct these problems and deficiencies."

In the legislative history of the Health Planning Act, the bill's authors state that goals and objectives represent quantifiable statements. Clearly, if something is to be quantified, some sort of data must be available. On the other hand, the legislative history also expresses some concern over the possibility that agencies collect data as an end in itself. For this reason, the laws are written to discourage the initiation of data systems by health system agencies and to encourage the use of existing data sources.

The executive branch of government initially was responsive to the needs expressed in this and similar legislation. For instance, the U.S. Department of Health, Education, and Welfare (DHEW) forward plan for 1977-1981[4] included the following:

In order for government to make informed decisions for policy development and planning, to assess the impact of those decisions, and to operate its program effectively, we need to focus on the information base. . . .We need reliable, timely, pertinent, and comparable health data and their analysis at all levels which will describe the health status of the population, the availability of resources, the accessibility of services, the costs of services and resources, the resources of funding, the utilization of present services, and the quality of care. The lack of such statistics severely limits the capacity of the health industry to plan, manage, and evaluate our tremendous investment in health resources and delivery systems.

---

[3]U.S. Congress, House, Interstate and Foreign Commerce Committee. *National Health Policy Planning and Resources Development Act of 1974.* House Report 93-1382. 93rd Congress, 2nd Session. September 26, 1974, p. 59.

[4]U.S. Department of Health, Education, and Welfare. *Forward Plan for Health FY 1977-1981.* Washington, D.C., U.S. Government Printing Office, 1975.

Similar statements can be found in the DHEW forward plans for 1978–1982 and 1979–1983.[5] The comments and proposals in these plans move toward more specific and focused action recommendations.

As a reflection of health planners' need for data, the National Center for Health Statistics (NCHS) and the Bureau of Health Planning and Resources Development issued a formal agreement on December 10, 1975 for a work program. The work program was designed to establish a symbiotic relationship between the providers and users of data, with NCHS representing the technical concerns of providers for collection and storage and the health planning bureau representing user concerns related to analysis and interpretation. Recently, however, there has been a drastic reduction in executive branch support of activities that would provide the data required for rigorous analysis of policies, planning, and evaluation of the results of policy and planning decisions. This is reflected by the data in Table 5, which were extracted from federal budgets.

In the meantime, there has been an equally dramatic increase in the emphasis on and investment in institutional information systems. Until recently, most health services organizations had diverse and incompatible clinical, financial, and administrative systems that were uneven in their sophistication and quality. Now, as the result of the new system of reimbursements, hospitals are frantically seeking to develop and implement integrated information systems. The urgency of this activity is reflected by the introduction of a regular section on information systems in the journal of the American Hospital Association.[6]

The initial articles in this series indicated that in 1983, hospitals in the 201- to 500-bed range had an average of 32 computer-based systems (16 financial, 7 patient-related, and 9 management). Data collected just 15 years earlier indicated that only 54 percent of hospitals in this size group were using computers and that more than 50 percent of them relied on a service bureau or some other external computer. Of even greater significance is the fact that these hospitals had only a few applications. Approximately 20 percent of all users had only a single application; roughly 80 percent confined their applications to a single functional area; and 4 percent had systems that combined data from

---

[5]U.S. Department of Health, Education, and Welfare, *Forward Plan for Health FY 1978–1982*, Washington, D.C., U.S. Government Printing Office, 1976; _____, *Forward Plan for Health FY 1979–1983*, Washington, D.C., U.S. Government Printing Office, 1977.
[6]"Focus on Information Systems." *Hospitals, 58*(9):83–86, May 1, 1984.

TABLE 5   Statistical Budgets for Fiscal Years 1974–1985 (millions of dollars)

| Fiscal Year | Department of Health and Human Services | | National Center for Health Statistics* | |
	Actual Obligations (FY82 = 100)	Constant Dollars	Actual Obligations (FY82 = 100)	Constant Dollars
74	93.6	121	18.7	95
75	93.2	110	20.3	93
76	109.1	118	25.0	105
77	114.4	115	29.3	114
78	139.6	131	37.3	137
79	145.8	130	38.9	135
80	162.8	132	43.3	136
81	157.8	113	33.7	94
82	163.0	100	37.7	100
83	168.0	110	40.8	104
84	165.7	104	46.6	114
85†	160.3	97	42.8	101

SOURCE: Office of Management and Budget, Statistical Policy Office. *A Special Report on the Statistical Programs and Activities of the United States Government, Fiscal Year 1985.* Washington, D.C., U.S. Office of Management and Budget, April 1984, pp. 55, 60.

*The National Center for Health Statistics was selected to represent the federal commitment to general statistical programs because it is responsible for general (nonprogram) statistics and because its allocations include support for the Cooperative Health Statistics System, a major effort to assist in the development of information systems to meet needs at state and local levels. Also, the total obligations for DHHS include NIH data activities, which contribute very little to planning analyses and which generally have continued to grow while other DHHS programs have been cut back.
†Estimated amounts.

several functional areas.[7] A survey of representative hospitals led to the prediction that the $2 billion spent by community hospitals in 1983 for computer products and services (an increase of 23 percent over 1982) would increase to $4.5 billion in 1988.[8]

The development of better information systems in both the public and private sectors should permit substantial improvements in the prac-

[7]Philip N. Reeves. "A Study of the Adoption of Electronic Data Processing in the Hospital Industry." Unpublished dissertation. The George Washington University, Washington, D.C., 1970.
[8]"Increased Data Needs Seen as Trigger for Rise in Computer Expenditures." *Hospital Week,* 20(24):3, June 15, 1984.

tice of planning. The availability of data, however, is a necessary but not sufficient condition for successful planning.

There is a temptation to refer to information-based planning as a concept that supports the need to acquire large quantities of data. But, in reality, the need for data is a nonissue in deciding between information-based planning and some other type of planning, because information of some sort is always used in making choices. The distinction, then, lies in how much hard data are to be used and to what degree they are depended on in the decision-making process.

Hard data are reported facts, systematic opinion surveys, and quantitative estimates; soft data represent the opinions of decision makers, based on intuition, ad hoc comments, testimony at public hearings, and similar sources. Planners will never use only hard data in the decision-making process, because social values and political considerations also enter into the calculus of the decision maker. Consequently, any discussion pertaining to decision making must focus on a mix of hard and soft data (see Figure 14).

Although exclusive use of hard data in decision making, represented on the left side of the continuum of Figure 14, is unattainable, the greater the use of hard data in the decision-making process, the more likely that analysis of decisions can be more rigorous; there can be more precision in estimating outcomes; decision makers can arrive at mutually acceptable choices; the public can be effectively informed of the rationale and can thus be persuaded to support decisions; there will be fewer challenges to decisions, and there will be less difficulty in a legal defense of decisions when challenges do arise.

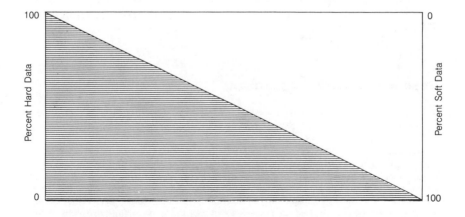

Figure 14 Data mix in decision making.

DATA AND PLANNING APPROACHES

There is a danger that planners will be overwhelmed by the quantity of data produced by some information systems. This is true for several reasons that relate to the quality and heterogeneity of the data and/or the fact that those involved have no appropriate models for using statistics. In other words, it is essential to have a conceptual model to transform raw data into useful information. The following discussion focuses on four planning models or approaches, examining each in regard to its relationship to data.

Problem-Oriented Approach

The problem-oriented model usually relies heavily on soft data, such as testimony given at public hearings, which may or may not be representative of the entire community, or the unsolicited comments of special-interest groups affected by a particular problem. This approach does not foster the development of a comprehensive data base because each problem is treated as unique. It focuses only on immediate outcomes without regard to costs, especially opportunity costs[9] elsewhere in the system. Furthermore, since a systematic data base is not available, the model usually concentrates on a single solution rather than choosing from several alternatives.

The problem-oriented approach is generally quite weak in evaluation, because interest in the specific problem does not persist over an extended period of time, except in the case of special-interest groups that benefit from continuing expenditures and that consequently are not supportive of evaluations that might jeopardize continuation of the program.

Resource-Oriented Approach

The resource-oriented model uses more hard data than the problem-oriented model and tends to perpetuate current activities because of

---

[9]*Opportunity costs* are the value of alternative services or products that are foregone because a decision has been made to use available resources to provide a selected service or product. For instance, available physician working hours could be used to provide health prevention services, diagnosis and treatment, or rehabilitation services. If the physician working hours are used for diagnosis and treatment, opportunity costs can be expressed as the value of the preventive services or rehabilitation services that cannot be provided because of the nonavailability of physician working hours for these purposes.

the interest of resource owners; that is, a special-interest group has a specific reason for acquiring, maintaining, and presenting facts that demonstrate the efficacy of its activities.

The hard data base used in this model tends to be very limited and focuses on the supply of resources and services, giving little consideration to the effects of resource utilization. The model typically assumes continuation of historical use patterns and seldom considers either interaction between subsystem decisions or the continuity of patient care. It also frequently assumes that the only solution to a problem is more of the same response rather than a new response. The resource-oriented approach usually is based on the aspirations of individual institutions or organizations rather than on the benefits to the general population, because the facts used in decision making have been generated by those whose interests dictate continuation and expansion of their own activities.

Market Approach

The market approach emphasizes identification and satisfaction of the needs of those served. Consequently, it requires substantial amounts of data that reflect both the availability of resources and services and the needs of those who reside in the service area. To satisfy needs adequately, the organization must have information on the characteristics of the population and the services currently offered. In some instances, special information gathering and analysis—market research—will be required.[10] This will be true, for instance, when psychographic data are to be included in the planning process. On the other hand, a great deal of marketing data can be obtained from existing information systems and health-related research reports. For example, epidemiologic data will become increasingly important as managers seek to do strategic planning based on clusters of homogeneous clinical programs.[11]

Systems Approach

A systems model maximizes the opportunities to use hard data. It establishes a set of decision variables for each aspect of the system and

---

[10]Roberta N. Clarke and Linda Shayvitz. "Marketing Information and Market Research—A Valuable Tool for Managers." *Health Care Management Review,* 6(1):73–77, Winter 1981.

[11]Philip N. Reeves. "Uses of Epidemiologic Data in Strategic Planning." Paper presented at the annual meeting of the American Public Health Assn., Dallas, Tex., November 15, 1983.

thus defines in advance the relevant data elements, thereby eliminating the need to collect large amounts of data as a precautionary measure when the types of statistics to be used are not known in advance. The model identifies the factors necessary to estimate the values of the decision variables and reflects interactions among these variables so that first-, second-, and third-order impacts can be anticipated and estimated.

The systems approach includes both individual and community costs and benefits when estimating impacts and thus provides an opportunity for explicit recognition of soft data. The model helps planners identify and analyze alternative courses of action. It also maximizes productivity, because the data elements collected are frequently relevant to several aspects of the system's functioning. Thus, in effect, the systems approach incorporates the major elements of the other approaches and also considers the interactions among these elements.

The system illustrated in Figure 5, which is derived from the perspective of planning as a control function, shows the flow of data (feedback and feedforward) into the control element for decision making. Input data are statistics on the quality, quantity, productivity, and costs of resources. Similarly, process-related data cover costs, accessibility, acceptability, and continuity. Intermediate outputs (i.e., services) can be described in terms of availability, quality, and effectiveness. Data on the final outputs are measures of health status, and external forces include population characteristics and data describing the system's economic, social, political, and physical environments.

USES OF DATA

Figure 15, a schematic model of an information system, shows that data sources contribute facts to a data base used for three purposes or processes, one being proactive decision making. The first step in this process is to describe, forecast, and analyze a system's activities. The description typically will include both the current and historical situation and usually will be based on recorded "facts."

The forecast or prediction is essential, because planning requires knowledge of future circumstances to choose proper alternatives. Historical patterns provide a basis for an initial forecast; however, it is imperative that such a forecast be validated in light of information collected as feedforward data. The person preparing the forecast or prediction must ascertain whether historical patterns reflected by the feedback data will persist in the future. If not, appropriate adjustments must be made in the prediction.

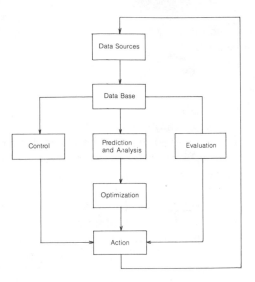

Figure 15   Schematic model of an information system.

Analysis implies combining data on inputs and process to estimate what outputs will be obtained. This requires knowledge of the productivity, as well as the quantity of inputs, and data on external factors that could affect the utilization and productivity or effectiveness of the outputs. For instance, a population's income may affect the use of health services, and age may limit the effectiveness of those services in changing health status.

Optimization, the next step shown in the model in Figure 15, implies choosing the best of several alternatives, considering interaction with other parts of the system. Once this process has been completed, the decision maker takes whatever steps are necessary to implement the decision. This stimulates the data source to modify the data base by reporting those actions. The new information is then used in the control and evaluation processes.

Control is the short-term monitoring of a plan's implementation and ordinarily will focus on the availability of resources and services. It ensures that day-to-day activities are occurring as intended and that they are relatively efficient. Evaluation, on the other hand, is a long-term assessment of the system's performance. It requires that all decision variables be considered, and, in particular, it focuses on effectiveness. This is important because it is frequently impossible to assess system effectiveness in the short run. Evaluation is also important because it permits examination of the accomplishments of the planning organization in improving the community health care system or the performance of its parent organization.

FILES REQUIRED

A data base is a group of files. Each file is a set of standardized records, each of which contains predetermined and comparable data elements on a set of similar subjects (e.g., people, organizations, or service transactions). A major consideration in establishing file requirements is the time periods to be encompassed. Of course, current data should be available. Historical data are important because of their value in forecasting. Futures or feedforward data describe the circumstances in which a system will be operating. Futures data might include such items as projected population size and composition or projected resource inventories.

Various files will be used in combination with one another (e.g., population data as the denominator and vital statistics data as the numerator in computing incidence or prevalence rate). Thus, it is important that the files established be based on comparable time frames to the greatest extent feasible.

Once time periods have been established, the file content should be determined. Although an entire book could be written on the detail of the data base for the health planning process, it is sufficient here to say that the files must cover resources described in terms of quantity, quality, productivity, and costs. Other elements of the files should be a description of services by the site or setting in which they are provided and information on accessibility, acceptability, availability, continuity, quality, and cost.

Health status files should include information on natality, mortality, morbidity, and disability. They also should contain information enabling selective identification of high-risk subgroups within the population. The file on external factors should include data on population characteristics and on the economic, social, political, and physical environments in which the health system is functioning.

INFORMATION SYSTEM COMPONENTS

Each information system consists of four sets of components: procedures and documentation, people, equipment, and communication. The first set, procedures and documentation, tells what the system is to do and how it should be done and includes performance standards for evaluating the system. Procedures must be clearly and fully documented, since they will provide an important basis for training new users and operators of the system and will facilitate communication among those already familiar with it.

Although an information system may vary from a pencil-and-paper operation to one that is completely automated, people will inevitably be involved in its operation and use. Because human beings are the most variable part of any system, particularly when the system's procedures have been clearly outlined, it is important that a substantial investment be made in ensuring that both users and operators can function in an informed and intelligent fashion. It is also important for systems designers to consider carefully the possibilities of substituting people for equipment or vice versa (e.g., automated [mechanical or electronic] recording devices rather than clerks for transcription of data onto paper forms and/or magnetic media). Opportunities for performance improvement and cost reduction through such substitutions must not be overlooked. Possibilities for equipment range from pencils to computers. Computers depend on programs—software—to carry out assigned functions. The user of an information system should be aware of the potential problems and benefits that can arise from choices involving software. A particular concern should be the amount of programming effort required to extract useful information from the available files. Each request for information can be treated as a unique problem to be dealt with by a special set of procedures developed by a trained programmer. This process can be very expensive and time-consuming but can yield the precise information the user wants. On the other hand, sets of programs can be stored within a computer that will take a few simple instructions from the user, incorporate these instructions into a general processing program, and produce results that are more-or-less tailored to the needs of the user. The advantage here is elimination of the programmer's costly effort and the time required to prepare a unique set of instructions. The trade-off may be that the output is only approximately what the user would like to have, rather than a product tailored to fit his needs precisely. In most cases, however, the general-purpose software will provide decision makers with adequate results and can often make the information immediately available.

Three recent trends have greatly expanded the options available for equipment for information systems: decentralization and miniaturization of equipment, differentiation of software, and diffusion of knowledge.

Decentralization of hardware has been the result of dramatic reductions in the size and cost of various pieces of equipment. The most apparent example is the micro computer, which can cost as little as $2,000 but has the computational capacity of the full-scale computers of 20 years ago. It is approximately the size of an electric typewriter and thus fits easily into an office environment.

Differentiation of software simply means that it is now feasible for the user to choose from a wide variety of products those items that are most suited to his needs. Moreover, these products are designed to meet the needs of nonexperts. This characteristic is termed *user friendly*.

The advent of user-friendly software has emerged concurrently with a diffusion of knowledge about the operation of computers, for a synergistic effect. Not only is the equipment easier to use, but the number of people in the general population who have adequate knowledge to operate a computer is increasing geometrically. The consequence is the evolution of a new form of information system called the *decision support system* (DSS). The function of a DSS is to help decision makers deal with complex situations that cannot be routinized and delegated to lower level employees. In effect, a DSS permits the partial automation of the decision-making processes of analysis and optimization that were described earlier as information system functions.

Certain important characteristics of the DSS distinguish it from the management information system (MIS). The DSS increases ease of access to the data base and provides greater flexibility in the use of data. It is a personal tool under the direct control of the users. It is evolutionary, becoming more sophisticated and more focused as its users gain experience.[12] The first of the four components of a DSS is a data base management system that allows the manager to select and organize facts from a comprehensive data base containing both organizational and environmental information. The second DSS component is a set of statistical analysis programs that can be used to convert the data into information. The third component is a system that allows the decision maker to create models to predict the outcome of decisions under a variety of conditions. Currently, these models are limited to quantitative analyses, either deterministic or probabilistic. In the future, however, as the branch of artificial intelligence called *expert systems* develops, it will become easier to incorporate nonnumeric factors into these models. Finally, the DSS includes a capability to create verbal, numeric, and graphic displays of the results of modeling and analysis.

---

[12]Jacob W. Ulvila and Rex V. Brown, "Decision Analysis Comes of Age," *Harvard Business Review*, 60(5):130–141, September–October 1982; Efraim Turban, "Decision Support Systems in Hospitals," *Health Care Management Review*, 7(3):35–42, Summer 1982; Richard M. Denise, "Technology for the Executive Thinker," *Datamation*, 29(6):206–216, June 1983.

Of equal importance is the capability of the DSS to work in an interactive mode with the decision maker. In other words, the decision maker should be able to ask "what if" questions and obtain virtually instantaneous responses.

Since the data base, data sources, analysts, and decision makers are unlikely to be located proximately, an information system must provide the means by which data can be communicated from one functional area to another (e.g., from the place where analyses are prepared to the location of the decision maker). When the DSS is being used, communication will often include transfer of selected data from mainframe computer files to personal microcomputers for modeling and analysis. It may also involve transmission of results between executive work stations. Furthermore, provision must be made for transfer of data between sites within a function (e.g., when errors are detected during the validation function, the erroneous data must be transmitted to the data source, which then returns the revised data for reentry into the system).

INFORMATION SYSTEM FUNCTIONS

Data Collection

An information system must perform seven generic functions. The first of these is data collection. The system designer must take particular care to ensure that the methods selected for data collection minimize the opportunity for errors to creep into the system. For example, he must ensure that persons reporting hospital discharges are professionally competent to determine diagnostic codes.

Data Validation

The importance of this function is indicated by a term commonly used in the data processing industry: GIGO, meaning garbage in, garbage out. This term implies that the product of an information system can be no better than the quality of the information introduced into the data base. Thus, it is important that action be taken to detect and correct errors before they are permitted to enter the system. When secondary data are used (i.e., those collected by another agency), a transaction validation function, although important, is insufficient, because it merely analyzes individual items of data entered for compatibility with the system and therefore can overlook significant deficiencies. Consequently, there also must be analysis or evaluation of the method by which the data were collected.

Data Operation

Once the new data are ascertained to be as correct and error-free as possible, they must be added to the files as additional records or corrections to existing ones. For example, if a file contains records based on experiences such as hospital discharges, a data transaction might either add or amend a record, depending on whether the person concerned had a previous hospital admission.

Data Storage

After a data transaction has been completed, the amended data must be stored in a safe and accessible place until they are needed. From the decision maker's point of view, storage-cost considerations must be weighed against the important characteristics of an information system: responsiveness, flexibility, and comprehensiveness. For instance, in an automated system, reels of magnetic tape are the least costly means of storing data, but the use of such a medium makes the data far less accessible than immediate-access storage, such as a disk file.

Data Transformation

Generally, decision makers will have little interest in the entire content of a single file. Rather they will require selection of a subset of records or a set of specific items from all records for analysis, or a combination of material from several files for a complete analysis. For instance, they might wish to combine data from both vital statistics and population files to compute mortality rates.

Information Retrieval

Once the data have been transformed into an appropriate configuration, the next step is to convert them into information, that is, to develop answers to specific questions. This is the point at which the decision maker has a great deal at stake. In the past, it was common practice to create many data tabulations that would provide general descriptions of the items of interest. These tables, however, seldom could be used as direct answers to the questions confronting decision makers. Consequently, a great deal of manual manipulation of the data displayed in the tables was necessary to arrive at the information needed. (See the discussion on flexibility as a systems-operating characteristic on pp. 145–146.) Still, this method has been widely used because it is considered a relatively inexpensive way of providing information to multiple users. An alternative that considers the cost to the user, as well as to the provider, is to leave the data in storage until the decision maker has a specific problem, then to extract the relevant material and arrange it in the most suitable manner for that problem. This option is more feasible with an automated system than with a manual system. Ways in which the data can be organized to respond to questions include listings of individual records, cross tabulations, scatter diagrams, and statistical summaries. Software designed to develop this kind of information is known as a data base management system.

Information Presentation

This is the last step in getting information to the decision maker. It involves the choice of whether the information display should be temporary or permanent. For instance, a television-like device known as a cathode ray tube (CRT) could be used for temporary display. In some situations, this is quite adequate, provided the decision maker will have no reason to refer to the same data at a later time or at some location not convenient to using the display device. Another choice involved in information presentation is whether to use a printed format or a graphic format such as a chart, graph, or map. Many believe that graphics convey a much more effective message than a printed page does. Once again, the choice usually involves a trade-off based on cost factors.

INFORMATION SYSTEM MATRIX

The discussion thus far has focused on the issues involved in designing an information system. Figure 16 represents a schematic integration of the concepts heretofore presented, providing a basis for the design of information systems. Each cell in the matrix requires a decision before

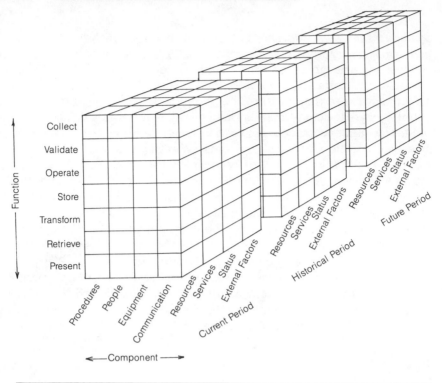

Figure 16   Information system design matrix.

the system can be completed. It is possible, however, to design partial information systems that will be very useful in the health planning process; to do so, each file (e.g., a hospital's current inventory file) must be considered a subsystem.

For each subsystem, all the cells represented by the intersections of the function and component axes of the matrix must be considered. In other words, the design of a hospital facility subsystem should consider all the procedures involved in collection, validation, operation, storage, and transformation; the personnel who would perform each of these procedures; what equipment would be used; and the communications to be established.

More specifically, it is possible to imagine a system with a procedure wherein data are collected by an annual survey, validated by computer edits, organized as new records in a file, stored on magnetic tape, transformed and retrieved by computer processing (using standardized programs such as the *Statistical Package for the Social Sciences*), and presented as computer printouts. The persons involved might be hospital employees collecting the data; representatives of a state center for health statistics performing the validation, operation, and storage functions; and individual users carrying out the data transformation, retrieval, and presentation, since the procedures for these functions are designed to minimize the intervention of trained programmers.

With regard to equipment and communication, the data collection could take place through a sample survey instrument and mailing process, and a terminal data entry operation could put the material into the system. The remaining collection functions would be performed by a central computer, and the communication involved in validation, operation, and storage would be internalized in the computer.

Users need a way to make their requirements known to the system. This could perhaps be done by sending a set of instructions to the state center for health statistics either by mail or via telephone lines using a modem. The remaining processes for transformation, retrieval, and presentation would be performed by the central computer. Through a final communication link, the material developed in the presentation function would be transmitted to the ultimate users.

OPERATING CHARACTERISTICS
REQUIRING DESIGN DECISIONS

Most decisions involve trade-offs between desirable characteristics and increased costs. Thus, an overall strategy is required at the beginning of the design process even though the system may be developed on an incremental basis. If this advanced planning has been done, some characteristics can be upgraded later. For example, responsiveness and flexibility can be improved by going from a few fixed programs to a general-purpose statistical system. To achieve this, however, the record layout must initially be designed to be compatible with a later system. For instance, redesign of the initial record to save a few seconds in processing might make the record incompatible with a general-purpose program. Specific operating characteristics that should be considered include

1. *Responsiveness.* This represents the time lag between the initiation of a request for information and its receipt by the user.
2. *Flexibility.* Flexibility involves two major considerations: the structure of the information produced (it should be as close as possible to that needed by the user) and the level of aggregation. Data can be grouped, for instance, in a highly aggregate form, which can conserve

storage space and thus reduce costs. Once the data are aggregated, however, it is virtually impossible to disaggregate them for an analysis that requires a different organization of the information.

For example, one could store data on persons in the age groups 0–14, 15–45, 46–65, and over 65. Such an arrangement would probably be quite satisfactory for hospital-use information. On the other hand, if one then wanted to use the data for a problem connected with substance abuse among school children, it might be desirable to compile data on persons in the age group 8–18. If the data have been stored in summary form for the age groups previously described, a reanalysis based on school years would be virtually impossible; if, however, the data were stored either in single-year groups or as individual records for each person involved, then the aggregation in a different arrangement would be completely feasible.

3. *Comprehensiveness.* This relates to how much data the system should include, whether it be the minimum essential information or additional items that might be useful at some point in the future.

4. *Accuracy.* Accuracy involves data validity (i.e., are there any errors in the recorded information?) and data completeness (i.e., has the system succeeded in gathering all the information that is eligible for inclusion in the file?). Although it is unlikely any file will ever be 100 percent accurate, the degree of accuracy necessary to satisfy the purposes of the decision makers must be determined. Since many decision makers seem to believe that nothing less than perfect information is acceptable, it is important for systems designers to emphasize to users the impossibility of achieving this objective and the extraordinarily high costs of even approaching that level of accuracy.

5. *Timeliness.* Timeliness relates to how current information must be and how frequently it should be updated. Data can be changed continuously to reflect the most current situation, but this is well beyond the requirements of any planning decision, although there will be great pressure on decision makers to have very current statistics, especially in situations where an agency's data are being used in an adversary situation (e.g., a disputed application for a certificate of need). Cost-benefit questions must be answered when aiming to achieve a very high level of timeliness.

6. *Compatibility.* Because different files will frequently be used together to provide information, they must be compatible. For instance, when calculating incidence or prevalence rates, numerator and denominator data should be from the same time period; also, when two files contain comparable elements, definitions of data elements should be the same.

7. *Consistency*. File data should be consistent over both time and space. In other words, comparisons should be possible between historical and current data and between political jurisdictions or geographic areas.

8. *Linkages*. When data are to be combined from different files, a common element in the records of each file is essential. For instance, an analysis of hospital activity by different medical specialists might require the use of both personnel and hospital discharge files. In this particular instance, a number would be needed to identify individual physicians both within the personnel file and for each of the hospital discharges for which the physician was responsible.

A common type of linkage is *geocoding,* in which individuals, organizations, or transactions are linked to a specific area about which the decision makers have a certain amount of information. For example, planners often wish to relate hospital discharges to the socioeconomic characteristics of the area in which the patients reside. (See Chapter 9 for a discussion of geocoding.)

9. *Security*. A discussion of linkage raises the question of security for two reasons. First, operators and users of information systems have both moral and legal obligations to protect the privacy of individuals about whom information has been collected. Second, linkages make it possible to use data in ways not anticipated when the affected persons reported information about themselves for a specific purpose. For instance, using discharge data to identify individuals for inclusion in psychographic surveys can be regarded as a breach of patient record confidentiality.

In addition to concern for the protection of individual rights, an information systems designer should also take steps to protect the system from physical damage due to events such as fire or flooding.

10. *Costs*. Information is a commodity, not a free good. Therefore, all decisions on systems design must be based on a cost-benefit analysis. For example, does increased accuracy or inclusion of additional data result in improvements in decision making, and are those benefits worth more than the costs involved?

DATA SOURCES

A troublesome problem for all planners is the location of specific sources of data that will permit them to assess the environment to identify opportunities and threats that should be addressed by their plans. Analysis of strengths and weaknesses focuses on issues that are internal to the organization and, consequently, are described by its own information system.

The availability of external data can be considered by contrasting national systems with state and local systems. In the Federal Government, statistical systems that are of particular interest to health planners are operated by the National Center for Health Statistics (NCHS) and the National Institute of Mental Health (NIMH). These agencies conduct surveys on health status, use of services, and inventories of resources. The Bureau of the Census in the U.S. Department of Commerce is the primary source of data on population and on housing as an environmental factor, and the Bureau of Health Insurance and its intermediaries collect a large amount of data (primarily financial) on organizations that participate in the medicare program.[13]

A variety of other organizations operate data collection systems that are uniform throughout the country. The American Hospital Association performs annual hospital surveys, and data on physicians are collected by the American Medical Association. A publication by NCHS, *Selected National Data Sources for Health Planners,*[14] contains a comprehensive inventory of data available from national sources. These sources offer a useful set of comparable data that have been carefully collected and processed, so that the quality of the information is high.

Information created and stored by state and local organizations frequently lacks the uniformity across jurisdictional boundaries that would be necessary to create a useful catalog of data available from these sources. As an alternative, NCHS has authored a publication entitled *Guidelines for Conducting an Inventory of State Data Sources for Health Planners,*[15] which describes a process that groups of planners may follow to identify the data resources available within their respective states.

---

[13]The content of this data system is explained fully in Alpha Center for Health Planning, *A Planner's Guide to the Medicare Statistical System,* Washington, D.C., American Association for Health Planning, 1981. For an excellent description of the potential of cost-related systems for providing a large amount of the data required for planning, see Katharine G. Bauer, "Hospital Rate Setting: A Potential Information Resource for Health Planning," in: *Papers on National Health Guidelines: The Priorities of Section 1502,* Washington, D.C., U.S. Government Printing Office, 1977. (HRA 77-641)

[14]U.S. Department of Health, Education, and Welfare, National Center for Health Statistics. *Selected National Data Sources for Health Planners.* Washington, D.C., U.S. Government Printing Office, 1976. (HRA 76-1236)

[15]U.S. Department of Health, Education, and Welfare, National Center for Health Statistics. *Guidelines for Conducting an Inventory of State Data Sources for Health Planners.* Washington, D.C., U.S. Government Printing Office, 1976. (Health Planning Methods and Technology Series No. 5)

DATA ANALYSIS

Data are of little value in and of themselves. To be useful, they must be transformed into information, a process that requires an explicit or implicit model. Some of these models have already been alluded to. In this chapter, we first describe a generic model that reflects the relationships between health services and health status. Next, a more specific flow model, which indicates the series of decisions that must be made to plan health services, is outlined.

Figure 17 shows that desired outcomes, goals, or objectives are affected and effected by a set of policy variables that the planner can influence and a set of nonmanipulable variables that are beyond the control of the system but that nevertheless have a significant influence on the level of goal achievement. Frequently, the desired outcomes will feed back to the nonmanipulable variables and change them in a significant way. Also, implementation of programs affecting policy variables will often produce both primary side effects and secondary effects arising from changes in the goal status. In turn, these side effects may feed back to change the goal status and the nonmanipulable variables.

This is clearer in Figure 18, where health terms have been substituted for the abstractions in Figure 17. The diagram shows that the goal—health status—is the product of health services, which a planner can vary, and population and environmental characteristics, over which a planner has virtually no influence. It also shows the feedback from the goal to the nonmanipulable variables (e.g., as health status im-

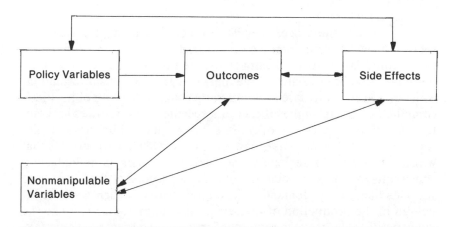

Figure 17   A generic model reflecting the relationships between variables and goals.

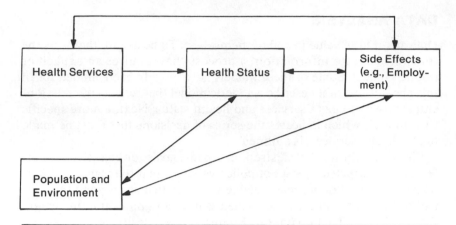

Figure 18   A model reflecting the relationships between health services and goals.

proves, the population will have a larger proportion of elderly people). The side effect shown in this diagram is employment. As health status improves, employment may increase, and an increase in employment levels may reinforce the improvement in health status. In this case, there would be interaction between the side effect and both the policy and nonmanipulable variables. For instance, if the number of health services produced is changed, employment will change, and, as employment changes, the circumstances under which health services must be offered also change.

In Figure 19, the process begins with population data for the entire region. First, those market segments that are to be served must be determined. Measures of health status are then selected to determine objectively the health status of the market segments. This information, which is usually a measure of illness rather than a measure of health, is combined with data on the efficacy of a specific health services program to determine the quantity of those services needed by these market segments. It makes no sense, however, to provide health services that will not be used. Consequently, the next step is to examine budgetary constraints to reduce the quantity of services needed to the quantity of services likely to be demanded. The productivity of each resource involved in the production of the service is determined to estimate the quantity of each resource required. Finally, the market data are reexamined to learn the spatial distribution of the population to decide where the resources should be located.

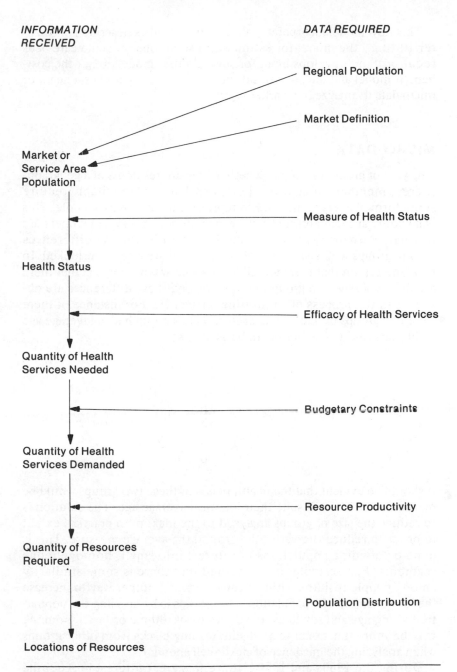

Figure 19 Flow model indicating the decisions involved in planning health services.

This flow model incorporates a number of models described in Chapter 10 (e.g., the model for estimating the number of acute care beds required) and develops input for several other models (e.g., the cost-benefit model and the priority-setting model). It also implies a need for micro data to analyze the market segments.

MICRO DATA

Analyses of groups of people, whether they are residents of a geographic area, members of an age cohort, or whatever, inevitably require some form of average measure to represent the group as a whole. This is a widely accepted practice with which all health service planners are familiar. Perhaps they are too familiar with it, for the differences among groups with a similar average measure are often overlooked. In fact, the reason that there are differences between groups is that there are differences within groups. Unfortunately, these differences are obscured in the process of computing an average. For instance, if there were two groups of five people each and each group had an average age of 40 years, the actual ages might be as follows:

Group A	Group B
30	10
30	10
40	10
50	80
50	90

It should be evident that the health needs of these two groups would be markedly different despite their identical average age. The solution is to reduce the size of groups analyzed to the maximum practical extent in order to reduce the variability around the average measure. This is done by dividing populations of interest into small, homogeneous segments. For example, it is assumed that there is some similarity among people residing within a census tract. Another way to increase the homogeneity of a population's subgroups is by dividing the population along age and sex lines. In certain cases, ethnic or racial grouping may be more functional (e.g., distinguishing blacks from other groups when analyzing the incidence of sickle-cell anemia).

During the 1960s and 1970s, there was great interest in acquiring data that would be sufficiently detailed to permit analyses of different population subgroups. Unfortunately, the more detailed a file, the more expensive it is likely to be. Furthermore, most files of this sort are available only from governments because of the large investment required to establish and maintain them. (Corporations often have such data, sometimes extracted from government files, but because of the effort and expense of developing the data, it is often treated as proprietary information). In an era of increasing budgetary pressures, some reductions must be made, and it is much easier to reduce expenditures for analysis and research than expenditures for the direct provision of patient care even though the analyses, if they were available, might lead to far more effective use of patient care dollars. This phenomenon, together with the efforts of the Carter and Reagan administrations to curb federal expenditures for health services, has led to the halt and sometimes to the abolishment of many data-related programs that may have yielded a far better understanding of the functioning of our national health services industry.

FUTURES DATA

A chapter in William E. Rothschild's[16] book, *Putting It All Together, a Guide to Strategic Thinking,* is entitled "Looking Backward with One Eye on the Future." This succinctly describes the nature of most forecasting processes and the job of the health planner. Planning can be defined as making current decisions in the light of future expectations. Hence, a planner must have some idea of what the future will be.

When discussing forecasting, the question is frequently asked, "Can the future be predicted?" Most knowledgeable authors agree that the value of forecasting far outweighs the pitfalls.[17] The following quote, attributed to Albert Olenzak, Director of Corporate Planning and Economics at Sun Company, Inc., characterizes the value of forecasting:

Forecasting might be thought of as analogous to the illumination provided by the headlights of a car driving through a snow storm at night. A bit of what lies ahead is revealed, not always clearly, so that the driver may find his way. It is not necessary for the driver to recognize every landmark and road sign, but merely to avoid danger and pick out enough detail so that he may arrive at his planned destination.[18]

---

[16]William E. Rothschild. *Putting It All Together, a Guide to Strategic Thinking.* New York, AMACOM, 1976, p. 15.
[17]Edward Cornish, *The Study of the Future,* Washington D.C., World Future Society, 1977, pp. 93–95, cited in Terry W. Rothermel, "Forecasting Resurrected," *Harvard Business Review, 60*(2):147, March–April 1982.
[18]Terry W. Rothermel. "Forecasting Resurrected." *Harvard Business Review, 60*(2):146, March–April 1982.

A forecast consists of two elements: content and rationale. The specific situations or phenomena being forecasted comprise the content. Examples are the demographics of a market, the use of a service, and the adoption of a new technology. The rationale of a forecast seeks to explain how the situation will evolve from its current state to the future state. The application of a rationale to the content results in an outcome or in the description of alternative futures.[19] For example, the content of a forecast might project that the percentage of persons over 65 years of age in a given community will increase dramatically over a period of 10 years. The forecast rationale might go on to state that this increase will occur because of an economic decline within that community. Such a decline would reduce job opportunities, driving out persons normally found in the labor force and leaving the community with a residual of elderly persons. The net effect of this change would be to reduce the absolute size of the population and increase the proportion of persons over 65 years of age. Much of the criticism of forecasting focuses on inaccuracies in the outcome, but to the planner, the value of forecasting is frequently contained in the construction of the rationale.

Forecast Content

The planner must have a solid understanding of all reasonable alternative futures. Thus, the forecast content must be comprehensive. It should contain both quantitative and qualitative data and should be based on the best available information, whether that is the average expected condition or a range of expected conditions. Parts of the forecast content frequently are combined into sets of alternative futures to be considered by the decision makers.

The process of forecasting in health planning begins with the identification of forecast content. Next, the current status of each content item is measured, and the basis for determining rates of future change is laid out. Finally, the rates of change are applied to the current status to forecast the future. In carrying out this process the planner must analyze

---

[19]The term *alternative futures* implies that the planner is more interested in identifying reasonable alternatives than in the precise state of the future. See David C. Miller and Ronald L. Hunt, *Advent Future Studies and Research Curriculum Guide,* San Francisco, DCM Associates, 1973, p. A3. In addition, use of the term *futures* implies that no specific time is to be planned for but that planning is an ongoing process.

facts and data and interpret them in conjunction with qualitative judgments to determine a rationale for a forecast.

The content most appropriate for a community's health plan generally consists of six major components, outlined in Table 6. The items listed under each component are intended to be suggestive rather than comprehensive. A brief explanation of each component follows:

Political: Describes the decision-making individuals, organizations, and processes—both official and unofficial

Social: Provides a description of the community's population

Economic: Includes geographic and communications information, as well as traditional economic factors

Technological: Considers the state of technology that will prevail in health, environmental management, economic activities, and services

Personal health: Covers the health status of the population, the health resources available, and health services—both existing and required

Environmental health: Contains a separate discussion of each major component of the physical environment, with relationships between components also described

The content of a forecast most appropriate for an institutional planner will include several of these elements; the political, social, and technological components are critical external variables to the institution. The planner will be concerned with linking these with market variables for the institution. For example, the forecast of demographic variables will need to be constructed in relation to those market segments most important to the institution. If the institution is providing services to an "aged" market segment, the forecast will need to focus on the demographics of that market segment and portray the changes that will occur within it.

Geography, political boundaries, psychographics (social, life-style), and the need/demand for services are also examples of important variables related to market segments. Their use is discussed in Chapter 7. Beyond the external variables concerned with the forecasting process, the planner must address internal variables such as management capacity, institutional resources, and the capacity to accept new technology. He or she must construct a forecast of the critical variables used in the marketing of the services provided by the institution. In addition, the forecast must be sufficiently broad to help the planner identify new market potential and to provide information to help the institution determine if it is meeting its social obligations to the community.

TABLE 6   Outline of the Forecast Content: Specific Forecast
           Components

A. Political
    1. Jurisdictions*
    2. Governments
        a. Official Health
            Agencies

B. Social
    1. Population Size and
        Composition
        a. Age, Race, Sex
    2. Education
    3. Housing
    4. Ethnicity
    5. Mobility

C. Economic
    1. Major Sources of
        Employment
    2. Occupations and Income
    3. Natural Resources
    4. Transportation Systems
    5. Land Use

D. Technological
    1. Health Services
        Technology
    2. Environmental
        Management Technology

E. Health (Personal)
    1. Health Resources
        a. Facilities
        b. Manpower
            (1) Education and
            Training
        c. Funds

2. Health Status
    a. Mortality
    b. Morbidity
3. Health Services
    a. Existing Services
        (1) Availability
        (2) Utilization
        (3) Effect
        (4) Adequacy
        (5) Efficiency
    b. Needed Services

F. Health (Environmental)
    1. General Subject (e.g., water
        quality)
        a. Current Status and
            Impact
        b. Existing Programs
            (1) Criteria
            (2) Procedures
            (3) Resources
            (4) Constraints

*The general content of this and each specific component outlined should be current
status, trends and other bases for determining rates of change, and the expected future
state or states.

Forecast Rationale

When preparing statements about alternative futures, the planner must identify the specific rationale that leads to each statement. The rationale is essential because it clarifies the result of the forecasting process. Without it, it is impossible for the decision maker to understand or evaluate a given forecast. For example, a decision maker may be given a forecast stating that the population of a community will increase from 800 to 1,000 persons in the next two years. If there is no rationale for that forecast, the decision maker is forced to accept or reject it on intuition. But when he is given the rationale that this population increase will result from added jobs created by a new industry in the community, he then understands why the change is predicted and is able to evaluate whether the level of change is appropriate to the circumstances involved.

Not only does the forecast rationale provide a basis for evaluating the strengths of the forecast, it also helps clarify the decision maker's expectations for the future. After studying the rationale on which a forecast is based, the planner and decision maker can more readily increase or reduce those expectations as the situation requires.

General Forecasting Methods

Techniques for looking at the future fall into two broad categories.[20] The first, identified as *authority methods,* uses experts to predict the future. The second, *conjecture methods,* uses some logical approach to identify the current state, rates of change, and future states based on those rates of change. The major difference between these two approaches is that with the authority methods, the planner does not try to create or evaluate the forecast rationale but merely accepts the rationale proposed by authorities. By contrast, the conjecture methods require the planner to become involved in developing and evaluating the forecast rationale.

Authority Methods

Authority methods of forecasting are based on the planner's ability to identify and secure the services of experts. The prospect of finding

---

[20]A more expanded version of this taxonomy, with some differences in the definitions of the conjecture methods, is presented in David C. Miller and Ronald L. Hunt, *Advent Future Studies and Research Curriculum Guide,* pp. A13–A16.

knowledgeable people depends on the subject matter. For example, identifying several experts or authorities in the use of diagnostic ultrasound techniques would not be difficult; however, the prospect of finding an expert in "the American way of life" is another matter. Although many individuals would claim expertise, it would be difficult to identify a single, generally accepted expert. The problem lies as much in the diffuse nature of the topic as in the number of individuals claiming expertise. In general, the more narrowly defined and/or scientific the subject matter, the more easily one can identify an expert.

There are certain characteristics of experts that the planner must be aware of. First, expertise does not always equate with education. In the sciences, the two are often linked, but in other spheres, that is not always the case. For example, the best expert on a local political situation is not likely to be the university political science professor but the local mayor. Second, an expert can more easily be prescriptive than descriptive about the future (i.e., generally he can identify what *should* occur more readily than what *will* occur). Third, it is sometimes difficult to persuade experts to identify the specific rationale behind their predictions. Experts with a great deal of knowledge in an area frequently assume that major portions of their rationale are generally accepted or well-understood assumptions. The planner must make a determined effort to force experts to be specific when discussing their rationale.

The advantages of using authority methods relate primarily to time and money, since these methods tend to be quick and inexpensive. In addition, they lend themselves better to qualitative than to quantitative subject matter. The main disadvantage of authority methods is that equally qualified authorities may develop very different views about the future. If a forecast uses only one expert, it is difficult to know whether that individual's views are consistent with general thinking. On the other hand, if several authorities are used, there arises the problem of resolving potentially diverse opinions.

Some specific authority methods follow. This list is not exhaustive but represents a series of techniques that can be used by most agencies or institutions in the health planning process.

1. *Single expert:* Uses a single individual who is highly knowledgeable in the forecast's content
2. *Task force:* Brings together a group of experts who can provide collective input into the forecast content
3. *Delphi panel:* Gathers information from a group of dispersed experts (a more detailed explanation of this technique appears on pp. 167–168)

4. *Delbecq panel (or nominal group process):* Maximizes the input of a group of experts gathered in one place (a further discussion appears on pp. 168–169)

5. *Questionnaire:* Gathers the responses of a large group of experts to a list of questions

6. *Permanent panel:* Identifies and maintains a group of experts who can be used for several studies of the future

7. *Essay writer:* Obtains a group of experts to write essays on the forecast content (this approach is especially useful in identifying the forecast rationale)

Conjecture Methods

Conjecture methods of looking at the future always involve the three-step process of (1) identifying the current state, (2) identifying rates of change, and (3) drawing conclusions based on the two elements. These techniques tend to be especially suited to manipulating quantitative data but are by no means limited to that activity; some are also very useful in manipulating qualitative information.

Within the category of conjecture methods is a hierarchy tied to the forecast rationale: The simpler methods are limited in their rationales, whereas the more complex methods have well-developed rationales.

The major advantage of conjecture approaches is that the rationale tends to be more highly developed and better understood than with authority approaches. The major disadvantage is that conjecture approaches are usually more expensive and more time consuming. Following is a list of specific conjecture methods that are useful to health planners:

1. *Simple projection:* This approach measures the current state, makes assumptions about rates of change, and draws conclusions based on both. It seeks only to discover what will happen if the assumed rates of change are realized. Although assumptions are clearly stated, the simple projection approach does not critically evaluate these assumptions. Such techniques as time series analysis fall under the category of simple projection. Projection is most closely associated with quantitative phenomena, although it may be qualitative as well.

2. *Analytic projection:* These methods identify the current state, seek to identify and evaluate the most probable factors affecting the rates of change, then draw appropriate conclusions based on the three elements. With these techniques, the forecast rationale is developed more completely. Specific techniques within this category include

a. *Scenario writing:* Primarily suited to qualitative forecasts, scenario writing consists of a narrative statement defining some specific alternative future based on a series of background facts and assumptions that are clearly identified and examined.

b. *Cross-impact matrix:* This evaluates the interactions of a series of possible future developments. The specific developments under consideration are arrayed in a matrix—once in columns and once in rows. The cells of the matrix act as points of interaction, which the forecaster describes. Evaluations can be performed both quantitatively and qualitatively.

c. *Modeling and simulation:* A model is a representation of reality that usually embodies only the most important factors or variables of the environment; thus, it is normally a simplification of the real world. By modeling or simulating a phenomenon, the effects of a wide variety of changes may be explored. A discussion of the use of modeling in health planning is included on pp. 170–177.

d. *Forecasting:* This method not only identifies a series of possible changes and arranges those changes in a set of alternative futures but also identifies a rationale under which each alternative can be realized. It seeks to make specific quantitative estimates of the probability of each alternative taking place. Although forecasting is a very complete approach to looking at the future, it is also extremely complex and expensive and rarely lends itself to use in the health planning field.

The preceding outline of general forecasting methods is not comprehensive. To further expand the technique of forecasting, Bell[21] has outlined 12 modes of prediction, and Jones[22] has identified 5 approaches to forecasting.

Specific Forecasting Techniques

The following techniques are useful when forecasting some of the community dimensions outlined in Table 6.

Economic Forecasting

Economic projection methods have been thoroughly described in both professional and popular publications; an overview of the five most common techniques is presented here.

---

[21]Daniel Bell. "Twelve Modes of Predictions—A Preliminary Sorting of Approaches in the Social Sciences." *Daedalus, 93*(2):847–868, Spring 1964.
[22]Martin V. Jones. *Technology Assessment Methodology: Some Basic Propositions.* Vol. 1. Washington, D.C., Mitre Corp., 1971.

1. The first category of economic projection could be called the *naive model,* which can take one of several forms. In its most simplistic form, the model assumes no change. When planning without a forecast, an assumption of no change is implied; however, a no-change assumption also could be the result achieved after careful analysis of an environment. Another form of the naive model assumes a proportional change — that is, everything increases by *x* percent per year.

2. The second method, *time series analysis,* is a more sophisticated approach to economic forecasting. The analysis of a time series of data indicates trends, cyclical variations, seasonal variations, and residual irregular events. Two of the specific techniques used in time series analysis are moving averages and least squares.

3. The third method of economic forecasting is the *barometric technique,* which is based on the use of data associated with the phenomenon being considered. Thus, one finds that certain indicators or events tend to precede changes in the area of interest and that some happen at the same time as (coincident indicators) or lag behind (lagging indicators) the change in the variable of interest.

4. An example of the *opinion poll* is the McGraw-Hill capital spending projection, which is based on an opinion poll of industrial leaders throughout the country.

5. The fifth economic projection technique is the *mathematical model,* which can be simple, single-equation models; more complex, simultaneous-equation models; or dynamic models that permit a study of the effect of each period of activity on the following period. A useful but complex economic projection device is the input/output model, which divides the economy of a region into production and consumption sectors. By varying the coefficients in this table, it is possible to see how a change in one sector could affect other sectors throughout the region.

Since complex mathematical models generally are costly and difficult to develop, very few health planners have the opportunity to use them. Usually, health planners can expect to have appropriate data available to them only when another agency has developed mathematical models for its own purposes. This might occur when the health planning area has boundaries that are coincident with a regional body, such as an economic development district. For the most part, however, the health planner will have to make economic forecasts on the basis of less-sophisticated techniques.

Social Forecasting—Population Estimation and Projection

Social forecasting uses a combination of qualitative and quantitative approaches. Qualitative approaches deal with attitudes, values, social systems, and the like. The techniques used to deal with these factors are limited; the Delphi technique, discussed on pp. 167–168, is one of the few methods that can be applied to qualitative factors.

Quantitative social data are available primarily on population and housing — the same areas for which data ordinarily are gathered by the U.S. Census. Because population is usually the key independent variable in the health planning process, this section concentrates on the quantitative approaches to projection and estimation.

The methods used to create current population estimates and those used to project the population are frequently similar, but the difference between these two activities must be understood. A current estimate of population is derived by applying postcensus ratios to data derived from the last census. For example, the 1985 population of a city is estimated by adjusting the 1980 census data for births, deaths, and net migration that took place between 1980 and 1985. Birth and death data for that period are available through the Vital Registry System and can be used to calculate the 1985 population estimate. In contrast, a population projection is technically an estimate made for future dates; thus, the data used for a projection are of a predictive, rather than observed, nature. Following are five major methods used to estimate and project population:

1. The least complex method of population projection is simple *extrapolation.* This can be done on an arithmetic basis, which involves equal amounts of change throughout each period, or on a geometric basis, which allows for constant rates of change. This technique should be used only for rough estimates or projections of population that do not consider age and sex.

2. Another technique is known as the *ratio method,* which relates the total population with some regularly measured variable (e.g., school enrollments, utility hookups, automobile registration) that is assumed to be constantly proportional to the total population.

In the ratio method, the historical relationship between two populations is used as the basis for determining the projection. For example, if a subpopulation has consistently been 25 percent of the larger population, then 25 percent of the latter's projected size is used to approximate the subpopulation's projected size. This method can be applied in a number of different ways and situations but only with populations that have been stable over a period of time.

3. The third approach, *correlation methods,* can be simple or multiple. It is a more sophisticated variation of the ratio approach and uses statistical correlations of variables in the projective process. This approach

tends to give better results than the ratio approach, since the implied relationships can be measured and tested; however, the following problems can arise when these techniques are used:

a. There is the possibility of omitting certain variables, even when using multiple regression.

b. Multicollinearity, in which the independent variables also are correlated with each other, may yield an accurate outcome, but the effect attributed to each variable cannot be determined. This can be overcome by stepwise multiple regression.

c. Autocorrelation, in which the dependent variable (projected population in the latter year) is most closely correlated to its previous value (e.g., population in the first year), can be solved by differential equations.

d. Identification, in which there are two curves—such as supply and demand—either of which can shift so that neither can be identified by points of intersection between a stable curve and a moving curve, can be overcome by making one of the curves more variable than the other by adding an extra independent variable to one equation. For example, weather could be added to agricultural supply, but not to demand. This would make the supply curve sufficiently variable to show how it moves along a stable demand curve.

e. Spurious correlation or causality occurs because forecasting models frequently are based on a consistent relationship between variables without considering the causes of that relationship. Such a situation can be very misleading; consider, for instance, a case in which academic salaries and the consumption of liquor are positively correlated. This problem can be avoided by using a structural model that is based on a theoretical causal relationship rather than on the simple outcome of mathematical manipulations.

4. A fourth approach to population forecasting is the *component method*. This can be used to forecast total population or to measure the outcome for subgroups (e.g., age, sex, race), which can be summed to give an overall total. The component formula is simple and straightforward:

$$P_{t+1} = P_t + B - D + M$$

where

P_{t+1} = the population after the completion of one period
P_t = the population at the beginning of the period

B = the number of births during the period
D = the number of deaths during the period
M = the net migration during the period

With this method, the death rate is assumed to be constant. No one really looks for dramatic changes in mortality rates, since most major diseases have now been conquered. This is true, however, only for the overall population, because it may be possible to decrease the mortality rate of specific subgroups, particularly infants and children. The birthrate is not so predictable; therefore, low, medium, and high fertility rates are used to generate a range of outcomes. The migration rate is very difficult to identify and often varies substantially from place to place. Net migration can be roughly estimated by applying the residual net migration to data acquired from previous censuses. The formula for residual net migration,

$$M = P_{t+1} - (P_t + B - D)$$

assumes that the data on births and deaths are accurate; unfortunately, such an assumption is seldom completely justified.

These four population forecasting methods usually do not meet the requirements for health planning population projections. A display of changes in individual cohorts[23] is needed; a simple assumption that the aggregate projections can be broken down into the same proportions as the base population is inadequate. Each cohort has special population growth and health characteristics; therefore, the projection should be made according to these subgroups and should include adjustments for any changes in health status that may be likely to occur (e.g., a survival rate for a given cohort may change as new health programs are added).

5. The fifth approach to population forecasting, the *cohort survival method,* appears to meet the preceding criteria for a population projection method for health planning. Furthermore, the sum of the cohorts yields a more accurate projection than the aggregate projections described in the other approaches to population forecasting. Following are the steps involved in the cohort survival (cs) method:

a. The population should be broken down into appropriate subgroups. The interval covered by each age group should be equal to peri-

---

[23] A cohort is a group of people with similar characteristics born in the same time period. For example, all white women between 15 and 20 years of age form a race-sex cohort.

ods of projection; for example, for 5-, 10-, or 20-year projections, use 5-year age groups (10–14, 45–49, . . .).

b. Multiply each subgroup by the appropriate survival rate, which is the complement of the death rate for the cohort. If the death rate is 10 per 10,000, the survival rate will be 9,990 per 10,000.

c. Multiply female groups in the 15–44 age cohort by the appropriate birthrates to obtain the number of births.

d. Multiply the total number of births by the proportion of male births and the proportion of female births to obtain the number of male and female births.

e. Multiply male and female births by the appropriate survival rates.

f. Add surviving births to the youngest cohorts.

g. Adjust each group for net migration.

h. Adjust each cohort for the percentage that will advance to the next cohort due to age increase during the year. This should be based on the number of survivors rather than on the initial number of individuals in the cohort.

In Table 7, column $t + 1$ *(cs)* illustrates the computations by the cohort survival method. Note the following for the male cohort in the 0–14 age group:

970 of the original 1,000 survived

70 (approximately 1/14 of 970) moved into the 15–44 age group

50 male babies survived the 90 births to the 1,000 females in the 15–44 age group

Column $t + 1$ *(95.5%)* illustrates the results that would have been obtained had the total population been decreasing at a rate of 4.5 percent over the past decade. The aggregate projection would be the same as that obtained by the cohort survival method, but when this aggregate is broken down into age groups on the basis of the age distribution at time *t,* it does not reveal the shifts in age and sex distribution, which are of critical importance in estimating health service requirements.

MIGRATION

One of the constant problems of population estimation and forecasting is the measurement of net migration. Two factors should be noted: Net migration is a function of both in-migration and out-migration; and, although actual net migration may be zero, changes might have occurred

TABLE 7 Example of Cohort Survival and Constant Rate Methods of Population Projections

Age Group	Mortality Rate, in percent	Number		
		t	$t + 1$ (cs)	$t + 1$ (95.5%)
Male				
0–14	3	1,000	970 − 70 + 50 = 950	955
15–44	1	1,000	70 + 990 − 30 = 1,030	955
45–64	4	1,000	30 + 960 − 50 = 940	955
65 and over	22	1,000	50 + 780 = 830	955
Total Male	8	4,000	3,750	3,820
Female				
0–14	2	1,000	980 − 80 + 40 = 940	955
15–44	0.5	1,000	80 + 995 − 35 = 1,040	955
45–64	2	1,000	35 + 980 − 50 = 965	955
65 and over	11	1,000	50 + 890 = 940	955
Total Female	4	4,000	3,885	3,820
Total Male and Female		8,000	7,635	7,640

Natality rate = 9 percent
Male:female baby ratio = 55:45

in the makeup of a population. Even though a planner may find little or no net migration and no change in total numbers, he should be careful to identify any major population shifts within those numbers.

Methods of social forecasting other than population estimation and projection techniques have also been used, including a group of techniques based on economic data; these approaches typically view population migration as a function of employment. Land use also has served as the basis of population projection in a number of cases.[24]

Technological Forecasting

Although both demographic and economic forecasting have become commonplace in many health planning agencies and health institutions, few organizations have undertaken technological forecasting. This type of forecasting often is seen as lying outside the abilities or direct interests of planning organizations and thus is not attempted. As noted in the discussion on economic forecasting, if no attempt is made to forecast, then an assumption of no change is implied. But such an assumption is clearly inappropriate given the recent rate of technological change in the health industry.

There are two basic approaches to technological forecasting. The first involves the prediction of new or expanded applications of existing technology, and the second forecasts a potential that does not now exist.

Generally, health planners lack the expertise needed to make a technological forecast and must rely on the knowledge, opinions, and judgments of experts. It is not unreasonable, say, for a hospital administrator to rely on a radiologist to help anticipate the types and uses of radiological equipment during a period five years in the future; however, the radiologist's opinion alone is not sufficient basis for this type of forecast. To be meaningful, the prediction also must consider technical and economic feasibility, as well as acceptability by users. In a case such as this, some variation of the Delphi technique, involving inputs from a variety of viewpoints, is most likely to yield a useful, valid forecast.

DELPHI TECHNIQUE[25]

Regardless of the approach taken in technological forecasting, the planner still faces the problem of advancing from the opinion of an individu-

---

[24]Richard Irwin. *Guide for Local Area Population Projections.* Washington, D.C., U.S. Government Printing Office, 1977. (U.S. Bureau of the Census Technical Paper No. 39)
[25]Olaf Helmer. "Analysis of the Future: The Delphi Method." In: *Technological Forecasting for Industry and Government.* Edited by James R. Bright. Englewood Cliffs, N.J., Prentice-Hall, 1968, pp. 116–122.

al to a more systematic forecast. One of the best known techniques for achieving this has been given the name "Delphi" by its developers, the Rand Corporation staff. In its original form, this method probably exceeds the resources and requirements of most health planners; however, it can be readily adapted to meet the needs of almost any organization.

Briefly, the steps in this procedure are as follows: First, a panel of experts on a particular problem is drawn from within and outside of an organization. Each expert is asked to make an anonymous forecast. Each panelist then receives a composite feedback of the answers of the other panel members. (The feedback is designed to maintain the anonymity of each forecaster.) Armed with this additional information, the experts then make a second round of forecasts. This process may be repeated three, four, or as many more times as necessary, until some consensus has been achieved and the decision maker is satisfied that the outcome is sufficiently refined. By maintaining the anonymity of forecasters rather than assembling the experts in face-to-face interaction, the decision maker allows the panelists more freedom to change their minds after reading other opinions. In a face-to-face session, they might be more concerned with defending their own forecasts than with making good predictions.

In short, Delphi refines the judgments of experts. The first round of forecasts is not expected to produce a definitive answer, but, with successive rounds, responses gradually become more refined and eventually result in a better group judgment. This improvement results from giving each panelist the benefit of the other participants' knowledge, without allowing the participation of the other panel members to add social or emotional biases in individual judgments.

The Delphi technique need not be restricted to technological problems. It has been successfully used to make forecasts in political and social areas and, therefore, might reasonably be expected to be useful in the health planning field.

DELBECQ TECHNIQUE[26]

The Delbecq technique, like the Delphi technique, has proved useful in technological forecasting and in other cases where group generation of ideas is important. Also known as the *nominal group process,* it seeks

---

[26]The Delbecq process is fully described in André L. Delbecq, Andrew H. Van de Ven, and David H. Gustafson, *Group Techniques for Program Planning: A Guide to Nominal Group and Delphi Processes,* Glenview, Ill., Scott, Foresman, 1975.

to accomplish many of the same goals as the Delphi technique; however, it brings the panel of individuals together in a face-to-face meeting. The panel proceeds according to the following sequence of small-group activity:

1. Participants are given a clear statement of the task they are to accomplish.
2. The individual participants write down their ideas.
3. Following this period of idea generation, the participants, in round-robin fashion, list their ideas on a flip chart. No social interaction occurs in this step, so that all individuals will be encouraged to participate and contribute their ideas to the process.
4. Each idea can then be discussed to ensure that everyone clearly understands the intent of each point.
5. If a ranking of the list is desired, this could be done individually, in silence, and then reported in round-robin fashion. Normally, ranking is done in two rounds to generate a final priority listing of the ideas.

Like the Delphi technique, this approach seeks to inhibit social contact between participants at the critical point of idea generation. Two key factors in making the Delbecq process work are agreement among the participants to adhere to the rules of the process and a well-trained leader capable of managing the group process.

The Delbecq technique has proved useful in areas other than forecasting technology and is particularly useful in establishing priorities and in setting criteria and standards for the operation of an institution or health delivery system.

Political Forecasting

Current political forecasting is almost entirely lacking in formal forecasting methods other than the Delphi and Delbecq techniques. Dror[27] has suggested a process for estimating political feasibility that uses the Delphi technique with politicians, business executives, and citizens who are considered politically astute. He also has suggested a methodology for forecasting the domestic political situation that includes the use of matrices; however, there are at present only a few cases in which Dror's matrices have been applied.

---

[27]Yehezkel Dror. *Ventures in Policy Sciences.* New York, Elsevier/North-Holland, 1971, pp. 69–92.

MODELING FOR HEALTH PLANNING[28]

Planning agencies and health institutions are using quantitative modeling and simulation more and more frequently when considering the future. The advent of small business and personal computers, supported by data base and electronic spread-sheet software, has made modeling and simulation much easier. With that development in mind, we identify the functions of models, their application within the planning process, and a set of criteria for evaluating the use and technical aspects of models (see Tables 8 and 9).

The Functions of Models

A quantitative model must fulfill at least one of these three general functions:

1. *Description.* A model can be developed to describe the current state of a system or an environment. It shows the critical factors of that system, their interrelationships, and, sometimes, the system's interaction with the environment beyond its boundaries. A descriptive model can elucidate the complex interactions of health care system components.

2. *Prediction.* A model can be designed to forecast a specified future state of an environment. It can predict health manpower requirements, the need or demand for various types of health care services, facility occupancy rates, patient waiting time, and other factors for a specific time in the future. The forecast might assume that two variables are correlated in a constant relationship so that as the number of houses built in an area increases, the number of potential patients will increase at the same rate.

3. *Prescription or evaluation.* A model can analyze the relevant information and, considering the constraints and objectives of the planner and/or the system involved, recommend an optimal policy, goal, or strategy. Such a model might, for example, recommend an optimal number of operating beds based on the goal of reducing community health care or facility operating costs or of increasing the use of beds and related services. Other models may evaluate the potential effects of alternative goals or policies without choosing a single optimal solution.

---

[28]This material appeared previously in David F. Bergwall and Stephanie A. Hadley, "An Investigation of Modeling for Health Planning," Washington, D.C., The George Washington University, 1975. Mimeographed.

TABLE 8   Criteria for User Evaluation of Health Planning Models

I. Practicality and Appropriateness

    A. Does the model address an agency problem? Is this problem sufficently understood by the planner and the model author?
Do both the planner and the model author understand the problem well enough to create a useful model?

    B. How will the response generated by the model help in decision making? What additional information will be needed to make this decision?

    C. To what extent will users of the model be involved in its development and/or application?

    D. Is the model acceptable (in terms of constraints, assumptions, etc.) to
        the community at large?
        the board?
        the staff?
        other interested parties?

    E. Is the model sensitive to the variables under study? Is it flexible? Can the model contribute to decision making on multiple problems?

    F. Is the model adaptable, and can it be easily modified? Can the model be used with other models or be the basis for future models?

    G. Is the model comparable to other known models in terms of the problem addressed and output? If the model is very similar to another model, which is preferable? Why?

II. Clarity

    A. How easy is it to understand the model in terms of the
        planning staff?
        board?
        other decision makers?

    B. Is the model's output easily understood by
        the planning staff?
        the board?
        other decision makers?

    C. Does the documentation indicate the complexity of the model?

    D. How well is the model documented for
        the planning staff?
        the board?
        any required technicians (e.g., statisticians, computer programmers, etc.)?

III. Validity

    A. What are the model's assumptions?

TABLE 8   (Continued)

B. Can the validity of the model be demonstrated in a practical manner? If so, has it been demonstrated?

C. Has the model been used before? Where? By whom? With what results?

D. Is the developer or someone else working to improve the model? Will these changes be available to the user?

IV. Use of Resources

A. What are the input parameters? Do they require empirical data or estimated data? Does the user supply the values of the parameters or does the model generate them internally?

B. What parameter estimation processes are required to make the model operational? Are they required each time the model is applied? Are parameter estimation processes explicitly defined in the documentation? Are they reliable?

C. What empirical data does the model require in terms of
types of data?
amount of each type of data?
data management?
frequency with which data must be updated?
freshness of data?
constraints on data?
historical data (number of years, detail, etc.)?
reliability of data?
What hypothetical data are required? Can hypothetical data be substituted for empirical data? How does this affect the validity of the results?

D. Are the data required by the model accessible?

E. How is the model applied?
by hand?
with a computer?

F. Can the model be made operational and applied
with existing staff?
with existing data?
with existing computer capabilities?

G. What are the time requirements in terms of person-hours, elapsed time, and computer-use time to
gather required data?
prepare the data?
make the model operational?
apply the model?

H. Are the model and/or computer program developers available to consult with those interested in using the model?

TABLE 8   (Continued)

V. Cost

A. What investment is necessary to determine the model's usefulness?
B. What is the total cost of using the model in terms of
    feasibility study cost?
    development and/or modification costs?
    consulting costs?
    manpower costs?
    equipment costs?
    data costs?
    operation costs?
    application of output costs?
C. Is the model cost-effective in relation to other available decision-making tools and the problem under consideration?

Because models usually are created to fulfill one of these three purposes, any individual model can be classified as descriptive, predictive, or prescriptive-evaluative. Nevertheless, a model can be used for other than its primary purposes, although such use often requires greater effort. For example, a model that uses current enrollment figures to forecast demand for services at a health maintenance organization (HMO) might also be used to determine an optimal enrollment figure by predicting the demand for various services, using hypothetical enrollment figure alternatives. The model user then could compute the costs of and revenue from these service mixes and determine an efficient enrollment goal for the HMO.

Models Within the Planning Process

Theoretically, models and the modeling process can offer a number of advantages to the health planner. This section covers these potential advantages and places them within the functions of the health system decision-making process. In effect, these models are important components of the decision support system described on pp. 140–141.

An Aid in Understanding the Health Delivery System

To create a model of health delivery system components, one must first understand that system. Because building models forces one to

TABLE 9   Criteria for Technical Evaluation of Health Planning Models

I. Model Validity

    A. What does the model attempt to provide?

    B. Is the model directed toward the analysis of a meaningful problem?

    C. Does the model realistically capture the essence of the problem?

    D. Is the problem modeled correctly? Are the assumptions used in the model realistic? Are any critical components of the problem omitted in the modeling process? Is there a modeling approach more appropriate for this problem than the approach used?

    E. Has the model been validated with a real-world application?

    F. Does the model provide reliable solutions that can be used in decision making?

II. Technical Errors

    A. Are all equations used in the development of the model correct?

    B. Are there any errors in programming or calculations?

    C. Is the solution technique correctly applied?

    D. Is each component of the model logically sequenced and integrated?

    E. Are appropriate statistical tests used to validate assumptions and conclusions?
Have the results of these tests been properly interpreted?

    F. Are all data and equations used in other studies accurately transferred to this model?

III. Appropriateness and Availability of Data

    A. What data are needed to implement the model?

    B. Do the data appropriately represent the system or problem modeled?

    C. What sources are available to the user for each data element? Are these sources reliable?

    D. Are any data elements not available? What are these?

    E. Can unavailable data elements be estimated? Are guidelines for making these estimations provided in the documentation?

IV. Implementation and Operational Considerations

    A. Has the model ever been implemented?

    B. Where was it implemented?

    C. How successful was the implementation?

    D. Were any decisions made as a result of the implementation?

    E. How easy is it to update the model?

    F. How often should the model be updated?

TABLE 9   (Continued)

V. Transferability and Extendability

    A. Is technical documentation complete, accurate, and understandable?
    B. What flexibilities are available in using the model?
    C. Are there computational limitations relative to computer type, programming language, and the ancillary equipment required?
    D. Is the setting of the original implementation unique?
    E. Can the model be extended to perform analyses that were not originally intended by design?
    F. What are some possible extensions of the model?
    G. What types and levels of personnel are required to adapt or extend the model?

VI. Cost

    A. Is there a cost to acquire the model?
    B. What is the cost of personnel necessary to adapt the model?
    C. What is the cost of data acquisition?
    D. What computer or other equipment costs are involved in making the model operational and applying it?
    E. What is a feasible time horizon for implementation?

examine the system closely, identify its critical factors, and differentiate these factors from the less-important ones, the process promotes an understanding of health delivery. The completed model also can aid users in understanding the health delivery system, because it may reveal the interactions of health delivery system components.

When a model is used as an aid to understanding the workings of a system, both its user and its developer must have the same assumptions about that system. For example, if a model developer assumes that the demand for a hospital bed is predicted on a patient's illness, but the health planner trying to use the model thinks that bed demand is controlled by the physician, the model might define relationships that seem untenable to its prospective user.

An Aid in Experimentation and in Considering Alternatives

Quantitative models can help the planner choose among alternative policies or programs. They can help reveal the results of various goals, policies, or strategies when real-life experimentation with these options is impossible because it is too costly, time-consuming, or disruptive of existing services or delivery modes.

A quantitative model may aid experimentation with new modes of delivery, reimbursement schemes, staffing policies, bed allocation, or a host of other possible changes. Thus, policy and/or goal alternatives can be compared more easily. Each option can be tested on the model, and the expected outcomes can be predicted.

If the model is computerized and the necessary data are available, the outcomes of alternative options can be estimated very quickly. Because computerization adds to a model's expense and complexity, however, it is important to analyze the model's data needs, methodology, and function, as well as the user's resources, to determine if the model should be computerized.

An Aid in Providing "Objective Criteria" for Decisions

A prescriptive-evaluative model may recommend a solution to a problem, and other models may predict the potential effects of possible decisions. If a planner agrees with a model's responses, these responses can then be used to support the planner's decision.

Many people seem enamored of this and other kinds of quantitative documentation, which seem more convincing to them than qualitative information or opinion. This could result in models aiding health planners as "selling tools."

An Aid in Forecasting the Future of the Health Services Delivery System and the Population It Serves

Some predictive models can be used to forecast the population of a health services area and its sociodemographic, economic, and health characteristics. Others can forecast numbers and types of health manpower. These models, a specialized subset of all health planning models, may provide planners with valuable information and forecast data required to use other models in an experimental mode.

An Aid in Identifying Trends in Health Care Systems

Certain models can help identify trends. For example, the use of a single descriptive or predictive model with different sets of historical data might help health planners recognize trends more quickly than would analysis of the data without a model. Computerized models allow large amounts of data to be examined and often are able to combine these data for examination in different aggregations. The sheer mass of data might hide the same conclusions from the health planner attempting an analysis without a computerized model.

SUMMARY

Information is an essential ingredient for a valid planning process. This need has been recognized by both community planners and organizational planners. Recently, the organizational need for information has been highlighted and reinforced by changes in the system for reimbursing hospitals. Ironically, federal support for state and local data collection programs that are primary sources of environmental data for institutional planning has been reduced just as organizations are seeking to develop more comprehensive information systems. This raises serious problems for state and local health program managers, too. At a time when these individuals are being given greater responsibility as a result of federal efforts to decentralize decision making, other federal decisions are preventing them from obtaining the data they will need to carry out their new tasks. The decline in federally supported information systems also poses a serious threat to community planning, policy analysis, and program evaluation.

Data alone, however, are not sufficient. A valid planning process must be based on a conceptual model that will suggest how the data should be transformed into information. A systems model that considers both internal and environmental (particularly market) data is recommended.

Once the model has been selected, data are used to predict the effects of alternatives and estimate the costs and benefits of available options in order to aid decision making. After decisions have been made, the data reflecting the results of the actions taken are used to control the process and to evaluate the system's accomplishments.

Design of an effective information system requires special care in identifying the content of files and in selecting the system components. The choices must be made with a view toward the accomplishment of six generic functions. The resulting information systems design must be evaluated in terms of 10 operating characteristics. Often a trade-off between two or more of these characteristics will be required to achieve a balanced systems design.

Institutional planners should be able to obtain the necessary data on internal functions from their organization's systems. There are numerous sources of community data that provide environmental data for institutional planners and systems data for community planners. Many of these sources, however, are in jeopardy because of current and projected reductions in federal support.

A flow model (see Figure 19) depicts the sequence of critical decisions required in designing alternative health services delivery programs. The model can be far more useful when small area data are available so that the model's outputs will reflect accurately the heterogeneity of the population to be served. The national effort to increase the availability of small area data is one of the many aspects of the federal statistical programs that has suffered from reductions in federal spending for nonmilitary domestic programs.

Since planning is for the future, the planner must have some method for predicting what the future will be like. Without adequate estimates of what the future holds—with or without change—it is impossible for the decision maker to select choices that will move the community or institution in the desired direction.

Forecasting is one of the processes by which planners transform data into information. Its outcome is not only data but a developed rationale that provides the context for understanding and interpreting the data. All forecasts are composed of content and rationale. *Content* is the variable or set of variables being forecast, and *rationale* is the set of assumptions that are applied. In most cases, the rationale is of major importance to the planner. A variety of forecasting methods are available and can be classified according to the level of development of their rationale.

Forecasting of the demographic elements of a community or market is the usual starting place for the planning process. Because health services are delivered to people, it is essential that the planner know the numbers and composition of the population/market. In addition to demographic data, geographic, psychographic, economic, social, and technological data may need to be forecast as part of the planning process.

This chapter discusses forecasting in relation to community components. It covers specific methods for forecasting some of these components and reviews general methods that can be applied when specific ones are lacking. In many instances, general techniques can be adapted to the planner's needs; in some cases, they exceed his needs or resources. Nevertheless, it is important that the health planner understand the general methods of forecasting to be able to judge the results of those who are using these techniques.

7

ANALYSIS OF THE ENVIRONMENT

One step in the strategic planning process, outlined in Figure 11, is environmental analysis. This chapter focuses on those factors that are external to the organization or community undertaking the planning process; such factors are not directly or immediately impacted by the community or institution for which the planning is being undertaken. Chapter 6 examines more closely factors directly affecting the planning process, including the industry and the institution or organization.

Many of the approaches presented here for environmental analysis can be applied to either a community-based or an institution-based planning effort. Because of the introductory nature of this book, the concepts considered basic to the health planning process are discussed in greater depth.

In some cases, the purposes and applications of community-based and institution-based planning are the same. Often, however, the community planner and the institutional planner are forced to analyze the environment or organization differently because their purposes and goals are different. The community planner is usually working toward the goal of a rationalized health delivery system within an extended series of political boundaries encompassing a number of individual service providers. The institutional planner, on the other hand, is usually seeking to compete and gain financial viability in a much more narrowly defined market.

There are philosophical and ethical dimensions contained in the issue of how planning in both the community and institutional perspective relates to decision making. These include the role of consumers in health, the degree of altruism motivating the provision of health services, the profit and nonprofit motives, the impact of government reimbursement, and the use of technology. These conflicts strongly affect the desired outcome of the planning process (discussed in Chapter 8) and the manner in which both the environment and the institution are assessed. Planners must be aware of the prevailing value systems to gather the proper data and develop the needed information for an environmental or internal assessment.

ENVIRONMENTAL ASSESSMENT

The term *environmental assessment* often is used to represent an analysis of all factors outside the organization's direct control that could affect its activities significantly during the time covered by the plan. The factors addressed in an environmental analysis usually include the economy, technology, sociocultural considerations including basic demographics, and political/legal issues. The health planner may wish to include an additional factor, personal health status, which is more likely to be used in community-oriented processes than in institutional planning processes.

A description of the current status of each of these factors and a forecast of each are required for the planning process. Because of the broad nature of the factors, descriptions and forecasts tend to be readily available from secondary sources, especially for the economic and sociocultural areas. The important task for the analyst is to determine and focus on those elements of each factor that are most likely to affect the organization for which the planning process is being undertaken. Table 10 presents a general model of an environmental assessment involving the factors identified. The elements included in the dimensions are only examples of what might be appropriate for an environmental assessment. The planner must analyze which elements are most appropriate to the organization and industry with which he is dealing. Table 11 presents an approach to an environmental assessment that might be appropriate for a home health agency. In this example, the assessment is undertaken at two levels. The first seeks to identify broad trends on a nationwide basis; the second attempts to identify the local or regional experience for those same trends.

Identification of national trends and local or regional trends is useful when good secondary data are available at the national but not the local level. Because regional experience can differ greatly from national experience in such areas as population demographics, employment pat-

TABLE 10   Summary of Environmental Assessment*

Society	Economy	Political /Legal	Technology

Values and beliefs about
  Health
  Life-styles
  Cost controls
  Services
	Income levels
	
	Employment patterns
	
	Inflation
	
	Interest rates
		Regulation of
		  Health services
		  Workers
		  Reimbursement
		  Certificate of
		    need
		  Zoning
			Medical
			  New equipment
			  New drugs
			  New procedures
			
			Environment

Expectations
  Goods
  Services
	Growth rates
	
	Local indus-
	  trial base
		Government
		  reimbursement
		  policy
			Health services
			  organizations

Demographics
  Age trends
  Mobility
  Birthrates
  Mobility
  Education
  Religion
	Investments
	  and savings
	
	Wage levels
		Changes in the
		  offing
		
		Taxation policy	

*The elements included in Table 10 are examples of the information that might be included in an environmental assessment. This table would serve as a summary of the environmental trends and would be backed up by substantial narrative.

terns, and general income patterns, it is important to reflect the proper level of experience in the environmental analysis. The two-tiered national/regional approach allows the planner to clearly identify the degree to which macro-environmental trends will, in fact, affect the local experience.

The purpose of environmental assessment is to develop information that will permit the identification of threats and opportunities. The assessment should establish the political decision-making processes, key actors in the health delivery system, target markets and segments, consumer behavior, and need and demand. It also should seek to explain the causal relationships between the environment and these factors.

The process is a continuous scanning and monitoring of the environment that should identify changes as soon as they occur and, in a competitive sense, before other organizations can react. Because organizations maintain their viability by being responsive to their environment, this process is one of the most critical, ongoing parts of the planning activity.

TABLE 11 Environmental Assessment of Factors Affecting Home Health Agencies

Society	Demography	Economy	Technology	Politics
		Nationwide		
Increased awareness of sense of limits	Increase in aging of population	Decrease in percent of the GNP for health	Decrease in technological imperative	Increased conservatism in all levels of government
Increase in change of life-style to improve health	Decrease in birthrate	Growth likely over short run	Technological advances for the future	Decreased governmental regulation
Desire for alternatives to hospital care	Increase in chronic illness	Inflation will continue at a low rate	Ability to predict disease	Increased interest in home care
	Decline in the 15 to 44 age cohort	Reimbursement will stress lower cost care	Cure for cancer	Federal monies will be made available to home care field
			Improved nutrition of population	
		Locally for Community X		
Better health education will make people aware of home health services	Population will continue to grow slowly	Growth will have lessened impact on local community	No short-run changes seen	County council will support home care
Home health will become accepted as an alternative type of care	Increase in incoming older population	Energy problems will cause increased costs		State will cut funding of all health programs
	Decline in the birthrate	Insurance will cover more home care services		Local officials will promote home care but not with dollars

The following discussions of each of the major factors in an environmental assessment suggest elements that are most important for the health planner. The purpose is to present a potentially useful range of elements rather than to identify specific elements related to various portions of the health services industry.

Society and Consumers

Social characteristics of interest to the health planner include societal values and beliefs and basic population demographics. These descriptors help identify the direction in which society is moving. The beliefs and values of society and consumers directly affect the way in which we seek and deliver personal health services. The role of the planner is to understand the decision-making process and the important variables in that process in order to make the institution or community health system responsive to the population it serves.

Both society and consumers place demands on all our social structures and systems. They specify the limits of acceptability, accessibility, and demand for health services. Hence, the planner needs to monitor the pulse of society and the consumer to be able to include these factors in the planning process.

The methods used to identify societal changes generally are not highly sophisticated. Most frequently, the simple process of reading the newspaper and being aware of other news media will give major clues to societal change. Polls and studies of societal expectations are especially useful. Infrequently, the planner may engage in polling or interviewing major community agents, although the environmental assessment process usually does not require this level of activity.

Patients or consumers of health services are becoming increasingly sophisticated in their use of the health system. They are demanding more input in the decision to consume specific health services, are more knowledgeable about health and the delivery of health services, and are paying an increased percentage of the health care dollar. These trends have forced the planner to become more aware of consumer behavior.

The approach to understanding consumer behavior is largely related to the psychographics and "use behavior" of consumers. Psychographics relates to the social class, life-style, and personality dimensions of the consumer. Use behavior focuses on consumer attitudes, knowledge, use, and/or response to specific products and services. These approaches, along with the standard demographic and geographic approaches to examining consumer behavior and traits, serve as the basis of market segmentation — the division of markets into distinct groups of consumers who will need, want, prefer, or use different products or services.

Increasingly, organizations and trade associations are publishing environmental assessments for their constituents. A good recent example is the effort of the Hospital Research and Educational Trust in publishing its environmental assessment for hospital executives.[1] The interest and pressure for better planning will make these reports more readily available in the future.

In addition to changes in societal and consumer beliefs and values, basic demographic trends are important to the planner. Because the demand for health services will change according to the demographics of a population, these trends are vital to the environmental assessment process. The internal assessment process places much greater emphasis on detailed analysis of demographics than does the environmental assessment process. The basic trends are of prime importance here.

The specific population descriptors that are most useful in health planning will vary with the organization doing the planning. A nursing home, for instance, is more interested in the aged than a children's hospital would be. Some of the specific demographic characteristics of a population that might be of interest include

1. *Population size* (i.e., the community's total population). This provides a basic indicator of the demand on which planning is based.

2. *Age distribution,* or the proportion of the population within each age group. This is usually studied in five-year cohorts. Mortality and morbidity vary considerably within different age groups, as do acute and chronic diseases.

3. *Sex ratio* (i.e., the proportion of males to females in the population). This ratio has a direct effect on marriage, birthrates, and family structure. It also is linked to occupational patterns and longevity.

4. *Racial, ethnic, and cultural characteristics* measured as proportions of the total population. Mortality and morbidity vary with different groups, as does the use of health care services.

5. *Mobility,* measured in terms of immigration and emigration over a specific time frame. Mobility data are important in tracing population changes and also indicate community stability.

---

[1]Hospital Research and Educational Trust. *Environmental Assessment Overview: 1984.* Chicago, Ill., American Hospital Assn., 1984.

6. *Education data* for persons 25 years of age and older. The level of education affects both the use of health services and individual behavior in preventing accidents and illness.

Housing characteristics may be important to the health planner because of their link to the general health status of the population. Such factors as inadequate, overcrowded, or high-density shelters are closely related to the onset of certain diseases and mental health problems. Housing also is related to the economic base of the community; such data as median home value and average rent yield useful economic information.

Within any given geographic area there may be several subcultures or societal groups. These groups may have conflicting beliefs and values and, therefore, very different patterns of seeking care. Such situations require the planner to examine each segment of the community or market to understand the service needs of the community and the buyer behavior associated with these needs.

Political/Legal Characteristics

Our political/legal systems mirror many of our societal beliefs. It is through the political/legal process that we attempt to implement many of the values we hold in society. Government has made many direct inroads to the health delivery system and seems to be increasingly involved in the regulation and financing of health services. In most cases, these political/governmental actions are beyond the direct reach of health providers.

Political jurisdictions are key characteristics for health planners, because they have lawmaking, law enforcement, and taxation powers, which frequently influence the delivery of health services through regulation, financing of health services for certain populations, or direct delivery of services to a broad population. Unfortunately, the patterns of health services delivery rarely coincide with the boundaries of political jurisdiction. Most health planners—whether community or institutional—must assess multiple jurisdictions and multiple levels of government.

The political direction and climate of the jurisdictions in which the organization is planning can often be assessed through the analysis of newspaper articles, interviews with key political actors, examination of polls taken within the area, and the like. A problem arises when the political directions of several adjacent or overlapping jurisdictions conflict. For example, a state may be moving politically in directions that differ from a county or city, yet may affect the planning process. This situation requires careful analysis to predict a general direction of the future political climate.

The health planner is especially interested in several categories of government action: provision and regulation of health services, regulation of workers, taxation and regulation of organizational structure, and zoning. Because the government regulates, finances, and provides health services, its actions have a major impact on all sectors of the health delivery system. Small changes in any of these areas can have a major effect on an institution or a community. These changes occur most frequently at the federal and state levels and are relatively easy to chart. There are numerous publications that perform "government watching" services in the health arena.[2]

Regulation of what for-profit and not-for-profit organizations may or may not do as corporate entities has become increasingly important to the planner. The corporate structures being used by health services delivery organizations have diversified and become more complex in recent years. The trend toward corporate restructuring of the health industry has opened many new avenues and opportunities to health care providers and has made the job of the planner more complex. The community planner must be aware of the numerous forms that providers have adopted, whereas the institutional planner must be prepared to analyze many new markets and segments. As these trends continue, however, governments will become more concerned with the competitive practices of the restructured industry.

Regulation of the worker is important from two perspectives: its impact on the health of the population being served and its impact on the way in which health services can be delivered. The governmental agencies that regulate workers have become increasingly concerned with the health of the American worker. Occupational health and safety requirements have placed demands on health services delivery organizations to meet the needs of employees in industry. Likewise, many health workers are highly regulated through licensure, certification, and other governmental and nongovernmental regulatory processes.

A final factor that is important to planners within specific communities is zoning. The ability to locate health facilities in specific areas has major implications for the success of those facilities and the health of

---

[2]Two examples are *Washington Report on Medicine & Health,* Washington, D.C., McGraw-Hill, and *"The Blue Sheet,"* Chevy Chase, Md., Drug Research Reports, a Division of F-D-C Reports, Inc.

the community. Frequently, concerns for the nature of a neighborhood conflict with the needs for health services. Trends in this area are an especially important issue for facilities planners.

The actions of the Federal Government in providing health care services for portions of the population are of major importance. The recent trend of shifting more of the cost of health services to consumers, physicians, and institutions is causing a substantial change in the health services delivery system. The shift from fee-for-service approaches to prospective payment systems and the requirement for higher copayments under medicare and medicaid may constitute the most important government actions in the next few years. The reactions of state and local governments to these moves will likewise be important trends for planners to track.

Economic Characteristics

The economic characteristics of interest when conducting an environmental assessment include the general vitality of the economy on a national or regional level, as well as the economic condition of the population being served by the organization undertaking the planning process. Economic analyses that focus on interest rates, growth, inflation, and expenditure of income are readily available from many sources.[3] Government, universities, and industry make these forecasts and predictions frequently and with various levels of detail. The planner's job is to find the one or two most appropriate analyses for use. These broad economic characteristics are of less importance to the planner in a community that is financially insulated from the cost of health care as a result of employment or insurance coverage. To the extent that the cost of care is shifted more directly to the consumer, these measures will become more important.

Economic characteristics of the population can be further categorized into income and employment. Specific income characteristics that are important to the health planner include per capita income, median family income, and number of persons below the poverty level or receiving public assistance. All of these are closely related to a population's ability to buy and use health services and, hence, are directly linked to certain jobs. Other key economic characteristics are major sources of employ-

---

[3]Sources for the reports include the U.S. Department of Commerce and most economics journals. Most major newspapers publish an economic forecast edition for the local area in early January of each year.

ment;[4] the natural resources available (e.g., water and land); and trans-portation systems, which affect the success of health care services.

Data on the economic characteristics of a community, as related to individuals, are frequently used as a surrogate measure of community health status and often help predict use of a community's health services. Traditionally, income and volume of health services consumed have had a direct relationship. Recently, however, financing of health services programs for the poor has complicated this relationship. Variations in the relationship between income and use also depend on the type of service and the extent to which it is covered by third-party reimbursement mechanisms such as medicare or private insurance. For example, since general hospitalization is covered by most third-party payers, the relationship between income and hospitalization is weaker than that between income and dental services, which are not as frequently covered by third-party payers.

Items related to the financing and investment markets and the cost of capital are of prime importance to the institutional planner. The fact that almost 70 percent of the funding for hospital construction now comes from debt or sale of equity indicates the need for substantial analysis of these factors.

Technology

Two types of technology are most important to the health planner: medical technology and environmental management technology. Medical technology can change a community's health services delivery system, as well as affect the quality of services rendered within the system. Medical technology, especially new technology and high technology, tends to be costly.

There are three major types of medical technology of interest to the planner: equipment, drugs, and procedures.[5] Most planner's interest in and needs for information will focus on equipment and, to some extent, drugs. It is important to be aware of the potential impact a change

---

[4]This factor also is important in terms of the health insurance provided by local employers. For example, if employers in a given area are competing for workers, they may use benefits such as dental or optical coverage as an incentive. Such coverage will have a definite impact on the utilization of these services in the community.

[5]Gary S. Whitted. "Integrating Technology and Strategic Planning in Hospitals." *Hospital and Health Services Administration, 27*(4):22–40, July–August 1982.

in medical procedures could have on the system and the practice of medicine, however. For example, the number of surgical procedures now considered appropriate for ambulatory rather than inpatient treatment has had a major impact on the delivery of health services.

In addition to being costly, implementation of new medical equipment technology might have secondary effects: The new technology itself may create health problems. For example, the introduction of computerized axial tomography (a computerized diagnostic x-ray technique) in the health delivery system brought a valuable diagnostic tool to the physician. The first impact of this technology was high capital costs, since the early models cost close to $750,000. A second immediate impact was the need to train or hire a new set of technologists to use this equipment. After the technology was used for several years, a new problem surfaced—the effect on health of the levels of radiation associated with its use.

Historically, most health planners have addressed this type of technology only from the cost perspective. But, clearly, the issues of the impact of technology on the productivity of the delivery system and on the health status of the community also are important. This can easily be seen in the computer revolution, which has drastically changed the cost of health services and the way in which they are delivered. Unfortunately, few sources of data or assessment techniques are available to help the planner deal with these considerations. One hopes that the field of technology assessment will provide methods for addressing these questions in the near future.

The second type of technology that the health planner is concerned with is environmental management technology. The specific technology used to cope with problems of air pollution, solid-waste disposal, water purification, and other environmental factors certainly can affect a community and its health needs. In this area, the health planner is dealing with issues of prevention rather than diagnosis and treatment. The costs and impacts of environmental management programs are often of a much longer duration than those of health services technology, and their results may be just as important.

Although health planners often have little jurisdiction over environmental management technology, they must attempt to address the issues arising from its development and use. They may find themselves confronted with issues related to environmental impact statements. Consequently, they should develop relationships with the environmental protection agencies in the community to enable them to assess the health impacts of environmental projects.

Health Status

As with the other dimensions of the environmental assessment, the planner's interest in health status depends on the organization and the perspective from which the planning is being undertaken. Because the health status of the community is usually the outcome that the planner is attempting to affect, it might seem inappropriate for inclusion in the environmental assessment portion of the planning process. In some cases, however, its inclusion is essential. Since individual health services delivery organizations may have limited impact on the overall health status of a community, it might be useful to include some general indication and forecast of health status in the environmental assessment. There also are important conceptual ramifications to the planning process, based on how the organization defines "health" within this process. Because these ramifications tend to help define the scope of the planning process and are not always within the direct control of the organization undertaking the planning, health status is included as a part of the environmental assessment portion of the process. In many cases, it will be included as part of the internal assessment.

Measuring health status is an elusive and difficult task because neither a generally accepted definition of health nor a generally accepted model of health status exists in the United States. For measurement purposes, health status historically has been defined as the absence of disease. This definition has been used even though it is generally considered inadequate.

The definition put forth by the World Health Organization in 1948 is more comprehensive: "Health is a state of complete physical, mental, and social well-being and not merely the absence of infirmity." Although this definition is more conceptually adequate, its breadth complicates the process of making operational measurements of health status.

Examples of four models that can be used to define health status are described in the following list, beginning with the model narrowest in scope:

1. The *medical model* focuses on individuals and emphasizes the absence of physiological malfunction or disease. This fairly narrow model of health status uses a physician to determine the status of individuals, with the total absence of disease being the highest obtainable level of health.
2. The *epidemiological model* focuses on groups of individuals and views disease as the result of disequilibrium among agent, host, and environment. In this model, the measurement of health status is ac-

complished by identifying incidence and prevalence rates, which reflect disease dynamics within a population. Again, this model establishes the lack of disease as the highest level of health.

3. The *ecological model* uses a methodology similar to the epidemiological model but examines a wider range of variables and interactions. This model focuses on preventing illness and shifts the responsibility for health more to the individual than to the professional. It is more readily adaptable to the study of mental health problems than to the epidemiological model.

4. The *Georgia model*,[6] an ecological model, views health status as a function of four major variables: human biology, environment, lifestyle, and the system of health care organization.[7] It is depicted in Figure 20 in more detail. The Georgia model provides one of the most comprehensive approaches to health status but is one of the most difficult models to use from a measurement point of view.

Regardless of the model the health planner uses in defining health and health status, measuring the absence of health is an important part of the process. The three major measurements are mortality, morbidity, and disability.

Mortality is described by crude or overall death rates or death rates adjusted for age and sex, as well as cause of death. Infant mortality generally is considered a useful indicator of a population's health level because it is responsive to many conditions within the community (e.g., nutrition, availability of prenatal care, and education).

Morbidity measures the incidence and prevalence of a disease and other conditions. *Incidence* is the number of new cases occurring during a specific period, usually one year. *Prevalence* is the number of cases in a given population at a single time (usually one day), such as the first day of the year.

Disability carries morbidity one step further by relating the effects of disease on the population. This usually is measured as either bed days

---

[6]The title, *Georgia model,* is used because it was in Georgia that the model's concepts were first applied within a formal health planning program in the United States. The general structure seems to have originated in the work of the Canadian Marc LaLonde (*A New Perspective on the Health of Canadians,* Ottawa, Government of Canada, 1974) and has been eloquently advocated by a number of authorities in the United States, most notably Henrik L. Blum. See: Henrik L. Blum, *Planning for Health: Generics for the Eighties,* 2nd Edition, New York, Human Sciences, 1981, and Henrik L. Blum, *Expanding Health Care Horizons,* 2nd Edition, Oakland, Calif., Third Party Press, 1983.

[7]G. E. Alan Dever. *Guidelines for Health Status Measurement.* Atlanta, Georgia Department of Human Resources, Division of Physical Health, 1977.

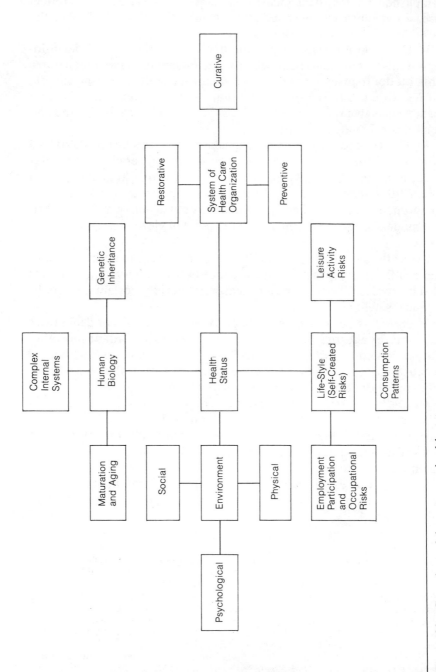

Figure 20   Georgia model to measure health status.

or restricted-activity days. A *bed day* generally is a day in which an individual is bedridden because of a certain condition. A *restricted-activity day* is one in which an individual must limit some portion of normal daily activity because of a health condition.

Few attempts have been made to measure the positive rather than the negative aspects of health status because of the difficulties in defining "positive health." Attempts made to date usually have relied on subjective judgment or observation.

Health status characteristics are used both as direct indicators and as tools to create indexes of health status. When used as indicators, this information becomes a general descriptor; that is, the statistics are used as numerator data to build rates and ratios for morbidity, mortality, and disability. These data are then compared with similar statewide or national data. The following example illustrates the use of mortality rates as a health indicator in the creation of the Unnecessary Death Index (UDI) for the community,[8] which can be defined as

$$\text{UDI} = \text{DRA} - \text{DRE}$$

where DRA is the actual death rate for the community and DRE is the expected death rate.

The DRE may be state or national data adjusted for the local population. The UDI can be calculated on the crude death rate, age-specific death rates, or cause-specific death rates; the index is simply a way to describe the local experience compared with state or national experience. The DRE also can be established as a normative definition of what is acceptable to the community. In this case, the UDI expresses the degree to which the death rate exceeds the standard desired by the community. It should be noted that when the index becomes a negative rather than a positive number, the community is doing better than expected.

Although health status characteristics have been used to develop indexes for aspects of health status, a generally accepted health status index, normally defined as a multicomponent composite indicator (i.e., a single number, such as the consumer price index, which attempts to express price increases), has not yet been developed. Several attempts have been made to develop a health status index, but none has gained wide acceptance in the United States.

Direct measurement is the ideal source of health status information. Health planners, however, may sometimes resort to proxy measures,

---

[8]L. Guralnick and A. Jackson. "An Index of Unnecessary Deaths." *Public Health Reports, 82*(2):180–182, February 1967.

of which hospitalization is the most frequently used. This proxy does not measure the actual health condition of the community in terms of a specific disease, but it does indicate the existence of conditions requiring care. Other proxy measures include patient days, number of physician visits, and number of medications or prescriptions issued during a given period of time.

Health status data often are available from the National Center for Health Statistics (NCHS) of the Department of Health and Human Services. NCHS publishes a *Monthly Vital Statistics Report* and an annual publication, *Vital Statistics of the United States,* which are the best sources of mortality and natality data (these data also are available from each state). The mortality data in these federal sources are very good in terms of total numbers of deaths, but their cause-of-death information is somewhat questionable. Morbidity statistics are available from several sources. Most state health departments gather some morbidity data in disease registries. The quality of these data varies greatly from state to state and according to the type of disease being reported. For example, venereal diseases and tuberculosis are among the most commonly reported diseases, but information on them is not always reliable. Hospital discharge data usually include morbidity information coded to conform with the international system for classifying diseases. Morbidity data also are available on a survey basis in the National Health Interview Survey, conducted by NCHS on a sample of the nation's population. The data from these two sources are good at the national level, but the samples are too small to provide local-area estimates of morbidity. (Disability data also are gathered as part of the NCHS health interview survey.)

SUMMARY

Environmental assessment is the process of identifying the trends in society, the economy, the political/legal arena, technology, and health status that are external to, but impact on, the organization for which planning is undertaken. The planner's role in conducting an environmental assessment is to identify and forecast those factors that are most pertinent to the process. Although much of the information needed for an environmental assessment is available from secondary sources, it may be necessary for the planner to fill in some gaps.

The specific factors chosen for the assessment depend on the focus of the planning process. Community health planning and institutional planning will use similar processes but quite different foci. Health status may not be included in all environmental assessments, but it is useful in some cases.

8

DESIRED OUTCOMES: POLICIES, GOALS, OBJECTIVES, AND ACTIONS

The purpose of planning is to create the future. The question at hand is, What sort of future will we strive to achieve in the process? In other words, who will specify the character of what we attempt to create?

Some persons believe that the sole responsibility of an organization is to maximize the benefits to the owners. Within this group, there are those who maintain that this will maximize society's gains through the workings of the marketplace. Others assert that even in the world of commerce and industry, organizations, as well as individuals, have social responsibilities that override the goal of maximizing economic gain for the owners. Thus, there are corporations in which the decision makers allocate some portion of the organization's resources to civic and philanthropic purposes, even though such action diverts profits from the accounts of the corporate ownership. In such firms, actions are taken in the interest of all stakeholders, not just the stockholders. This seems appropriate for organizations such as many health services providers, which are not owned per se. In other words, it is reasonable to expect a public corporation to be responsive to the interests of those who are affected by its actions, since no one has a proprietary claim to the "surplus revenues" generated by the organization's activities.

Nevertheless, it is not at all certain that some stakeholders do not act to serve their own interests, sometimes to the detriment of other stakeholders. In particular, there has been concern that health care professionals may give insufficient attention to other groups of stakeholders, especially consumers, when allocating resources available to the health services system and to individual organizations and agencies within the system. Consequently, efforts have been made to mandate consumer involvement in the decision-making processes of the health services industry, but these requirements have been met with very effective overt and covert resistance from those who see consumer involvement as a threat to their own interests and power. The resulting conflicts have diminished considerably the effectiveness of the community health planning movement. This is not because conflict is inherently destructive. In fact, dynamic tensions between stakeholders are inevitable natural occurrences and, if resolved by reasoned debate, will strengthen the system. On the other hand, conflict can be destructive when one (or more) of the parties involved views the situation as hostile and seeks to achieve its own ends by almost any means available. The result is usually a reduction in both the power and the effectiveness of all parties.

Two major developments arose as a consequence of the perceived ineffectiveness of government-sponsored planning agencies. First, large corporations, who felt that their own economic interests were at stake because of the ever-increasing cost of health services benefits for their employees, and some labor organizations, who realized that the welfare of their members was being rapidly eroded by the inflation of health care costs, began to use their power to ensure that the system was responsive to at least the concerns of major purchasers of health care. The business coalition movement is a major example of these efforts. Second, makers of public policy began to propose that unfettered competition would exert the needed control that had not been achieved through a regulatory approach. There was substantial doubt in some circles about the appropriateness of commercializing a human services industry, particularly when it was not clear that the customer had sufficient knowledge to make an informed choice. But a drastic reduction in the rate at which resources became available was occasioned by a nationwide recession, coupled with a major effort to reduce governmental expenditures for health and human services. The consequence was that, regardless of their philosophical stance on this issue, all health services organizations had to adopt an intensely competitive stance to survive. Since satisfaction of customers is a key ingredient of competition, it became necessary to pay unaccustomed heed to their wishes. In other words, a movement that had begun as a legislatively sponsored activity and that had met with only limited success became viable when the economic interests of a number of powerful stakeholders were threatened. The fate of the remaining consumers who lack economic power is as yet undetermined.

In any event, virtually all health services organizations are paying attention to the interests of a much wider variety of stakeholders. The relevant question is how these interests can be defined and reconciled as abstract values that in turn can be transformed into plans for specific actions that will lead to the achievement of the stakeholders' values and thus to satisfaction of their interests. This occurs through the sequence of activities depicted in Table 12. First, the organization determines what its mission will be. Then the stakeholders' values relevant to that mission are identified as megapolicies. The identified megapolicies *may* lead to a revision of the mission statement and *will* be used as a basis for specific policies that will guide all subsequent actions. The next action is an environmental assessment to identify the threats and opportunities on which the organization's goals are based. These goals, in turn, provide a focus for the development of a general strategy designed to accomplish the organization's mission within the bounds prescribed by policies. The general strategy is then expanded into more specific functional strategies for the achievement of objectives that will be steps toward goal attainment. Next, the organization will identify the actions that must be taken to achieve the objectives. Finally, the programs and projects that will comprise the actions are designed. In the final phase in particular, multiple options must be considered, and the selection of the preferred option will be based on criteria derived from the organization's policies.

POLICYMAKING

Metapolicy

Dror[1] identifies three levels of policy: metapolicy, megapolicy, and specific policy. The first can be defined as policy on policymaking. In other words, metapolicy sets the rules by which decision makers will establish all the policies within an organization. It includes such generic components as the policymaking system's mode of operation (e.g., its degree of stakeholder involvement), the system's organizational and personnel components (e.g., board/staff relationships), information inputs into policymaking (e.g., public hearings), policymaking methods (e.g., modes of policy analysis), and methods and criteria for evaluating policymaking. Metapolicy is important, but because it is complex and falls outside the scope of this book, it is not discussed further here.

---

[1]Yehezkel Dror. *Design for Policy Sciences*. New York, Elsevier/North-Holland, 1971, pp. 63–79.

TABLE 12   Antecedents of Program Design

Mission
Megapolicies
Policies
Environmental Analysis
Goals
General Strategy
Functional Strategies
Objectives
Actions
Programs/Projects

Megapolicy .

Megapolicy consists of a set of master policies that provides general guidance for the more discrete specific policies. The contents of a megapolicy document are illustrated by the following sample (not exhaustive) list of components:

1. Organizational roles
2. Basic values and their priorities (e.g., quality compared to cost)
3. Theory of health on which decisions will be based
4. Health system boundaries or organizational mission
5. Range of topics to be considered within the system (e.g., public sector only, services only)
6. Type of change sought (e.g., incremental or comprehensive)
7. Time values applied to decisions (e.g., relative value of immediate results in contrast to long-range changes)
8. Level of acceptable risk and controversy
9. Assumptions about availability of resources
10. Assumptions about the future
11. Acceptable instruments for implementing decisions
12. Threshold values (e.g., Will the goal levels set be the minimum acceptable or the ideal?)

This list indicates that the number of issues to be addressed through megapolicy is small and, furthermore, that the issues are couched in nontechnical terms that can be understood by any interested citizen. This simplicity and conciseness is essential because the number and complexity of discrete policies tends to be very great, and presenting all of those specific policies to the stakeholders is not in keeping with the principle of accountability in a public decision-making body.[2,3,4]

Accountability

The principle of accountability is intended to deal with a major problem of modern living: Few people can live in isolation from and independent of others. It is evident that the vast majority of stakeholders have neither the time nor the inclination to monitor or participate in all of the collective decisions required in a modern community. On the other hand, each decision may have a significant effect on many stakeholders and, therefore, should be based on consideration of the interests and values of all affected. The solution to this dilemma is to delegate decision-making responsibility to a small group that presumably is responsive to the values of the community as a whole. Thus, in the health field, accountability could mean that the governing body of a health planning agency or the board of trustees of a community health services organization would inform the general community of each decision so that stakeholders could indicate approval or disapproval of all actions taken.

In this form, accountability has two weaknesses. It assumes that stakeholders often are considering many decisions individually and that any advice given to the governing body or board can only be a reaction to a fait accompli. On the other hand, if the planning agency or health services organization adopts a set of generic rules to guide all future decisions, stakeholders can focus on a manageable number of major issues and provide long-range guidance that will be used in making all

---

[2]Clayton Medeiros takes a somewhat different view of accountability, but he also supports the idea that the plan is an essential ingredient in achieving accountability. See Clayton Medeiros, "Planning and Public Accountability," in: *Health Regulation: Certificate of Need & 1122,* edited by Herbert H. Hyman, Germantown, Md., Aspen Systems Corp., 1977, pp. 135–167.

[3]The definition of accountability intended here is comparable to the conception developed by Etzioni. He discusses symbolic, political-process, checks-and-balances, and guidance approaches to accountability. The guidance approach, which is espoused here, is a combination of the first three approaches plus an additional component that requires the accountable agency to take an active role in educating and mobilizing the stakeholders affected by its actions. See Amitai Etzioni, "Alternative Conceptions of Accountability: The Example of Health Administration," *Public Administration Review, 35*(3):279–286, May–June 1975.

[4]The decision makers of investor-owned health organizations should also be held accountable to each organization's stakeholders. Their level of accountability, however, is determined by their own inclinations and the working of the marketplace rather than by the ethics of public service.

future decisions. In other words, a governing body or board can become more accountable to the public by establishing clear, explicit megapolicies.

Policy

Just as megapolicies provide a means of achieving accountability, specific policies contribute to efficiency in the planning process. Without policies, the decision makers will be engaged in repeated debates over the same crucial issues. This wastes time and adversely affects an organization's ability to execute its mission. Furthermore, policies provide guidance so that the staff can perform its assignments without waiting for decision makers to ratify each step along the way.

Kerr's[5] description of the conditions for establishing a policy implies a useful definition: A specific policy constitutes legitimate authorization for a designated agent to act in a particular way whenever a particular condition exists. It is, of course, expected that the specified condition will occur frequently. Successful policy also must meet other conditions:

1. The implementing agent must have both the capability and the resources to carry out the policy.
2. The required action must achieve the goals of the authorizing agent.
3. The policy's purpose must be justified to the stakeholders and the costs and side effects of taking the required action must be less than the benefits involved.
4. Finally, an effective policy must be adopted by a fair process. At the very least, it must be made known to affected stakeholders prior to implementation.

Consumer Input

The members of the community as actual and potential consumers are important stakeholders in the health services system. In the past it often happened that consumer interests were considered only to the extent that they were known and accepted by professionals as valid

---

[5]Donna H. Kerr. "The Logic of Policy and Successful Policy." *Policy Sciences,* 7(3):351–363, September 1976.

criteria for establishing objectives. The professionals' assessments of consumers' knowledge of their own needs have ranged from complete knowledge to complete ignorance. At one extreme is the assumption that individuals are the best judges of their own welfare. Even though consumers cannot perform the services required, they do know when and how much service should be provided. At the other extreme is the implicit assumption that consumers simply do not know their own needs and therefore cannot evaluate the health services provided. Consider the issue of licensure of professionals. If one accepts the consumer-knowledge idea, one believes that licensure tends to create unnecessary monopolies. If, however, one accepts the consumer-ignorance idea, then one believes that licensure is necessary to protect the individual even though it might have certain undesirable side effects.

It is generally accepted that poor health persists in some areas because resources are applied in a manner that is inappropriate to a given situation. Usually, such misapplication is directly attributable to a lack of understanding between providers and recipients. It is natural— almost inevitable—that the optimal method of using available resources based on the assumptions and biases of providers is less than ideal from the standpoint of the consumer. When consumer input is not considered, the resulting consumer dissatisfaction is evident.

Sociologists have demonstrated that one group generally sees a situation quite differently from another group, even when members of the two groups are from the same socioeconomic stratum. Surely if there are disagreements and feelings of disenchantment between two groups that have many similarities, such as consumers and providers from the same socioeconomic level, then the likelihood of dissatisfaction will be far greater between groups with many differences, such as recipients of public assistance and professional providers of medical services.

The disparity of views was demonstrated by two large-scale national surveys conducted for the Equitable Life Assurance Society of the United States. These reported that physicians are "out of step with the nation on many key issues." The surveys showed that physicians are more accepting of the status quo and less willing to accept innovative service delivery arrangements than consumers.[6,7]

Dissatisfaction leads to avoidance. Thus, services predicated on inappropriate assumptions about the benefits and desirability of medical care become even less appropriate when those services are used only in

---

[6]"MD, Public Attitudes Differ on Health Care Costs, Study Finds." *Hospital Week,* 20(24):2, June 15, 1984.
[7]*Today in Health Planning,* 6(12):1, June 11, 1984.

crisis or last-resort situations. As a result, this use of resources tends to be ineffective even from the viewpoint of professional designers of the system.

An important factor relating to consumer participation in determining objectives for health services systems is the level of intellect, education, and experience of the consumers. Anyone who cavils at the determination of health needs by laypersons is confusing ends and means. The consumer knows well what the desired ends are and often has better insight into certain aspects of the means than does the professional. The insistence of the medical profession on maintaining the personalized doctor-patient relationship shows that medical services cover a broad spectrum of activities, ranging from technical to psychological. No one is suggesting that consumers have technical expertise, but they may be the only ones who truly know the proper choices for the social/psychological aspects of health care.

Two kinds of expertise, consumer and professional, must be recognized. They are not antithetical and, in most cases, are not even conflicting. There will be a few cases where these areas of expertise meet, but the vast majority of situations clearly will be on one side of this boundary or the other. The need, then, is to use the expertise available in both areas in a complementary fashion. This can be achieved if each group willingly accepts the contributions of the other. To rephrase this, there are six dimensions of medical care: quality, continuity, availability, accessibility, cost, and acceptability. In the traditional health care system in the United States, the first dimension has been dealt with by the system of licensure and peer review. The others generally have been left to economic regulation by the mechanism of the free market, but this has not always worked. Therefore, other mechanisms, such as consumer councils in health institutions, have been designed to provide for more effective input by the recipients of health care, giving them meaningful control over these dimensions.

Consumer participation has led to many problems and misunderstandings. Often there is a definite difference in the degree of commitment as perceived by consumers and providers. For example, providers may feel that they are using an optimum amount of resources to deal with a particular problem; on the other hand, recipients may believe that the providers are slacking off or shirking their responsibilities because the problem is not totally solved.

Some, however, feel that consumer involvement conflicts with the professionalism of the providers. Professionals are those who are responsible for making decisions for people who are not qualified to decide for themselves. Thus, professionals have a fiduciary responsibility for providing health services; any delegation or sharing of this responsibility subjects them to criticism for actions over which they do not have complete control.

Despite these and other problems that may arise, sufficient reason exists to justify consumer participation in determining policies for health systems:

1. It reduces alienation between consumers and the institutions intended to serve them.

2. It provides consumers with an opportunity to influence the decisions that affect them.

3. It improves communication among all groups within the community.

4. It reinforces the underlying principles of our system of government. This factor is sometimes difficult to accept, but it may be that the strengthening of democratic institutions is more important than the efficient delivery of health services.

It is evident that participation will occur and will be maintained only if it is effective. Certain conditions for effective participation exist on both the consumer and provider sides of the interaction. These are outlined in the following series of questions on resources, motivations, and structure.

RESOURCES

Consumer	*Provider*
Does the consumer have the intellectual and knowledge resources required to deal with the situation?	Is the provider dependent on the consumer for resources such as money or information?
Does the consumer have the material and economic resources required to participate effectively?	
Does the consumer have the social resources, including leadership, that are necessary for effective participation?	

MOTIVATION

Consumer	*Provider*
Do consumers believe that participation will be effective?	Do providers believe that consumers have power?

Do consumers have relevant interests?	Do providers believe that consumer participation is proper?
Do consumers feel that participation is personally satisfying?	

STRUCTURE

Consumer	*Provider*
Does the structure encourage participation rather than just permit it? For example, are there voting laws?	Is participation discretionary or mandatory?

On the whole, it appears that active consumer involvement in the policymaking process has had a positive effect; however, the potential for negative effects cannot be ignored. Cupps[8] identifies four categories of potential problems:

1. Decision makers may make short-sighted choices in an effort to be responsive to the demands of citizen groups (e.g., granting a certificate of need on the basis of accessibility considerations without regard to cost, quality, and availability).
2. Each advocacy group, however small, tends to assert that it represents the views of the entire community and that the public interest corresponds to the position it holds.
3. Some groups have resorted to tactics that have virtually paralyzed administrative systems (e.g., extending hearing and legal proceedings interminably in the hope that the frustrated majority will finally give up).
4. There is an absence of willingness to make, or even accept, balanced cost-benefit analyses. This leads to simplistic thinking that fails to consider that every benefit has a cost (e.g., total elimination of some form of water pollution may destroy the community's economic base).

The discussion of consumer input up to this point has focused on a relationship between professionals and laypersons, with the latter in a somewhat submissive role. Although this condition is still predominant, there has been a notable shift in consumer attitudes. Younger consumers, in particular, are taking individual and collective responsibility for more and more health-related decisions. This is reflected by the development of business coalitions representing large blocks of

---

[8]D. Stephen Cupps. "Emerging Problems of Citizen Participation." *Public Administration Review, 37*(5):478–487, September–October 1977.

consumers and by some employers' demands for private utilization review programs to ensure that they are charged only for essential services. For many large corporations, the costs of health care have become a major drain on profitability and thus a critical issue in contract negotiations. In particular, businesses are seeking arrangements that will overcome the bias toward uncritical use of health services.[9]

The greater independence of individual consumers is made evident by actions such as requesting second opinions, selecting nontraditional service delivery organizations (e.g., urgent care centers), and participating in wellness programs. Currently, Congress is considering legislation that would give consumers access to information on the prices and quality of care offered by individual providers. This is intended as another step toward reducing consumer "ignorance," one of the major barriers to effective competition.[10]

The marketing orientation in institutional planning is another clear recognition of the size and significance of this phenomenon. Marketing is an effort to develop products and services that are responsive to the consumers' perceived needs. Thus, it follows that a process that includes consumer input in policymaking will facilitate market-oriented planning, since the resulting policies will guide the establishment of the system's goals, strategies, and actions.

GOALS, OBJECTIVES, AND ACTIONS

Setting Goals and Objectives

The following is a useful definition of the term *goals:*

Goals provide the basic framework for the plan by focusing directly on particular health issues or areas of concern. They are unconstrained by the present planning horizon and are not stated in terms of community or provider action. Goals are expressions of desired conditions of health status and health systems, expressed as quantifiable, timeless aspirations. Goals should be both technically and financially achievable and responsive to community ideals.[11]

The reference to community ideals makes it clear that goals are derived from policies that represent stakeholder value statements. Thus, goal

---

[9]"Chrysler Exec Urges Automakers To Help Pare Health Care Spending." *Hospital Week, 20*(24):4, June 15, 1984.
[10]"Health Care Data Collection." *AHA Washington Memo #505,* June 15, 1984.
[11]U.S. Department of Health, Education, and Welfare, Bureau of Health Planning and Resources Development. "Guidelines Concerning the Development of Health System Plans and Annual Implementation Plans." Rockville, Md., 1976, p. 22. Mimeographed.

setting becomes a major subsequent step in the plan development process. Goals, however, do not establish specific thresholds that tell decision makers the level or range of acceptable status or system performance. Consequently, another term—*goal levels*—must be introduced. Goal levels are "quantified targets set to indicate the achievement of specific goals." There should be a process of deriving the goal level from earlier policy statements. For instance, a megapolicy statement might assert that a community will strive to achieve system performance equivalent to the national average, and a policy statement might indicate that one measure of health status is infant mortality. In this case, the national average infant mortality rate, as reported by the National Center for Health Statistics, would be used as the normative goal level against which the community's actual experience would be compared.

The normative statement is then contrasted with the current and projected status for the issue of concern, and that comparison becomes the basis for establishing an objective. An *objective* is defined as "a quantitative statement of what should be achieved within a specified time period." The level set for an objective may not be identical with the goal level; this depends on the decision maker's expectation of a system's ability to reach and/or maintain the goal level within the planning horizon.

Goal Indicators

A key issue in establishing goals and objectives is the selection of appropriate indicators. Adele Hebb,[12] formerly of Government Studies and Systems, has suggested that, at the very least, indicators must be measurable, they must permit comparisons over time and across geographic regions, and they must be clear with respect to the desired direction of change (e.g., use of medical services would not necessarily be a good indicator of health status, because increased use might indicate a greater degree of illness or, alternatively, it might mean that a greater number of people are being treated who previously had not received care).

Hebb suggests several specific indicator criteria: relevance, clarity, direction of improvement, precision of definition, data availability and precision, and susceptibility to action. These indicators must be estab-

---

[12]Adele Hebb. Presentation during Health Resources Planning Educational System, a course on health system planning, sponsored by the Educational Testing Service; the U.S. Department of Health, Education, and Welfare, Bureau of Health Planning; and the Health Planning Development Center, Inc.; Atlanta, Georgia, May 25, 1977.

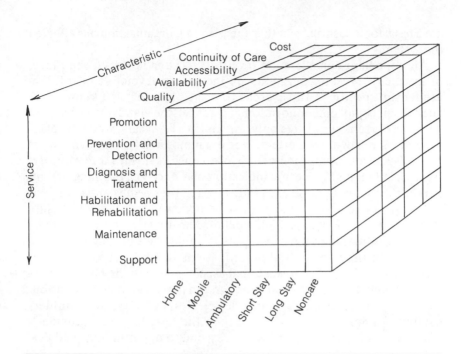

Figure 21 Indicators to be established for a health planning process.

lished for each service, setting, and characteristic within the taxonomy adopted for a health planning process. This array of indicators can be envisioned as the content of a three-dimensional matrix, as shown in Figure 21.[13]

Indicators are essentially criteria for decision making; that is, they are measures of the factors to be considered by decision makers. Indicators are those elements of the issue deemed particularly important; they do not represent a total or complete description, as this would overload the information-handling capacity of decision makers.

Indicator levels serve a number of purposes. They describe the health system. They inform managers within the system of what is expected of them (although they do not attempt to state methods of accomplishment). They aid in the determination of objectives and the setting of priorities. Finally, they are used to evaluate the performance of the system and of the planning organization itself. In other words, they

[13]Some service-setting combinations will not exist (e.g., cardiac surgery in a home setting); therefore, all cells of the matrix will not be completed.

are a basis for measuring whether the planning organization has affected the system.

An important consideration regarding these indicators is their level of specificity. Most organizations are inclined to develop standards that are far too specific in those areas that the planning staff knows well; such detail could stifle innovation and render the standards (which are based on current knowledge only) invalid in a few years, when the planning decisions will take effect. For example, in a field as dynamic as health services, technological obsolescence is always a possibility. Also, detailed, highly specific indicators may exceed a planning organization's capacity, because each indicator requires a substantial analysis before it can be accepted and must be reviewed frequently to ensure that it is current. Finally, a highly detailed health system plan would be counterproductive in the constraints it would place on the managerial activities of the persons and organizations to whom it applies. This might be described as a jurisdictional aspect related to the boundary between stakeholder accountability and internal management responsibility. In simplest terms, at some level of specificity, stakeholder-established norms will begin to impair the health service provider's management capability to innovate, respond to opportunities, and deal with problems.

Indicators and levels of specificity can be selected in several ways. The "single best way" approach is based on a theory or on some analysis of empirical evidence. For example, evidence that has shown that faster treatment of trauma victims has positive results implies that the emergency medical system (EMS) can best be improved by getting the patient to the hospital more quickly.

More often than not, there is no single accepted method of dealing with an issue. Consequently, it is frequently necessary to adopt what can be referred to as a "multiple perspectives approach," which attempts to determine all possible answers to problems and analyze how they overlap or complement one another. For example, physicians, parents, and teachers may have different views on mental retardation. Drawing on these varying perspectives, the modes of dealing with this problem are identified and some attempt is made to reach a consensus.

There are a variety of techniques for achieving consensus in a group setting. One of the best known and most effective is the nominal group technique developed by André Delbecq et al.[14] (The Delbecq technique

---

[14]André L. Delbecq, Andrew H. Van de Ven, and David H. Gustafson. *Group Techniques for Program Planning: A Guide to Nominal Group and Delphi Processes.* Glenview, Ill., Scott, Foresman, 1975. The nominal group technique is a carefully designed procedure to maximize the productivity of a heterogeneous group seeking to develop a mutually acceptable set of ideas in relation to a specified issue.

also is discussed on pp. 168–169.) Another method is to seek clarification and refinement of proposed measures by consciously establishing a conflict situation in which opponents will vigorously challenge one another's views. Through this process the "truth" may emerge. Although there are some obvious benefits to this sort of technique, its utility is quite limited because it requires an individual decision maker or an agency to exercise final judgment between the contending parties. If the planning process has become at all controversial, the hostility generated may remain after a decision has been made and will probably be far more costly than the value of resulting benefits.

Regardless of the method used, there are five phases or steps in the process of developing indicator levels. Phase 1 is the establishment of general values, accomplished in the policy-development phase. Phase 2 is the conversion of these values into operational measures—the selection of indicators. Phase 3 is the determination of a feasible range of outcomes for each operational measure (in other words, what is the extent of the possibilities?). Phase 4 involves the selection of an acceptable outcome threshold for each measure. This is the point at which goal levels are initially set and balance is sought among the conflicting indicators (e.g., a relatively high goal level for accessibility may contradict a low goal level for cost). In phase 5, measures and thresholds are validated in terms of values expressed in megapolicies.

Figure 22 displays in a three-dimensional matrix the possibilities for combining methods and participants in each of the five phases of indicator-level development. For instance, the governing body of a health organization might undertake phase 1 by using method B. Phase 2 might be carried out by a task force also using that method, whereas the staff might use method A for phase 3. Alternatively, this phase could be accomplished by a technical task force also using method A. Phase 4 could be undertaken by the governing body, using a method other than A, B, or C (i.e., a voting process), and the general community might carry out phase 5 in a series of public hearings.

The Action Phase

Actions can be defined as comprehensive collections of proposed programs aimed at achieving health status and health system goals and objectives. Actions describe the programs selected after consideration of alternative means of improving health and health system performance to desired levels. (See Chapter 10 for a further description of program development.) This definition makes it clear that actions are derived from objectives as another sequential step in the plan develop-

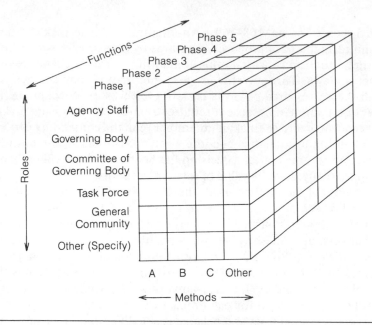

Figure 22   Phases in developing indicator levels.

ment process. An objective identifies a state or status to be achieved, whereas an action relates to some steps taken to achieve that state or status.

Some actions may affect numerous objectives; on the other hand, a single objective may generate multiple actions. For instance, the objective of achieving a reduced level of infant mortality might involve such actions as changing the availability and accessibility of obstetrical services or promoting disease-prevention subsystems, such as family planning services or prenatal care for mothers. Actions are important because they link status and services, services and resources, and resources and resource development plans. In other words, service actions are necessary to improve health status; resource actions are required to change services; and resource development actions are essential to alter the quantity and characteristics of resources.

Linkages

Linking Health Status and Health Services

Because the relationship between health services and health status is not well defined or well understood, the types of actions needed to achieve health status are not always apparent. Gradually, however, methods are emerging that will permit these linkages to be established. Some of the most important work in this area was done by the state of Georgia and by the Rand Corporation under contract to the U.S. Department of Health, Education, and Welfare.[15] There are distinct similarities between the approaches used in both cases; the following discussion draws heavily on each.

Both approaches involve a sequence of several steps. The first step is problem recognition achieved by analyzing the data that might result from comparing goal indicator levels and the forecast status of a community population or from compiling information on publicly expressed discontent.

Once a problem has been identified, the next step is to analyze it for causes and risk factors. For instance, with infant mortality, one of the causal factors might be low birth weight, which can be attributed to a number of risk factors such as maternal age, number of previous pregnancies, poverty, educational level, availability and quality of prenatal care, cigarette smoking, and diet.

After the risk factors have been identified, the areas of potential intervention must be examined. In Georgia, these are categorized as biological, environmental, life-style, and health services factors.

Next, the preferred potential intervention must be determined, which might be done on the basis of a cost-benefit analysis. The large number of alternatives that emerge from such a view of the system, however, would make a full-blown cost-benefit analysis infeasible. Therefore, other heuristic methods must be chosen for selecting a few key contenders from the large list of possible actions. Table 13 illustrates the risk factors for immature infants and the categories of appropriate intervention, with the likelihood of success indicated for each category. An obvious first approach would be to eliminate all types of intervention not categorized as having a high potential for reducing the problem. Beyond this point, other criteria, such as length of time required for implementation or community acceptability, will further reduce the contenders to one or two. These could then be subjected to a rigorous cost-benefit analysis to make the final choice.

---

[15]G. E. Alan Dever, *Guidelines for Health Status Measurement,* Atlanta, Georgia Department of Human Resources, Division of Physical Health, 1977; L. J. Harris et al., *Algorithms for Health Planners, Vol. 1, An Overview,* Santa Monica, Calif., Rand Corp., 1977 (see also other volumes in the set, which deal with specific health problems: *Vol. 2, Infant Mortality; Vol. 3, Breast Cancer Mortality; Vol. 4, Heart Attack Mortality; Vol. 5, Preventable Death and Disease; and Vol. 6, Hypertension)*.

TABLE 13   Analysis of Risk Factors of Immature Infants by Health Field Concept Components

| Risk Factors | Potential for Programs Aimed at Risk Factors | | | | Potential for Reducing Problems by Eliminating Risk Factors |
	Biological	Environmental	Life-Style	System of Health Care	
Maternal Age	Moderate	Moderate	High	Low	High
Previous Pregnancy	Moderate	High	High	Moderate	High
Poverty	None	Moderate	High	High	Moderate
Educational Level	None	Low	Moderate	Moderate	Moderate
Availability of Care	None	Moderate	Low	Moderate	High
Quality of Care	None	Moderate	Moderate	High	High
Cigarette Smoking	Moderate	Moderate	High	Low	Moderate
Diet	Moderate	Moderate	High	Moderate	High
Family Mores	None	Low	High	Low	High

SOURCE: G. E. Alan Dever. *Guidelines for Health Status Measurement.* Atlanta, Georgia Department of Human Resources, Division of Physical Health, 1977, p. 72.

Linking Health Services and Resources

The next linkage to be established is between services and resources. The organizational planner is concerned primarily with resource productivity and cost. The community health planner, however, must consider both supply and demand. In this case, development of a full description of a system would enable an aggregation of the data on availability (i.e., quantity of specific resources available) and a determination of the overall level of demand for the various resources required to provide health services. Since achievement of this development presently seems unlikely, the planning organization may resort to a somewhat simpler strategy, based on the traditional ratio approach to estimating resource requirements.[16]

Thus, the policy portion of the plan can establish widely accepted ratios, perhaps national ones, as an ideal supply level to be used as the goal indicator level for resource requirements until the actual need—based on desired total service availability—can be computed. With this indicator level, the current and ideal supplies can be compared. If the former is greater than or equal to the ideal, and a recommended action would increase the number of services in the community, then the total requirements of the community must increase by a sufficient amount to support the services to be added. If, on the other hand, the current supply is less than the ideal and recommended actions would once again add services to the community, then the increased services probably can be adequately supported, if the supply of resources is increased from the current level to the amount suggested by the resource goal indicator.

Linking Resources and Resource Development Plans

The recommended actions proposed to deal with resource shortages or surpluses provide an important link to plans oriented specifically toward resource development. This category includes the state medical facilities plan required by P.L. 93-641. It is also possible that a planning process for health manpower development eventually will emerge and that the recommended actions from community health system plans will provide important input to that undertaking.

---

[16]U.S. Department of Health, Education, and Welfare, Public Health Service, Bureau of Health Manpower. *Review of Health Manpower Population Requirements Standards.* Washington, D.C., 1976. (HRA 77-22)

SUMMARY

The aims of planning are achieved by a sequence of processes that move from abstract values to very specific actions. This chapter discusses a number of processes that represent different ways of expressing the desired outcomes and then describes how activities focused at one level are the linkages that lead to the achievement of the stated aims of the next level.

Policies, especially megapolicies, identify the values sought by the system. Actually, the values sought are those that arise from interaction among the people who are stakeholders in the system. The consumers as stakeholders are becoming more influential in the health services system, so planners must pay greater heed to the consumer point of view. This is the essence of a marketing orientation. Consumer input at the policy level is especially appropriate since most consumers lack the expertise to express their wishes in the technical terms required to define goals and goal indicators or to specify the details of program operation.

A *goal* is a measurable accomplishment in terms of the health status of the population and the characteristics of the health services system that is congruent with the values expressed by policies; it is an ultimate ideal that may not be fully attainable within the planning horizon. An *objective* is a step toward the achievement of a goal that is to be accomplished by a specific time. An *action* is a set of programs and projects that will lead to the achievement of one or more objectives. Actions provide the linkages between health status, health services systems, and health services resources.

9

ASSESSMENT OF CAPABILITIES
AND RESOURCES

The assessment of the organization and the market in which the organization operates is an internal assessment. For the community health planning agency, this combination is the agency and the community. For the organization providing health services, it is the institution and the population it serves.

The health industry has developed a great interest in marketing in recent years. Many of the concepts, techniques, and tools that health planners use are similar to and often the same as those of the marketer. For example, a planner may talk about the "population at risk" for a specific illness, whereas a marketer would discuss the "market segment" that is at risk for the illness. Although there are some minor differences between the two, the concepts are the same. This chapter uses terms and concepts from both marketing and traditional planning.

An assessment of the organization and market includes a description of the relationship between the organization and the market it serves. The market assessment is an examination of the industry of which the organization is a part and includes competing organizations and the structure of the market being served. As indicated in Chapter 1, the consumers or "market" for some health services can include both patients and providers (e.g., physicians, dentists). For example, physicians admit patients to hospitals; hence, physicians make the decisions to purchase hospital services. From the hospital perspective, then, the

217

market for hospital services could be defined as physicians.[1] In this text, however, the term *market* will refer to the final consumer of health services, the patient.

COMMUNITY/MARKET ASSESSMENT

Both community planning and marketing are basically oriented to the population or consumer being served. Therefore, this chapter begins by focusing on the market or community and by discussing a broad concept of community/market definition and ways to determine population service areas and markets. Facility location also is covered.

Identifying a health service community is not easy, but a useful approach is "the community of solution,"[2] defined by the National Commission on Community Health Services. It is not limited to a geographic concept but includes other types of groupings. This form of market definition is becoming more common and more appropriate as part of the task of market segmentation. The community of solution for any specific health problem tends to be a combination of the following seven subcommunities:

1. *Community of Identifiable Need.* An identifiable need is a factually substantiated lack that the overall society feels is both correctable and deserving of attention. A community of identifiable need is the specific group in need. Usually, this community is bound by a limited, geographically definable area; however, it might be a specific group without a fixed geographic location (e.g., migrant workers).

2. *Community of Problem Ecology.* Some problems have a clearly defined set of boundaries, since their causes occur only within a well-established and specified terrain. Where systems analysis of a condition or disease indicates relevant geographic, social, or other boundaries, these boundaries become significant for planning. In some instances, planning will have to embrace the entire nation, but more often, a subregion can be defined within which effective action can be taken. For some kinds of problems, however, particularly those of an environmental nature, the region becomes quite large. Taking the example of water

---

[1]For a discussion of derived demand, see Roice D. Luke and Jeffrey C. Bauer, *Issues in Health Economics,* Rockville, Md., Aspen Systems Corp., 1982, p. 337. Also see the discussion of physicians as a channel of distribution in the section on strategic planning in Chapter 5.

[2]National Commission on Community Health Services. *Health Is a Community Affair.* Cambridge, Mass., Harvard University Press, 1966, pp. 2–9.

pollution in Washington, D.C., one can readily appreciate that any attempt to clean only that part of the Potomac River that flows by the city would be virtually futile.

3. *Community of Concern.* This may include a much larger region than merely the area where a problem occurs, because of "spill-over" effects. Poor health in a ghetto neighborhood, for example, tends to raise taxes for non-ghetto residents and can lead to the spread of communicable diseases into more affluent areas. These factors, too, are part of the community of concern.

4. *Community of Special Interest.* This community seldom has specific geographic boundaries; rather it is based on a common interest among individuals or groups. A typical example would be a group of professionals and charitable associations interested in eradicating some specific illness, such as glaucoma or emphysema.

5. *Community of Viability.* A community of viability has enough clients to make the planned activity feasible. Thus, the viable communities for open-heart surgery and rubella vaccination will differ significantly.

6. *Community of Resources.* This community encompasses the area that has the resources necessary to perform a particular task. Obviously, there is no guarantee that the distribution of a problem and of the resources needed to solve the problem will be identical or even similar.

7. *Community of Action Capability.* This is the group of people who often have the potential for taking effective action to correct a problem. Frequently, because of legal and financial considerations, this community must be defined in terms of political subdivisions. Occasionally, however, groups can operate effectively without respect to political boundaries—for example, political subdivisions may unite into a common organization, such as a council of governments.

The community of solution defined by these seven factors clearly will be an ill-defined multidimensional entity. Conceptually, this is not unappealing; in reality, however, health problems are often within the purview of well-defined organizations or political jurisdictions that do not conform to the boundaries identified by the community of solution. Although this complicates application of the community-of-solution approach, it does not render the concept useless.[3]

Marketers use the concept of "publics" in a similar fashion. A public is a group of people or organizations that have a real or potential interest

---

[3]Philip Kotler. *Marketing for Nonprofit Organizations.* Englewood Cliffs, N.J., Prentice-Hall, 1975, p. 22.

or involvement with an organization or institution, and a market is the public that has resources to exchange with the organization or institution for benefits received.[4]

The broad concept of community determination can be useful as the basis for marketing activities undertaken by an individual institution. Marketing of health care services seeks to deal with the needs of the various constituents of a given institution. The community-of-solution concept is a similar activity in that it seeks to identify the constituencies for a given health problem. The concept is applicable at both the regional level and the level of an individual institution.

A region is the particular geographic area generally assumed to be the best territorial unit for coordinated economic and/or social planning.[5] An urban region will normally have a core city, suburbs, and an extended area, which is a part of the city's trade area. A rural region normally will have a series of well-identified trade centers and rural areas dependent on those centers.

As early as 1932, the Committee on the Costs of Medical Care urged the integration of primary and specialized care through regionalization. The idea was never used as the basis for a health delivery system, but the health system agencies (HSAs) established by P.L. 93-641 are an attempt to rationalize the existing system on the basis of a regional approach. For instance, HSAs must evaluate relationships between core cities and outlying areas and between primary and specialized care within the regions. The HSAs, however, do not fully meet the criteria for regionalization, because they are based on more arbitrarily defined areas than the regions defined naturally by patterns of use.

Community and market assessment requires the planner to define and gather information on the populations that make up those communities and markets. In the environmental assessment phase of the process, the planner identifies general directions and important trends. During this phase, he develops a detailed analysis of the populations being served.

Much of the data required for this assessment can be found in or derived from the U.S. Census and federal and state vital registries. Table 14 provides examples of statistics, sources of data, and uses within the

---

[4]For a more complete discussion of the relationships between geography and health, see John Eyles and K. J. Woods, *The Social Geography of Medicine and Health,* New York, St. Martin's, 1983.

[5]The definitions of "region" and "service area" are adapted from the Joint Committee of the American Hospital Association and Public Health Service on Area-wide Planning of Hospitals and Health Facilities, *Report,* Washington, D.C., U.S. Department of Health, Education, and Welfare, Public Health Service, 1961, p. 56. (PHS 855)

health planning process. The following sections discuss the U.S. Census and its use in communities, service areas, and markets. Because most census and health data are more useful when analyzed on the basis of small geographic areas, geocoding is covered.

Demographic Data and the U.S. Census

Population data provide the most useful information for describing communities and markets. They are used by health planners as general descriptors, denominator data, and reference data. One of the most important uses of population data is to describe the size and composition of the community where planning is taking place—*the* essential element in a population-based planning process. A community description can be simple or complex, depending on the individual planner's needs. An example of a complex description is the mental health demographic profile system created by the National Institute of Mental Health (NIMH),[6] which contains 130 demographic data items from the 1970 census of population and housing. The data are aggregated at the levels of census tract, county, and minor civil division for the entire nation, as well as for the 1,499 designated mental health areas throughout the nation.

This system gives the health planner a demographic data base for analyzing a community in several ways (e.g., in terms of its percentile rank compared with all other mental health areas or in terms of comparative norms using total national data for the comparison). In addition, the system can be used to focus on a number of target populations such as the elderly, families living in poverty, and other high-risk groups.[7]

Population data are used as denominators in calculating the rates and ratios developed to assess health status and resources. For example, hospital admissions per 1,000 population indicate the hospitalization rate within a community. In this rate, total admissions is the numerator and population size is the denominator. Population data of all types often are used in this manner; Table 14 shows examples of rates and ratios that use demographic information as denominator data.

Population data also are used as references for cross-checking other data to determine the extent to which various samples or studies are

---

[6]U.S. Department of Health, Education, and Welfare, Public Health Service, National Institute of Mental Health. *Demographic Profile System Description*. Washington, D.C., U.S. Government Printing Office, 1975.

[7]_____. *Typological Approach to Doing Social Area Analysis*. Washington, D.C., U.S. Government Printing Office, 1975.

TABLE 14 Pertinent Health and Demographic Information Derived by Combining Numerator Data from Vital Records with Denominator Data from the Census

Type of Statistics	Numerator Information Available from Most State and Local Registration Systems	Denominator Information Available from Census Data	Health and Population Information Basic to Local and State Health Program Planning and Administration
Demographic (population composition and distribution)	1. Births (by characteristics of parents) 2. Deaths (by age, sex, race, and so on)	1. Age groups 2. Sex 3. Race 4. In- and outmigrations	1. Population projections for state and by local areas 2. Population distribution variations by detailed characteristics and by detailed geographic areas

Natality	1. Births
	  a. Legitimate or illegitimate
	  b. Attendant
	  c. Institution
	  d. Plurality
	  e. Detailed characteristics of child and parents
		1. Marital status of females
		2. Age groups
		3. Sex
		4. Race
		5. Education
		6. Socioeconomic characteristics
			1. Illegitimacy rates
			2. Fertility rates
			3. Age/race-specific birth rates
			4. Birth rates by socioeconomic strata
			5. Birth registration completeness tests

Mortality	1. All deaths a. Causes by age group, sex, and race	1. Age groups 2. Sex 3. Race	1. Age-adjusted death rates 2. Age/race/sex-specific death rates

b. County and city allocations c. Occupation and industry 2. Maternal deaths 3. Infant deaths 4. Fetal deaths	4. Occupation and industry 5. Marital status	3. Cause-specific death rates 4. Education-specific perinatal death rates 5. Occupation-specific death rates 6. Life tables 7. Marital status/cause-specific death rates 8. Infant deaths by socio-economic strata
Morbidity		

1. Reported disease cases
  a. Cancer
  b. Venereal diseases
  c. Tuberculosis
  d. Contagious diseases
	1. Age groups
	2. Sex
	3. Race
	4. Marital status
	5. Occupation
		1. Age-adjusted morbidity rate
		2. Specific morbidity rates by age/race/sex
		3. Population at risk
		4. Prevalence rates

Social		
1. Marriages (age, race, previous marital status) 2. Divorces (age, race, number of times married)	1. Marital status 2. Sex 3. Education	1. Specific marriage rates by age and race 2. Specific divorce rates by age and race 3. Relative risk rates for marriages and divorces 4. Marriage and divorce rates by socioeconomic strata

SOURCE: Anthony Orgelia et al. *A Data Acquisition and Analysis Handbook for Health Planners.* Vol. 1. Washington, D.C., U.S. Department of Health, Education, and Welfare, Bureau of Health Planning and Resources Development, 1976. (HRA 76-14506)

representative. For instance, a planning agency that had sampled 10 percent of the population in a community health survey could determine whether the sample was representative by comparing the sample demographics of age, sex, and race with the same population demographics derived from the census. This approach also helps determine the comparability of communities.[8]

The major source of social data in the United States is the census of population and housing.[9] Although this effort is called a census, most of its data are gathered through survey sampling techniques, which have the advantages of economy, timeliness, and quality.

The U.S. Department of Commerce, Bureau of the Census has been conducting a decennial census since 1790. In the future, it may be supplemented with a quinquennial census.[10] Sampling was first used in the 1940 census, and, in the last three decennial efforts, a total population count was made for only five items: age, sex, race, relationship to head of household, and marital status.

The decennial census is an enumeration of population and housing and in the past was conducted by direct count. The 1970 and 1980 censuses were conducted primarily by mail, a trial run having shown that this method was effective and somewhat less expensive than direct count. Special groups, however, such as non-English-speaking or functionally illiterate people, are still counted physically by census takers.

Census data are available for 14 different aggregations of geographic areas—from regions, states, urban areas, and localities, to census tracts and blocks. Between decades, the census data are supplemented with current population surveys, which are monthly samples of households in the United States.

Partial or complete published census data are available in more than 1,000 U.S. libraries; of these, 137 are designated as census depository libraries. In contrast to the 1960 census, the 1970 census effort resulted in fewer published reports but more computerized data; this trend continued in 1980.

In addition to computer tapes, which are most useful for health planners, a few firms sell limited sets of census data on microcomputer

---

[8]U.S. Department of Health, Education, and Welfare, Public Health Service, National Health Planning Information Center. *Guide to Data for Health Systems Planners.* Washington, D.C., U.S. Government Printing Office, April 1976, p. 19. (HRA 76-14502)

[9]An excellent discussion of Census Bureau products can be found in Anthony Orgelia et al., *A Data Acquisition and Analysis Handbook for Health Planners,* Vol. 1, Washington, D.C., U.S. Department of Health, Education, and Welfare, Bureau of Health Planning and Resources Development, 1976. (HRA 76-14506)

[10]P.L. 94-521, signed in 1976, established the quinquennial census.

diskettes. Also, the Bureau of the Census provides a certain portion of its data in printed and microfilm form. These data are contained in libraries designated as federal depositories in every congressional district. It also publishes a series of ongoing tabulations and reports including the following:

1. Subject report series, which address special topics such as race and poverty
2. Monograph series, which include detailed analyses of such topics as changing characteristics of the black population
3. *Statistical Abstract of the United States,* a yearly compendium of statistical data on the nation and its population
4. County and city data books, which supplement statistical abstracts at the county and city levels[11]

Other demographic and related data, useful to health planners but not supplied by the census, can be obtained from the following sources:

1. *The Municipal Yearbook,* published by the International City Managers Association, gives independent population estimates and is especially good for small cities.
2. The F. W. Dodge Division of McGraw-Hill Publishing Company, as well as the R. L. Polk Company and other similar publishing houses, sell data on the socioeconomic characteristics of selected metropolitan areas. These are basically marketing research firms, and it is not unusual for them to use the census as the basis for their information.
3. Local organizations (e.g., school districts, utility companies, chambers of commerce, trade associations, government agencies) often tabulate population data. The quantity and quality of these data will vary, based on their intended use.

In short, data on a population and its health are available from a variety of sources, including the U.S. Census and publications of NCHS. No uniform method or model applies for using and analyzing community-based data, but the importance of these statistics is recognized by planners and marketers.

---

[11]See U.S. Department of Commerce, Bureau of the Census, *1970 Census Users' Guide,* Washington, D.C., U.S. Government Printing Office, 1970; ———, *Small-Area Data Notes,* Washington, D.C., U.S. Government Printing Office, issued periodically; also see Benjamin Gura, "Census Tape Delivery: Dates, Costs, Contents," paper presented at the Eighth Annual Conference of the Urban and Regional Information Systems Association, September 3–5, 1970, Louisville, Kentucky.

Geocoding

Service-area studies frequently require geocoding—that is, linking an individual or patient with a location in the community or attaching some geographic code to an individual record that is part of a data file. For example, attaching a census tract code to a hospital discharge abstract is a form of geocoding.

The lowest level at which health planning is likely to occur usually will establish the level for geocoding. It should be noted, however, that data geocoded to the level of small areas can be aggregated into larger areas but that data geocoded in large geographic groupings cannot be disaggregated. Hence, it is better to begin an analysis with data of a small area and aggregate, if necessary, rather than to begin with large aggregations and have to totally reconstruct the files for later analyses based on different areas.

A hierarchy of geographic aggregations that might prove useful to the health planner, beginning with the largest entity, includes state, region (HSA), standard metropolitan statistical area (SMSA), county, minor civil division, city, planning district, zip code, census tract, block group, city block, and specific address. Some of these aggregations are related to the U.S. Census and will be explained later in the chapter.

The level of aggregation used by a health planner can affect the results of a community analysis. A level that is too large might conceal important phenomena, whereas one that is too small may lack sufficient data to be reliable.[12]

Geocoding historically was done manually. To eliminate this tedious manual effort, the Census Bureau developed a computerized technique, ADMATCH, to place geocodes in machine-readable form.[13] ADMATCH is useful for individuals conducting service-area studies, but, unfortunately, it is available only in urbanized areas. Planners able to use ADMATCH gain benefits beyond the simple geocoding of records. Computerized geocoded data lend themselves not only to service-area analysis but also to other types of studies, such as those on population at risk and neighborhood health profiles.

After the 1990 census, planners will have much improved and more complete geographic coverage within the census data. The 1980 census made use of three different types of geographic reference tools: maps, geographic base files, and master reference files. The use of these ap-

---

[12]U.S. Department of Health, Education, and Welfare, Public Health Service, National Health Planning Information Center. *Guide to Data for Health Systems Planners,* p. 16.
[13]A good discussion of the ADMATCH system appears in Anthony Orgelia et al., *A Data Acquisition and Analysis Handbook for Health Planners,* pp. 106–123.

proaches resulted in some errors in the coding of the census data. To resolve this problem, the Census Bureau is creating a new system called the Topologically Integrated Geographic Encoding and Referencing (TIGER) File. This single file will eliminate the confusion created by the older system and will extend geographic coverage for the 1990 census.[14]

SERVICE AREAS

Historically, health services planning (especially facilities planning) has been based on the concept of service areas—those geographic areas having a population that can be expected to use the services offered by a specific facility. This is similar to the concept of defining geographic markets. In fact, many of the service area or market definition approaches have their roots in retail marketing theory.

The concepts of service areas and market segmentation are quite similar. Both seek to identify homogeneous subgroupings of people who are logical markets for certain services. Historically, the health planner has used "beds" as the service for which geographic service area analysis was conducted. This approach, however, has become inadequate, since consumers have become more sophisticated and the delivery system more complex. There is a service area or market for every product or service that a health delivery organization offers. The following methods do not specify a service or product as the focal point of the analysis. The reader should keep in mind that one of these techniques would be used for each specific service.

General Service Area or Market Definition Methods

Two methods can be used to determine the service area for a given facility. The first is the *boundary approach,* which seeks to establish a single continuous line around the service area of a given facility. This approach usually identifies the equiprobability boundary between two facilities—that is, the line identifying the point at which a patient has equal probability of visiting either facility. Figure 23 illustrates the boundary, or equiprobability, approach. The arrow pointing to contour 7 indicates a 70-percent probability that a person living along that line

---

[14]Robert W. Marx and John D. Loikow. "Digital TIGER: All Census Maps from One Digitized File." *Government Data Systems, 13*(1):22, January–February 1984.

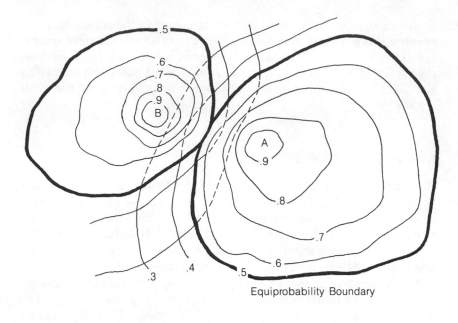

Equiprobability Boundary

Figure 23   Equiprobability boundaries.

will use the services of facility A and a 30-percent probability that he will use a different facility. The equiprobability lines are the heavy ones; they signify that people living along these lines would be equally likely to use facility A or facility B. Although equiprobability is the most frequently used boundary-setting approach, not all boundary methods use it.

The second approach to establishing service areas is the *nonboundary approach,* in which the patient load for a given facility is defined and described in terms of geography but no specific boundary is established for that facility. Figure 24 illustrates the relationship of two facilities using the nonboundary approach. The shaded part represents the geographic area from which facility A draws its patients, and the hatched area represents the territory for facility B patients. Patients in the overlap area may visit either one.

Neither of these approaches is inherently preferable to the other. The nonboundary approach best describes reality, but it does not provide a mechanism for allocating specific geographic areas to a facility. On the other hand, the boundary approach, if used in the equiprobability sense, does not identify the total area from which a facility's patients are derived.

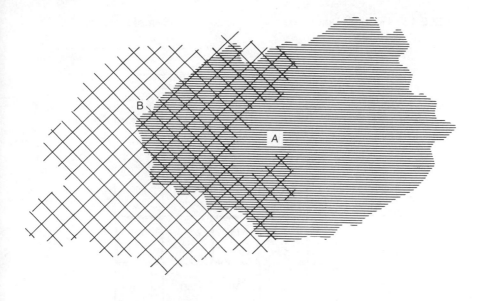

Figure 24 Nonboundary service area.

If a boundary is drawn at the outer fringe of the area from which a facility obtains its patients, the description of that area is complicated by the fact that many patients inside it will cross the boundary and use other facilities. Thus, in the process of conducting service-area studies, the planner may first use the nonboundary approach to describe the total area from which a patient load is derived and, then, place boundaries on that service area to identify major subareas.

Whenever possible, service areas should be established on the basis of patient-origin data, since they directly reflect the geographic area from which a patient load is derived. For example, a hospital would use either admissions or discharge data as the basis of a service-area study, with the latter preferred because it is more complete and more likely to be accurate. Occasionally, patient-origin data are not available to conduct service-area studies; when this occurs, alternative geographic information, such as patient travel time and distance, can be used.

Relevance and Commitment Indexes

Service-area studies can be conducted from two perspectives: that of the community and that of the facility. The first—relevance—seeks to identify the degree to which a community depends on a facility, whereas

TABLE 15   Hospital Discharges by Census Tract (Sample Community, 1984)

| | Hospital | | | |
Tract	A	B	C	Total
1	40	40	10	90
2	70	60	30	160
3	30	D 50	20	TT 100
4	60	30	40	130
5	100	20	50	170
Total	300	HT 200	150	650

the second—commitment—looks at how much a facility depends on the community.[15]

Indexes have been developed that measure both of these perspectives. The data required to compute a relevance index involve a community-wide patient-origin study. Both indexes show a relationship between a specific tract or area in the community and a specific hospital or facility.

The process for calculating relevance and commitment indexes can be illustrated by a specific example. The first step in the process is to construct a hospital discharge matrix similar to that shown in Table 15. The matrix arrays hospitals in the columns and tracts in the rows, with

---

[15]John R. Griffith. *Quantitative Techniques for Hospital Planning and Control.* Lexington, Mass., Lexington Books, D. C. Heath and Co., 1972, pp. 75–78.

each cell indicating the number of discharges from a specific hospital to a specific tract. For example, according to Table 15, there were 50 discharges from hospital B to tract 3.

The relevance index indicates the percentage of all discharges from a specific hospital to a certain tract. Using data for tract 3 and hospital B, the relevance index can be calculated as follows:

$$R = \frac{D}{TT} = \frac{50}{100} = 0.5(100) = 50\%$$

where

R = Relevance index
D = Discharges from hospital B to tract 3
TT = Total discharges from tract 3

The relevance index for tract 3 and hospital B is 0.5 or 50 percent, which means that half the discharges to that tract came from hospital B. The index also implies that 50 percent of the population of that census area depends on hospital B for care.

The commitment index is calculated as follows:

$$C = \frac{D}{HT} = \frac{50}{200} - 0.25(100) = 25\%$$

where

C = Commitment index
D = Discharges from hospital B to tract 3
HT = Total discharges from hospital B

The commitment index of 0.25 indicates that one-fourth of hospital B's discharges were to tract 3; in other words, hospital B derives 25 percent of its patient load from that tract.

With these two indexes, one could conclude that tract 3 is fairly dependent on hospital B for services; however, hospital B is not so dependent on tract 3 for its patient load. Table 16 shows a complete set of relevance and commitment indexes for this example.

The relevance index should be used in service area studies. This index, however, can be calculated only when a full set of discharges for each hospital in the community is available. In contrast, the commitment index, although not so useful in establishing service areas, is still an important planning tool, especially to the individual hospital. The institutional planner will find this index particularly useful in conducting marketing activities. The impact of marketing on this type of analysis can be seen in a number of recent articles.

TABLE 16   Relevance (R) and Commitment (C) Indexes (Sample Community, 1984)

	Hospital						
	A		B		C		
Tract	R	C	R	C	R	C	
	Percentages		Percentages		Percentages		Total Percentages
1	44	13	44	20	12	7	100
2	43	24	38	30	19	20	100
3	30	10	50	25	20	13	100
4	46	20	23	15	31	27	100
5	59	33	12	10	29	33	100
Total		100		100		100	

The relevance index can also be called a market share analysis. Folland[16] makes this observation in his approach to predicting market share. He also includes other variables in the analysis, such as distance, physician availability, and alternative trade opportunities. This type of approach is more frequently used in an institutional planning process than in a community planning process. It is important because it includes multiple variables to establish market share.

---

[16]Sherman T. Folland. "Predicting Hospital Market Shares," *Inquiry*, 20(1):34–44, Spring 1983.

Other Methods of Service Area Definition

A number of other approaches have been used to develop service areas. The following examples are representative:

1. McGibony[17] suggested a service-area approach that involves seven steps: (a) Plot the location of existing facilities on a map; (b) outline tentative service areas based on political boundaries and distances; (c) check travel flow based on highways; (d) check for physical barriers to travel (e.g., a river); (e) determine existing trade areas; (f) check the use patterns of other health facilities (patient residences may be obtained from hospital records, but often this source is inadequate; location of doctors' offices also must be considered, because it is the doctor who typically directs the patient to a hospital); and (g) determine population characteristics, including age, income level, racial composition, and ethnic groups. Unfortunately, no rules are provided for the use of these data once they are collected, except to apply them in a commonsense manner. The value of McGibony's approach lies in cataloging various factors that affect the establishment of health services.

2. In mental health planning, the concept of a "catchment area" evolved. Since no universal definition of a community has been developed, mental health authorities adopted a range of population size — namely, from 75,000 to 200,000 — to define a community. This notion presumes that everyone in the area has easy access to the facilities. It ignores political boundaries and assumes that mental health problems are fairly evenly distributed among all population groups. Because of the looseness of this definition, it has been applied in a variety of ways and to a variety of services. For example, Illinois bases its catchment areas on the distances from mental health hospitals, whereas Pennsylvania's areas conform strictly to county boundaries. In Arizona, the catchment area is based on both geographic area and distance from a mental health center.

The catchment-area concept has many problems. Census data are based on political boundaries; thus, it becomes difficult to determine the boundaries of a population-based catchment area. Population shifts, of course, require an adjustment of boundaries. There is also the matter of what should be done when the population is very sparse or very dense. For example, 75,000 people could be spread so widely that one community mental health center would not be accessible to everyone within the catchment area.

---

[17]John R. McGibony. *Principles of Hospital Administration.* New York, G. P. Putnam's Sons, 1969, p. 29.

3. A third, somewhat different, approach to the service-area problem is that taken by Anthony Rourke[18] in one of his Nebraska studies, in which he proposes three service areas and defines them on the basis of patient-origin data. The first area is called a *base service area*. It contains hospitals able to service most medical needs. In the second, or *peripheral,* service area are hospitals that serve as base service areas, but, more important, they provide some of the more sophisticated services not generally available in base service-area institutions. The third service area is regional. It concentrates on those hospitals that, to some extent, are used for both base and peripheral services but primarily focus on providing highly specialized services for persons normally treated at other base and peripheral service hospitals.

4. Another approach to the service-area concept is to designate census tracts as service areas and allocate them to various institutions, based on the proportion of patients served from any one census tract. Thus, if four hospitals received patients from a single census tract, the responsibility for that entire census tract would be assigned to whichever hospital received the highest proportion of patients.

This approach is inaccurate and somewhat misleading, but it does identify a means of dealing with an area that is dependent on a number of facilities for service. Obviously, caution is needed in applying it.

5. The patient-flow matrix proposed by Morrill and Earickson[19] is a highly sophisticated approach. It assumes that use of the nearest hospital is an ideal and then measures the deviations from this ideal. Their Chicago study clearly shows, first, that the service areas, as normally defined, are gross misrepresentations of the facts. For example, 35–40 percent of all patients crossed boundaries. Second, service areas cut across normal community boundaries, thus making a population forecast nearly impossible. Recent developments in small-area data beginning with the 1970 census should make it easier to define service areas on the basis of patient origin. Few communities, however, have the geographic base file necessary to convert ordinary maps into locational grids and then to plot residential addresses on these grids.

6. Another approach that has worked well in areas of low population density is the application of Reilly's law of retail gravitation.[20] This technique identifies the breaking point between service locations on the

[18]Anthony Rourke. Personal communication.
[19]Richard L. Morrill and Robert Earickson. "Locational Efficiency of Chicago Hospitals: An Experimental Model." *Health Service Research,* 4(2):128–141, Summer 1969.
[20]Laurence S. Klugman. "The Law of Retail Gravitation (Reilly's Law) Applied to Eastern Shore Hospital Service Areas." Philadelphia, Health Planning Research Services, 1975. Mimeographed.

bases of the distance between locations and the size or capacity of the services involved. The boundary point is identified as follows:

$$B = \frac{M}{1 + \sqrt{S}}$$

where

    B = Boundary between facilities X and Y in miles from Y
    M = Miles between X and Y
    S = Size or capacity of X divided by the size or capacity of Y

This technique merely identifies the breaking point between facilities X and Y and does not circumscribe a complete boundary around either. It thus provides useful information with a minimum of data for low-density population areas.

7. One of the simplest approaches to delineating service areas is to set travel-time standards for specific services and then to establish boundaries around a facility based on these standards. This approach differs from the others in that it is based on a description of what should exist within a community rather than what actually does exist. The approach, however, is consistent with the accessibility and availability criteria that a health system agency may establish for a given community.[21]

8. Poland and Lembecke[22] apply a method similar to that described in item 4 in that they use census tracts, townships, or minor civil divisions as the basic units of analysis and then allocate these to various facilities. The allocation is done by computing the percentage of total admissions from a unit that went to each facility and then drawing a single continuous equiprobability line around each facility. If the facility under study has a clear majority of the patients from a certain unit, the boundary line is drawn through that unit on the basis of transportation networks and population centers. This technique avoids some of the inaccuracies identified in the approach outlined in item 4.

9. The approach defined by Griffith[23] is based on relevance indexes and uses the census tract, township, or minor civil division as the unit of analysis. A relevance index is computed for each facility, and the ser-

---

[21]Robert Marrinson. "Hospital Service Areas: Time Replaces Space." *Hospitals,* *38*(2):52–54, January 1964.

[22]E. Poland and P. A. Lembecke. "Delineation of Hospital Service Districts: A Fundamental Requirement in Hospital Planning." Kansas City, Mo., Community Services, 1962. Mimeographed.

[23]John R. Griffith. *Quantitative Techniques for Hospital Planning and Control,* p. 75.

vice area for a given facility is determined by plotting its location on a map and shading the various units, based on the relevance index. An arbitrary definition of relevance could be made, such as high relevance equals 75 percent or more, moderate relevance equals 40–74 percent, and low relevance equals less than 40 percent. The concept is quite flexible and can utilize the ideas of primary and secondary service areas. In addition, the total population being served by the facility can be computed by multiplying the relevance index for each unit by the total population of the unit and summing the products of all the units. This approach is one of the most useful for a service-area analysis.

This list of methods is by no means exhaustive, but it does represent the approaches that can be taken to determine service areas. The availability of data frequently will determine which method can be used, but the planner should use the relevance index approach whenever possible, because it most clearly defines the service-area concept.

Facility Location

The health planner's concern with geography and space also is based on the need to evaluate the location of new health services. Since accessibility is one of the major criteria for evaluating the location of new health services, this discussion will deal primarily with accessibility criteria.

Accessibility can be broken down into four major components, with each affecting desirability of a location for a given health service. Often, the decision to locate a health service at a given point is a function of trade-offs among these four aspects of accessibility.

1. *Spatial accessibility* is measured in terms of physical distances. The distance a patient is willing to travel for service depends on the urban or rural setting and the degree of specialization of the service involved. Patients are more willing to travel great distances for specialized services than for routine services. Individuals in urban areas tend to be indifferent to distances up to approximately two miles, while individuals in rural areas tend to be more sensitive to the distance factor.[24]

2. *Temporal accessibility* often is measured in terms of travel time. This factor seems to have a greater effect on outpatient and primary

---

[24]J. E. Weiss, M. R. Greenlick, and J. F. Jones. "Determinants of Medical Care Utilization: The Impact of Spatial Factors." *Inquiry, 8*(4):50–57, December 1971.

care than on hospital care; however, it may affect the choice of the hospital when more than one facility is available.[25] Another temporal factor, waiting time, may be as important a factor as travel time in the selection of a facility.[26]

3. *Social accessibility* is measured in terms of the population characteristics that may affect use of a given facility. For example, religion, race, and social status have been shown to affect accessibility to given facilities.[27] These factors, however, are at best difficult to measure, and no generalizations can be drawn as to how they affect the location of health services. They are nonetheless important.

4. *Financial accessibility* refers to a facility's rates, provisions for free care, and third-party payer agreements. The more a service population depends on public sources of financing for care, the more these considerations become important in deciding where to locate a facility.

These factors are important in locating health facilities, but no uniform theory describes how they should be applied in a location decision. One methodology that attempts to take accessibility into consideration was developed by Health Planning Research Services, Inc. of Philadelphia. This model consists of a five-step procedure based on temporal and spatial accessibility:[28]

1. Determine the service areas of present facilities or services, based on travel-time standards. This step establishes the percentage of the population within the acceptable travel time of each service or facility.

2. Determine the best location for a new service — "best" being the point that will minimize the average travel time or distance for the residents of the area under consideration.

3. Determine the service area for a new facility or service located at the "best" location. This is accomplished by using the travel-time standards established in step 1.

4. Determine the impact of the proposed facility or service on the aggregate travel time of the total population. Aggregate travel time is defined as the total amount of time a population would travel if each individual made one trip to the nearest service site.

---

[25]M. S. Blumberg. "The Effects of Size and Specialism on Utilization of Urban Hospitals." *Hospitals,* 39(10):43–47, May 16, 1965.
[26]James Studnicki. "An Analysis of the Spatial Behavior of Obstetrical Patients in Baltimore City." Doctoral dissertation. Baltimore, Md., Johns Hopkins University, 1972.
[27]Health Planning Research Services, Inc. "A Guide for Evaluating the Location of a Health Service." Fort Washington, Pa., 1976. Mimeographed.
[28]Ibid.

5. Determine the impact of the proposed facility or service on the total aggregate travel distance of the population, defined as the total distance traveled if each individual in the population made one trip to the nearest service or facility location.

This methodology has proved useful in rural and suburban settings but tends to break down in urban areas because of the close proximity of facilities and service settings.

Although this discussion has focused on accessibility as the major factor in determining facility and service locations, other factors must also be considered. Facility location often is affected by such factors as zoning; availability of desirable sites; political and legal constraints; availability of ancillary services (e.g., sewerage, water, power); cost of available land; and environmental, physical, and aesthetic factors.[29]

INTERNAL ORGANIZATIONAL ASSESSMENT

Internal organizational assessment focuses on resources and programs. Both community and institutional planning processes need to catalog, assess, and consider these two dimensions. The material presented here concentrates on community-level planning. Many texts on strategic planning and marketing present excellent descriptions of the internal assessment of institutions.[30]

Community Resources

The Health Planning and Resources Development Act (P.L. 93-641) requires each HSA to assemble and analyze data on the number, type, and location of an area's health resources. The law then defines these resources as health services, manpower, and facilities. This chapter views resources somewhat differently, defining them as the components used to *create* health services; thus, the services themselves are not regarded as resources.

A list of resources used to create health services would include both manpower and facilities; however, facilities should encompass not only buildings but also major equipment items. If the law's authors intended

---

[29]A discussion of specific site factors can be found in O. B. Hardy and L. P. Lammers, *Hospitals: The Planning and Design Process,* Germantown, Md., Aspen Systems Corp., 1977, chap. 8.

[30]See Philip Kotler, *Marketing for Nonprofit Organizations,* Englewood Cliffs, N.J., Prentice-Hall, 1975; George A. Steiner, *Strategic Planning: What Every Manager Must Know,* New York, Free Press, 1979.

this inclusion, their intention has not been made explicit. At any rate, HSAs should be knowledgeable about and include among their facilities resources the major pieces of capital equipment (e.g., magnetic resonance imaging [MRI]) available in a community. This requirement raises the obvious difficulty of distinguishing between what constitutes a major piece of equipment and what may be regarded as an ordinary component of a health services delivery facility (e.g., autoclaves).

The certificate-of-need laws may determine what constitutes a major piece of equipment for the HSAs. Currently, these laws focus primarily on expenditure levels as a means of measuring importance; this identifies the third resource to be considered in the planning process—namely, dollars. This last resource is a proxy measure for the other two and allows them to be considered in the aggregate. In other words, the wages and salaries paid to health services practitioners can be added to the cost of using facilities to arrive at a single aggregate number that represents the community's use of health services resources during a specified period. Thus, the discussion of financial resources will deal with the costs of the other two resources as separate entities, and discussions of personnel and facilities (including major equipment) will, inasmuch as possible, recognize the interrelationship of the three.

Manpower

A community is concerned with resources only to the extent that they can be used to produce health services. Acceptance of this notion of resource productivity as a primary criterion must include the recognition that such productivity is contingent on the availability of *several* resources. Thus, a multimillion-dollar hospital can contribute nothing to health services unless it is supported by adequate personnel. Also, attempting to increase the productivity of highly trained medical personnel by teaming them with people who can perform certain specialized tasks that do not require a high level of training depends on the availability of such people and on the cooperation of highly trained personnel.

A planner is concerned with not only the current supply of resources but a forecast of the future inventory. Consequently, he must consider possible changes in the current stock of resources during the period between the present and the planning horizon; his concern is with the current stock minus projected losses plus projected gains. This simple formulation is probably adequate for facilities forecasting. To forecast the supply of personnel, however, a more precise measurement is needed—one that considers the nature of various gains and losses (e.g., whether they are permanent or temporary).

Permanent personnel losses include those resulting from emigration and such occupational changes as movement from a less-skilled to a more highly skilled job. Temporary losses include people who leave the labor force intending to return later, such as persons who enter the educational system for additional training that will not change their occupational category or professionals who leave the work force temporarily to raise children. With the exception of people who enter occupations as trainees (e.g., medical residents), gains to the manpower inventory are relatively permanent. They result from immigration, new entrants to the field (usually through educational programs), and the return of persons who were temporarily out of the work force. Such gains and losses are the basis for estimating the gross number of people who can be included in the forecast supply of health services manpower. In the health services field, however, many occupations have a tradition of partial employment. Consequently, the aggregate number would suggest a misleading level of productivity.

A more precise estimate of the productivity anticipated from the number of people available can be obtained by multiplying the sum of persons in the inventory by a full-time equivalent factor. For example, if 100 people worked 200 days to produce a cumulative total of 18,000 days, the full-time equivalent factor would be 0.9 (18,000/[200 · 100]).

The heterogeneity of the people involved further complicates forecasting the manpower inventory. This lack of uniformity results in wide variation among groups in rates of attrition, movement in and out of the work force, and full-time participation. The planner, however, can develop a fairly precise estimate of the future manpower inventory by stratifying workers, making separate computations for each stratum, and then adding the results to obtain an aggregate forecast. An obvious stratification of a category of people (e.g., registered nurses) would be a division into separate age groups. This may reveal substantial intergroup differences within a particular category.

The method for developing a forecast of future manpower inventory can be summarized by the following formula: Forecast inventory equals Σ(current supply − temporary losses − permanent losses + temporary gains + permanent gains) × the full-time equivalent factor.

Building a Resource Inventory

The process of developing a resource inventory essentially involves four steps: deciding what to count, listing resource units, getting information on these units, and keeping data current.

STEP 1

In the first step, the planner must identify, for each type of resource, the specific type of service-producing unit to be counted. He must then define each unit to make it distinct from the others; for instance, among facilities, domiciliary facilities should be clearly distinguishable from extended-care facilities or skilled-nursing facilities. This definition process requires that the planner decide what information is necessary to describe the specific resource adequately or what unit characteristics are relevant for decision making. This decision relates very closely to determinations made during the plan development process, when planners operationally defined the attributes of services and resources.

STEP 2

For the second step, the planner must develop a list of the resource units identified. He should initially identify specific data sources (name and location) and should carefully analyze the definitions of resource units used by the person or organization compiling these lists to ensure agreement between the planner's and the compiler's definitions.

To the greatest extent possible, the planner should identify several lists for the same category of resources to provide a check for accuracy and completeness. This is important because many sources of information are not comprehensive. For instance, health practitioners are not necessarily members of all the professional societies that they are eligible to join; thus, any single membership list may be incomplete. On the other hand, since it is likely that most practitioners belong to at least one organization, lists from several groups probably would identify most of the practitioners in a community.

An obvious problem in using a variety of sources is duplication, which can be dealt with only if the individual units in the resources inventory are identified so precisely that one can unequivocally determine whether similar units appearing on more than one list are duplicates.

Licensing bureau data, if current, provide another excellent source of names of health practitioners, but, particularly in service areas that cross state lines, the likelihood of multiple licensure may be very high. This raises the problem of identifying duplicate items on the lists provided by several states.

Culling duplicate names from a list can be done effectively with some sort of common identifier. Comparison of names generally will work well, although certain variations, such as the use of a full name in one state and initials and surname in another, could be misleading. Use of a unique identifier, such as social security number, is far more reliable in making these decisions. Combinations of data, such as birth date and name, also are likely to be effective. Addresses are of limited use in this process, since some practitioners may report their residences and others their primary place of employment and also because some may be employed in several locations. Furthermore, because licensure files are a state function, a licensed individual may move outside the planning area but still be within the state; consequently, this fact might not be reflected in the licensure data for a long time.

STEP 3

The third step in the inventory process is to obtain information on characteristics of individual resource units. At this point, the planner also should decide on a medium for storing the data—punch cards, computer tape or diskettes, or printed book. This decision is critical, because the data-collection process should be designed to transfer data from the source to the storage medium as efficiently as possible.

The planner should examine existing sources to determine what data are available. He should review, in particular, any files used to prepare the list of resource units described in step 2, since it is likely that such files also will include much additional material needed for planning purposes.

In reviewing data, the planner can isolate those items not available from any current source. He should design the data-collection process to avoid duplication so the respondents are not asked to provide the same information twice and are assured that maximum use has been made of their previous contribution—an important factor in obtaining their cooperation.

To deal with the lack of uniformity and discrepancies between lists and other data sources that frequently occur because organizations collect data in different ways and at different times, the planner should consider using survey techniques to collect data. An effective approach might be to give each respondent a questionnaire that includes all known data about the resource unit and to ask the respondent to verify the accuracy of that data and supply any missing material.

A detailed discussion on how to conduct a survey is beyond the scope of this book, but the subject is very important. Failure to follow carefully the necessary survey procedures is likely to result in an unproductive and/or counterproductive data-collection effort. Therefore, interested readers should examine at least one of the many excellent texts on this topic before embarking on a data-collection survey.[31] In reading these materials, however, the planner should know that research by successful health data agencies indicates that a combination of approaches (mail questionnaires, telephone interviews, face-to-face interviews) frequently yields the best information.[32]

STEP 4

The fourth step in the inventory process relates to keeping data current. An inventory of most resources will be a rather volatile set of information, particularly in dealing with manpower resources. In most cases, the volatility of that information will be directly proportional to the number of units in the inventory. In other words, one may expect more changes in a manpower file listing 20,000 persons than in a facility file of 50 institutions.

On the other hand, the impact of any individual change is not directly proportional to the number of units. For example, closing one nursing home would remove a very substantial part of a community's total nursing home capacity, whereas adding or losing a single practitioner frequently would have little consequence.

The planner should consider such factors in deciding how often to update the inventory file. Changes can be made in the file by conducting a new survey periodically or by continuously posting changes as they occur. In most situations, a periodic survey, such as that described in step 3, will provide sufficiently accurate data for decision makers. In some rural communities, where the supply of physicians is small, planning agencies have been known to monitor constantly the local newspaper, especially obituary columns, to detect gains or losses in the supply of available physicians.

In many cases, an individual planning organization, regional agency, or specific institution will not have to conduct such update surveys on its own. In some areas of the country, planners are able to rely on regional or state systems for much of the data they need for resources

---

[31]A good introduction to this subject, with references to other useful texts, can be found in Chapter 2 of Anthony Orgelia et al., *A Data Acquisition and Analysis Handbook for Health Planners;* also see C. H. Backstrom and G. D. Hursh, *Survey Research,* Chicago, Northwestern University Press, 1963.

[32]Owen Thornberry, H. D. Scott, and M. Branson, "Methodology of a Health Interview Survey for a Population of One Million," paper presented at the annual meeting of the American Public Health Association, October 1973, San Francisco, California; see also U.S. Department of Health, Education, and Welfare, National Center for Health Services Research, *Advances in Health Survey Research Methods,* Washington, D.C., U.S. Government Printing Office, n.d., pp. 13–16. (HRA 77-3154)

inventory; however, they should be aware of the inventory process we have described, so that they can participate effectively in decisions about the design and operation of such systems.

In those states where a relevant data system component such as manpower or facilities has yet to be implemented, the planner may wish to collaborate with an ongoing data-collection process, such as the annual surveys conducted by the American Hospital Association, which contain much of the desired information. He should be aware, however, that some of these more-or-less voluntary efforts might have problems, particularly in terms of consistency in definitions and standardization of reporting periods.

Funding

Dollar resources pose some special difficulties for the planner. First, any group of dollars is almost impossible to identify as a unique set. Second, funds are much more mobile than the resources they are intended to purchase. Consequently, the points at which funding data can or should be collected are difficult to identify. For instance, many funding sources will be outside the geographic area covered by the planning activity; residents of a community may be participants in an insurance program with headquarters in some other state; or people may receive health services in a remote location, such as a state mental hospital.

In an effort to deal with this problem, the Federal Government supported the development of a process known as community funds flow (CFF) analysis. Its purpose is to identify both the sources of funds for health services and the purposes for which these funds are used.

Figure 25 is a diagram designed by SEARCH to illustrate the flow of funds within a particular community (in this case, the state of Rhode Island). As the figure shows, the consumer is ultimately the source of funds for health services. Since, however, the channels through which consumer dollars flow into the health system are diverse and often very obscure and because direct consumer expenditures are fairly small, persuading people that escalating health care costs have an impact on them as individuals can be difficult.

SOURCES AND USES

It is virtually impossible to directly link fund sources and the specific uses to which these funds are put. For instance, hospital bills often are paid by multiple sources such as the patient and/or an insurance company; the money paid to a hospital is used for patient care, research, and education; if funds are received from federal sources, they often

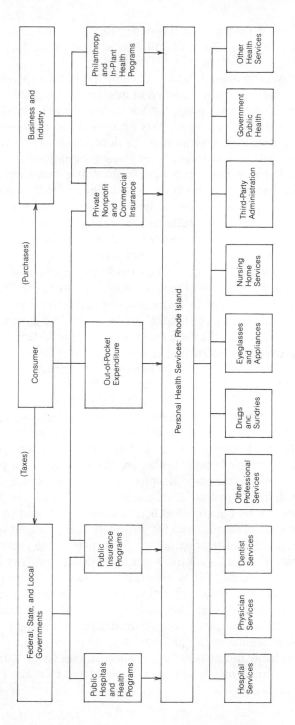

Figure 25   Funds flow diagram.

are combined with state and local funds to finance a single service; state or local budgets often fail to identify the sources of the funds; and so forth.

Some sources and uses of funds—notably, personal expenditures for prescription drugs—are not recorded in any accessible place. Some services are provided as joint products; for instance, the Federal Government provides medical care to military personnel and their dependents, but most communities assume that the dependents represent a legitimate demand on the local health services system. If one accepts this assumption, the question becomes, What dollar value should be assigned to the health services provided to dependents as part of the general military medical services activity so that this sum may be added to the other community expenditures for health care?

Table 17 illustrates the allocation of funds between sources and uses. Several examples of how to obtain data for the various rows in this diagram may be instructive. The total expenditure for hospital services is the sum of the expenditures of federal, state, and private facilities. Data for the expenditures of both private acute and federal hospitals are available from the American Hospital Association. The expenditures of state hospitals appear in the state budget, and states with rate commissions may provide an additional source of data on hospital services expenditures. Finally, the medicare system has amassed significant data that could be useful to the planner.

These expenditures are allocated to fund sources as follows: Federal funds for hospital services, which include direct expenditures for federal hospitals (assumed to be the total outlay for these institutions); expenditures for medicare, medicaid, and maternal and child health programs, as financed by federal taxes; and federal insurance programs. Data on medicare payments to hospitals and on federal insurance programs are available from the fiscal intermediary for the state. Medicaid expenditures can be documented by the state department responsible for that program; the same is true for other federally financed services.

State expenditures for hospital services include the cost of care in state hospitals, the state's contribution to medicaid, and any contributions to other service delivery programs. Data on state and local expenditures may be available from the same sources as information on federal expenditures. Private, third-party payments for hospital services include nonprofit and commercial insurance reimbursement. Usually, a Blue Cross association can provide data on most of these outlays. Since it is probably not possible to get specific data on the commercial insurance reimbursements, an agency may have to make estimates based on national data.

TABLE 17   Sources and Uses of Health Funds in Rhode Island During 1972, in dollars

Type of Expenditure	Public				Private				Total
	Federal Revenue	State	Local	Total Public	Federal Insurance*	Private Insurance	Consumer and Other	Total Private	
Services and Supplies									
Hospitals	71,534	29,013	51	100,598	4,821	65,419	19,871	90,111	190,709
Physicians	5,433	2,048	0	7,481	6,633	27,172	27,571	61,376	68,857
Dentists	638	631	0	1,269	0	366	26,304	26,670	27,939
Other Professionals	1,243	403	125	1,771	151	862	8,525	9,538	11,309
Drugs and Sundries	2,306	2,283	0	4,589	0	1,199	48,252	49,451	54,040
Eyeglasses, Appliances	212	210	0	422	0	101	8,925	9,026	9,448
Nursing Homes	7,782	7,123	0	14,905	565	0	13,878	14,443	29,348
Administration	0	264	0	264	0	20,174	0	20,174	20,438
G.P.H.A.†	2,421	6,148	599	9,168	0	0	0	0	9,168
Other Health Services	3,447	824	1,812	6,083	1,174	753	3,012	4,939	11,022
Subtotal	95,016	48,947	2,587	146,550	13,344	116,046	156,338	285,728	432,278
Research	4,424	0	0	4,424	0	0	219	219	4,643
Construction	1,900	0	0	1,900	0	0	4,000	4,000	5,900
Training	2,729	1,350	0	4,079	0	0	5,951	5,951	10,030
Total	104,069	50,297	2,587	156,953	13,344	116,046	166,508	295,898	452,851

SOURCE: Rhode Island Health Services Research, Inc. "Health Expenditures in Rhode Island: 1972." SEARCH Report No. 11. Providence, R.I., August 1974, p. 12. Mimeographed.

*Federal Insurance includes Part B, medicare financed by consumer premium payments, FEP, and CHAMPUS. The reason for including this in the private sector is discussed in Part I, B.
†Government Public Health Activities.

The final category—consumer out-of-pocket expenditures for hospitals—is "residual"; that is, expenditures from all other categories are subtracted from the total expenditures for hospital services to arrive at this figure.

The category of expenditures for physician services is defined as the gross business receipts of self-employed physicians—that is, their income. (Salaries paid by hospitals are included in hospital service expenditures.) Doctors' income is estimated by multiplying the number of self-employed physicians by the average gross business receipts of physicians. These figures can be obtained from such sources as the American Medical Association and the journal *Medical Economics.*

Information on federal payments for physician services is obtained from the fiscal intermediary. Data on local payments is obtained from the appropriate budgets. Blue Cross can provide data on its subscribers, and expenditures of commercial insurance funds are estimated from national data. Once again, out-of-pocket expenses are estimated as a residual category.[33]

CONTAINING COSTS

Information on the sources and uses of funds becomes a critical part of the health planner's contribution to the decision-making process, because there is much emphasis on the issue of containing costs. This is evident in P.L. 93-641, its legislative history, and its implementing regulations: The law's plan development guidelines include the statement that "attention to the cost of health care is an immediate national priority."[34]

Most of the pressure for cost containment is from federal and state levels. Although some individuals and organizations are actively concerned with cost containment, local emphasis is mostly on improving the health services system. (One could surmise that this attitude prevails because fund sources are so diffused that, to those asking for improved service, someone else always seems to be paying the bill.) Pressure for cost containment also is beginning to be exerted by private sector purchasers of medical care, such as large industrial purchasers, who are becoming anxious over the rapidly escalating expenditures.

---

[33]Rhode Island Health Services Research, Inc. "Methodology for Estimating Rhode Island Expenditures for Health Care." Providence, R.I., 1974. Mimeographed. (SEARCH Report No. 8)

[34]U.S. Department of Health, Education, and Welfare, Public Health Service, Bureau of Health Planning and Resources Development. "Guidelines Concerning the Development of Health System Plans and Annual Implementation Plans." Rockville, Md., 1976, p. 44. Mimeographed.

National data, citing billions of dollars expended each year on health, are far too abstract for the average person to appreciate. As mentioned previously, the ultimate source of all funds for health services is the individual, but how much each individual actually spends is not easy to identify. In addition, although the individual may vehemently oppose increases in federal and state spending, he also expects federal and state agencies to maintain—and frequently to increase—the quantity, quality, and accessibility of health services.

Howard Hiatt[35] pointed out that there is little hope in relying on medical professionals to help resolve the issue of cost containment because that would be contrary to the professional ethos of doing as much as possible for each individual patient. It is equally unlikely that managers will intervene effectively, since their constituencies are the ones demanding greater expenditures for health services and amenities.[36] Finally, most reimbursement mechanisms are unlikely to resolve the problem since they offer no incentives for cost containment.

Despite a continuing tension between the aggregate concern for containing health costs and the individual concern with improving the quality and quantity of health services, some efforts have been made to deal with this problem through processes such as certificate-of-need legislation, professional review organizations (PROs), and rate regulation. These programs, however, can be effective only to the extent that they receive widespread support—support that will emerge only when decision makers clearly understand the impact of their decisions on the community's total financial resources.

Without data on the availability and use of resources, people cannot be expected to support the kind of rational decision making implied in the planning process. Knowledge of a community's fiscal capacity and its present resource allocation would allow the decision maker to determine the size of the total health budget and what trade-offs should be made within it, but currently such knowledge and the documentation to support it are incomplete.

For example, the certificate-of-need process tends to limit capital spending, but the issue is presented simply as "Do we or do we not spend x thousand dollars on a particular project?" rather than "An x-million-dollar outlay at present will increase the total community health services budget for this and subsequent years (noting that capital

---

[35]Howard H. Hiatt. "Protecting the Medical Commons: Who Is Responsible?" *Trustee,* 29(10):14–17, October 1976.
[36]Stephen L. Tucker. "Introducing Marketing as a Planning and Management Tool." *Hospital and Health Services Administration,* 22(1):37–44, Winter 1977.

outlays imply later operating expenditures) by *y* percent." The former view of the cost issue does not encourage any consideration of trade-offs within the system, whereby planners could discontinue one service to provide the funds required for a new service without altering the community's total health services budget.

Another cost containment technique of limited effectiveness involves placing caps or ceilings on operating expenses of particular programs. This tends to be inequitable, and, since it focuses on a single program, it frequently results in the transfer of costs from a "capped" program to another program rather than actually eliminating costs. A cap on the medicaid program, for instance, would result in more charity care in hospitals. The cost of that care would then be added to the charges for hospital services, which, in turn, would lead to an increase in premiums paid to insurance companies. As a result, people would still be paying for the services, only the payment would be through the third-party insurance mechanism rather than through taxation.

Another approach similar to certificate of need involves placing a ceiling on capital spending. As of spring 1984, only one state, Maine, had enacted such a law, although five other states were expected to consider such legislation during the year.[37]

MEASURING FINANCIAL RESOURCES

The data made available through a system such as community funds flow (CFF) can be used effectively in health services decision making, particularly when the system has been in operation for several years. It is then possible to make longitudinal comparisons over time to learn whether programs have grown and whether changes in the resources allocated to a program can be associated with changes in its outcomes.

Data of this sort, which now are seldom, if ever, available to community decision makers, can also be used to develop a health system economic profile that would consider data on the service provided, the capital available, the population served, and revenues. Such a profile could then be used to develop aggregate and per capita revenue per unit of service within various types of hospital services. The use of the term *new revenue* illustrates the point that one of the many policy decisions to be made about health services is whether one type should subsidize another.

---

[37]American Hospital Association. "8 State CON Limits Above Federal Levels." *Hospitals*, *58*(8):24, April 16, 1984.

In measuring financial resources for decision making, a planner must take into account both capital financing and operating costs. For the first, he must consider the tax base, current bonded indebtedness, legal limits on taxes and bonds, past success of fund drives, and the possibility of large-scale contributions or endowments. As resources for operating costs, the planner must consider annual per capita and per family income; the volume and coverage of health insurance; the economic stability of the area (i.e., anticipated economic fluctuation and unemployment); and the public's attitude toward health services—notably, their willingness to use and pay for facilities and services.

Recently, discussion has commenced on the possibility of a shortage of capital. Should this prediction (by a number of experts) materialize, the pressures on a local community to provide capital for health services providers would grow significantly. The potential for this occurrence emphasizes the need for the planner to be aware of the community's capacity to finance its health care system.

The belief that the burden of health care payments should fall on those who directly benefit has shifted generally toward the concept that each citizen has a right to needed health care. Because financing health care through insurance contributions, sales taxes, or property taxes is either inequitable or inadequate, the tendency today is to rely increasingly on the government for general revenues. Therefore, it is necessary to assess the financing capability of a community, which, in turn, requires estimates of its tax capacity, its economic standing, and its economic stability.

The Georgia Study

To measure relative financing capability per capita, the state of Georgia analyzed intercounty differences in economic status.[38] The following procedures were used:

1. Several economic and demographic variables were examined for each county for citizens aged 21–64 (i.e., the appropriate working-age population): their effective buying income; their total adjusted gross income as shown by Georgia income tax data; the total assessed values for general property in the county, based on Georgia property tax data; and the number of persons receiving public assistance payments.

---

[38]E. Lamar White, *Provisional Affluence Ratings of Georgia Counties,* Atlanta, Georgia Department of Public Health, Office of Comprehensive Health Planning, 1971; Karen Butler, *A Method for Geographic Analysis of Target Areas,* Atlanta, Georgia Department of Public Health, Office of Comprehensive Health Planning, 1971.

2. Each county's data for each variable were compared with Georgia's population as a whole. Indexes were derived from these comparisons, and the counties were ranked according to the computed index numbers.

3. After ranking, the counties were distributed among seven groups, ranging from the most affluent to the least affluent. Georgia's statewide average was used as the standard of comparison for determining affluence.

ACIR Work

For many years, the Advisory Commission on Intergovernmental Relations (ACIR),[39] a federally funded agency, has been examining and testing ways to measure the relative financing capability of state and local governments and the extent to which they actually use this capacity. Improved measures of fiscal capacity and fiscal effort led the commission to recommend to both the Federal Government and the states that they place increased emphasis on equalizing local resources when distributing their grants among eligible jurisdictions. Also, the commission has urged state and local governments to make more effective use of their revenue resources and to encourage, in various ways, the mitigation of interstate and interlocal tax-load differentials.

Traditionally, two kinds of economic indicators have been used to measure relative fiscal capacity and tax effort: estimates of per capita personal income and estimates of taxable property values on the local-area tax rolls. These indicators, although useful, leave much to be desired. At the state level, for example, resident personal income fails to reflect accurately the potential of certain revenue sources such as severance, motor fuel, and gambling taxes. Locally, the property tax base pertains to only a portion of available financing resources. Nationally, approximately two-fifths of all own-source revenue of local governments is obtained from nonproperty sources.

The development of meaningful comparative measures of fiscal capacity and effort—that is, their actual or potential value for grant-in-aid use—was a major objective of ACIR studies. Although federal grants made directly to local governments had been multiplying in variety and dollar amount, these federal/local aid arrangements, unlike some important federal/state grant programs, do not provide for any differentiation between jurisdictions of relatively low capacity or high effort.

---

[39] Advisory Commission on Intergovernmental Relations. *Measuring the Fiscal Capacity and Effort of State and Local Areas.* Washington, D.C., U.S. Government Printing Office, 1971.

Because an organized body of statistics to reflect the relative fiscal capacity of local governments is lacking, it has been necessary to disregard such differences. If, however, meaningful comparative measures of fiscal capacity and effort can be developed for local jurisdictions, then new policy options might be available for the design and administration of federal/local grants. The commission has concluded that these measures can be developed.

The process of estimating the tax capacity of particular areas involves the following steps:

1. Determine the inclusiveness of the term *taxes;* decide which tax classes should be handled separately.

2. Review current state and local practices with regard to each type of tax to ascertain its predominant or representative form.

3. Locate tax-base data for each tax or, in the absence of such data, assemble quantitative information about some measure that could reasonably be taken to represent the actual base.

4. Obtain an average rate for each tax by dividing its nationwide yield by the nationwide base or its proxy.

5. Calculate the capacity (potential yield of each tax class for particular states, SMSAs, and counties) by applying the average rate to the base measure for such areas.

6. Add capacity figures thus developed for particular taxes in each area to arrive at the area's total tax capacity.[40]

Certain ACIR studies have led to the concept of "fiscal blood pressure," which uses a two-dimensional measure. The numerator, equivalent to the systole, is an indexed position on a ranked scale of current tax effort. The value for the median state is set at 100, and all other states are assigned an index number relative to that median value. For instance, if state A has a tax-effort value of 11.91 and the median state has a tax-effort value of 10.44, the index value of state A is 114.

The denominator, equivalent to the diastole, indicates the relative change in tax effort over a period of time. The index number for rate of change in tax effort is established by the procedure used for systolic indexing. Thus, if the rate of change in state A was 0.982, versus a median value of 0.685, state A's diastolic index value would be 143. As

---

[40]This procedure is described in detail in Advisory Commission on Intergovernmental Relations, *Measuring the Fiscal "Blood Pressure" of the States—1964–1975,* Washington, D.C., 1977; also discussed in the report are procedures for measuring revenue efforts and the capacity of nontax revenue sources.

a result, state A would have a fiscal blood pressure of 114/143. Table 18 illustrates these computations.

The important issue here is interpreting these data. A reading such as the one in the preceding example shows that state A is somewhat above the national median in current tax effort and that, over a specified period of time, the rate of tax-effort increase has been substantially above the rate of change in the median state. This latter time dimension is of considerable importance, since such a trend may cause local tax-payers and multistate corporations to perceive the tax burden in such a state as being much heavier than an equivalent current tax effort in a state with a downward trend.

These perceptions can influence policymakers concerned with the feasibility of financing additional health services activities. A state with a high fiscal blood pressure might be inclined to seek financial support from the private sector as an alternative to increasing public sector expenditures on health services delivery.

Programs

Health programs are compilations of resources directed at specific goals. In economic terms, this means that, in the long run, all programs can be viewed as manpower, funding, and facilities (land and buildings). For planning purposes, however, it is more useful to examine existing programs as programs per se rather than as resources. In the short run, programs cannot be broken into groups of resources that can be reallocated to other uses.

The assessment of programs for the planning process should consist of an inventory, a market service and competition analysis, and a centrality analysis. The inventory identifies those programs available to the community or in competition with the institution. The market service and competition analyses establish the linkage between programs and populations and identify those programs competing for service. The centrality analysis examines the programs against the community's or institution's health services delivery objectives.

Institutions need to identify programs as a part of their strategic planning and management process (as mentioned in Chapters 1 and 5). Likewise, programs tend to offer a limited range of related services and thus are the focus of market segmentation and service area activities as well.

PROGRAM INVENTORY

Perhaps the major problem encountered in the inventory of programs within a community or institution is the definition of what comprises a

TABLE 18   A Two-Dimensional Measure of Relative State-Local Fiscal Pressure Using Resident Personal Income to Estimate Fiscal Capacity (1964–1975)*

State	Own-Source Taxes as a Percentage of Income, 1975† (1)	Index (2)	Rank (3)	Average Annual Rate of Change in Tax Effort, 1964–1975 (percent per year)‡ (4)	Index (5)	Rank (6)	A Two-Dimensional Fiscal Pressure Index (7)
United States Median	11.10	100		1.033	100		
New England							
Maine	12.30	111	9	1.486	144	19	111/144
New Hampshire	10.25	92	38	1.565	152	18	92/152
Vermont	14.67	132	2	1.873	181	12	132/181
Massachusetts	13.86	125	3	2.935	284	2	125/284
Rhode Island	11.45	103	16	1.854	179	13	103/179
Connecticut	10.36	93	34	1.769	171	15	93/171
Mideast							
New York	16.17	146	1	3.069	297	1	146/297
New Jersey	11.18	101	22	2.670	258	5	101/258
Pennsylvania	11.13	100	25	2.134	207	11	100/207
Delaware	11.17	101	24	2.690	260	4	101/260
Maryland	11.70	105	15	2.536	245	7	105/245
District of Columbia	10.23	92	39	2.196	213	10	92/213

SOURCE: Advisory Commission on Intergovernmental Relations. *Measuring the Fiscal "Blood Pressure" of the States—1964–1975.* Washington, D.C., 1977.

*ACIR staff estimates based on U.S. Department of Commerce, Office of Business Economics, *Survey of Current Business,* various years; and U.S. Bureau of the Census, *Governmental Finances,* various years.

†Income is the average of resident personal income for calendar years 1974 and 1975.

‡Average annual rate of change in the ratio of total state and local taxes to resident personal income.

program. The problem is often one of scope. For example, it might be possible to identify a hospital as a program within the community. Yet that hospital is made up of numerous departments and services that might be identified as programs. Even a department within the hospital might comprise several programs.

The initial task for the planner, then, is to establish the level of program definition that is appropriate for the planning process being undertaken. This usually will result in a series of definitions that will vary in scope. In one case, acute inpatient medical care might be defined as a program. This definition is rather broad and includes a number of services. On the other hand, body scanning, which is limited to the application of two or three technologies, might also be defined as a program. The difference in these two cases is oriented toward the planner's concerns and objectives. Acute inpatient medical care might be an adequate definition for the planner to deal with inpatient medical beds. Because body scanning makes use of expensive high technology and because the community planning process includes some certificate-of-need requirements, the planner will define the program in a much narrower fashion.

Many of the definitions of programs within a community have been established through tradition, regulation, or previous planning effort. Certainly, these all are useful starting places, but the planner must constantly be aware of changes in the delivery system that might make it necessary to change definitions of "program." Changes in the methods of delivering services or changes in major technology that are identified in the environmental assessment will often suggest impending changes in program scope.

Having defined a set of services or programs, the next step is to identify where those services are available in the community. In most cases this is not difficult. Problems can arise, however, when tabulating some services or programs that might be located in private business or in physicians' offices. Some laboratory and radiology services are also a problem to locate. Unfortunately, there is no good method short of persistent investigation to identify these programs.

Market Service and Competition Analysis

The health planner needs to link specific programs to the populations they serve. The previous discussion on service-area definition is important here. Because the various programs within one institution may serve different populations, it is essential that these linkages be as clear as possible.

Many issues in community health planning revolve around access to services and the distribution of resources within the community. The market service analysis helps the planner focus on these issues. Unfortunately, the planner must consider more than the simple access or availability of services to the community. The institutions providing services must be concerned with economies of scale and cost considerations to remain viable. Thus, the community planner, like the institutional planner, must become concerned with market shares and competition.

Having identified the market and/or market segments[41] linked to the programs in the inventory, the planner should examine the competitive situation within the market. The purpose of this analysis is to make the planner and decision makers aware of competitive situations that could be or should be affected by implementation decisions. This information is important and useful in the action analysis phase of the planning process and in the marketing phase of the implementation process.

Centrality Analysis

A useful portion of the programs assessment process is the centrality analysis. In an institutional planning setting, this is the process of examining the degree to which individual programs are central to the mission, goals, and objectives of the organization.[42] The purpose of the institutional process is to determine whether scarce resources are being directed toward programs that are less central to the organization at the expense of programs that are critical (central) to the organization's mission. The analysis is usually combined with some form of viability measure, such as profitability or market penetration, to determine which programs should be eliminated from the organization and which should be promoted. The organization will want to keep programs that are highly central and highly viable and delete programs that are neither central nor viable.

This concept can be applied in the community setting by examining the degree to which various programs are central to the concerns, missions, and/or objectives of the planning body. The concept of viabil-

---

[41]Market segmentation is defined in many marketing texts. A discussion of segmentation in health care can be found in Richard M. Reese, William W. Stanton, and James M. Daley, "Identifying Market Segments Within the Health Care Delivery System," *Journal of Health Care Marketing, 2*(3):10–23, Summer 1982.
[42]Another similar technique is portfolio analysis. See R. E. MacStravic, Edward Mahn, and Deborah C. Reedal, "Portfolio Analysis for Hospitals," *Health Care Management Review, 8*(4):69–76, Fall 1983.

ity might be replaced with the degree of market penetration, allowing the planner to focus attention on those programs that are central to the planning agency's concerns and that consume significant amounts of resources.

Other strategies can be developed with this technique. Centrality could be compared directly with cost, and it could be compared with quality (assuming adequate measures were agreed on). Likewise, accessibility or acceptability could be used.

In Chapter 10, there is a discussion of priority setting. In some ways, centrality analysis is similar to priority setting in that it results in a determination of which programs are more central and, hence, more important to the planning process. As it is proposed here, it becomes a method for focusing the planner's analysis of programs.

SUMMARY

Internal analysis is the process by which the planner examines the community or market and the resources and programs serving that market. The desired outcome is an inventory and analysis of the relationship between a population and the services being consumed by that population. When this is combined with the environmental assessment, the planner has established the base of information needed to examine the alternative actions available to the planning agency.

10

DEVELOPING AND SELECTING ALTERNATIVES

DEVELOPMENT OF OBJECTIVES

Chapter 8, on policies, goals, objectives, and actions, described the sequence of events leading from policy planning (policies on policy-making, strategic policies, and operating policies), to strategic planning (mission, goals, general and functional strategies, and systems and subsystems), to operational planning (objectives, programs, and resources). As defined in that chapter, an objective is a measurable level of accomplishment that is to be achieved prior to some established date. Each objective is designed to support the eventual attainment of at least one of the organization's goals. If planners have successfully incorporated the concept of synergy, however, an objective will likely aid in the attainment of several goals. Just as goals may be supported by multiple objectives, objectives may be based in more than one program.

DEVELOPMENT OF ALTERNATIVE PROGRAMS

There is seldom a single best way to achieve any given objective. For instance, a reduction in the mortality rate among accident victims could be achieved by improving the response time of emergency vehicles, by enhancing the qualifications of the emergency vehicle crew members, by increasing the sophistication of the equipment in the emergency vehicles, or by some combination of these options. Similarly, there are usually several options for improving response time, such as increasing the number of emergency vehicles, dispersing the emergency vehicles, or improving the communications system.

The planner's challenge, then, is to design the full range of feasible alternatives and to choose a preferred alternative or combination of alternatives. The two general approaches to design are the synthetic approach and the analytic approach.

In the synthetic approach, the designer attempts to identify all of the possible components and then all of their reasonable combinations. Brainstorming and other "creativity stimulating" techniques (e.g., the nominal group technique[1]) are often used for this. A more systematic method, which is likelier to minimize the number of oversights that can occur with unstructured creativity exercises, is morphological analysis.[2] In either case, the designer must combine the basic elements to form subsystems that can be integrated into successively larger systems until the level of the program system is reached.

In the analytic approach, the designer begins with a general system to achieve multiple goals, which include the goal of the program that is being designed. The larger system is subdivided into the subsystems that achieve these multiple goals. This, then, provides the context within which the subsystem to be designed must function. In succeeding steps, that subsystem is divided and redivided into smaller and smaller subsystems until the designer reaches the level of the black box. The black boxes are then used as the building blocks that can be recombined in a variety of ways to form the alternative programs.[3]

Regardless of which approach is selected, the individual subsystems can be examined to determine their performance characteristics and their feasibility. This allows the designer to select a preferred configuration for each subsystem. At the lower levels, it is often possible to use relatively simple OR (operations research) techniques, such as transportation models, to assist in the identification of the "best" configuration. As more and more subsystems are combined, the relationships often become so complex that they require a different type of model. This is usually referred to as an operational flow model, which portrays the flow of resources from input, through the various transformation processes, to output as the good or service that the system is designed to produce.

---

[1]André L. Delbecq, Andrew H. Van de Ven, and David H. Gustafson. *Group Techniques for Program Planning: A Guide to Nominal Group and Delphi Processes.* Glenview, Ill. Scott, Foresman, 1975.

[2]Richard H. Turley et al. "Morphological Analysis for Health Care Systems Planning." *Socio-Economic Planning Science,* 9:83–88, 1975.

[3]Bernard H. Rudwick. *Systems Analysis for Effective Planning.* New York, Wiley, 1969.

Ascertaining Feasibility

The data developed from such a model are the first ingredient of the feasibility testing process. They tell the designer whether the system as structured is likely to achieve the program's objective. Following are questions that must be asked during the feasibility analysis:

1. Will this system clearly be unacceptable to the stakeholders? An alternative should not be rejected merely because there may be some objections to it, but if it would be illegal or obviously in conflict with local customs and mores, it should not be pursued unless it has some dramatic advantage over other alternatives, including the option of no action.

2. Will the required technology be available by the time of implementation? At the time of this writing, for instance, a system including a totally paperless office would have to be regarded as infeasible for an objective with a completion date of 1985.

3. Will the necessary staff be available? This involves an examination of both the quantity and qualifications of persons who could be recruited for the operation of the proposed alternative.

4. Will the cost be reasonable? The designer might not yet have data on what such a system would cost for a specific community, but it is usually possible to estimate the approximate cost per unit of output to determine that it will be below some threshold of reasonable charges for a good or service of the type being planned.

Estimating Requirements

Once the feasibility of various alternatives has been ascertained, it becomes worthwhile to prepare a more detailed analysis of how each would function within the environment for which the program is being developed. The first step is to estimate requirements. This encompasses both service requirements and resource requirements. The service requirements are determined from market analysis and then an estimate is made of the resources required to provide that level of service. Ideally, resource requirements will be expressed as life-cycle costs to ensure that the full impact of each alternative is recognized. These estimates of requirements then become key inputs to cost-benefit analyses, which allow the designer to discard those alternatives that would be detrimental to the stakeholders. The remaining alternatives are placed in priority sequence to determine how available resources should be allocated among them.

Definition of "Requirement"

The term *requirement* is used here to circumvent the problems that arise in describing the concepts of "need" and "demand" (which also are discussed here). Moreover, it is a useful term because it focuses on two key factors in health planning: services and resources.

Ideally, requirements are derived from goals and objectives, which flow from the general policy statements in a health system plan. The planning process should begin by identifying the services required to improve health status. When such an approach is not possible, the planners should define the health services that are consistent with a community's values and assumptions without regard for a causal link between health services and health status. In other words, they should look to the community to establish the standards it expects the health services system to meet. Those standards will include specific statements about the quantities of various services that are required, usually under the heading of availability. Whether the service requirements are based on an analysis of health status or are simply a response to community value statements, the level of these requirements should reflect the needs of the population to be served rather than the needs of a specific institution or agency.[4]

The resource requirements (personnel, equipment, facilities, and money) should be derived from the service requirements whenever possible. In community planning, however, it may not be feasible to aggregate the various resources needed to produce all of the services planned, either because the process is incomplete or because there is not enough information about resource productivity. In those cases, planners must somehow relate resource requirements to population characteristics. This usually is done through a ratio method as described in Chapter 8.

Finally, planners must translate the resource requirements expressed in numbers of people, facilities, pieces of equipment, and so forth, into dollar terms, since dollars are necessary to acquire and use the other resources.

Need, Demand, and Requirements

Need is usually defined as a professional determination of the health services or resources that a community or group of people should have

---

[4]John E. Wennberg. "Using Localized Population-Based Data in Evaluating Planning Problems." In: *The Priorities of Section 1502.* Washington, D.C., U.S. Government Printing Office, January 1977, pp. 78–91. (HRA 77–641.) Wennberg demonstrates the great variability in utilization patterns of institutions serving essentially similar populations.

to achieve and maintain adequate health status. Demand, on the other hand, is what consumers want, and effective demand is what they can and will pay for. These two concepts, need and demand, are often quite different, and utilization data, a common proxy for demand, actually reflect effective demand. The latter is the focus of the plans of individual health services organizations.

Figure 26 represents the relationship between need and effective demand. The shaded intersection of the circles is where need and demand are identical. In many situations, this overlap is nearly total; however, there almost certainly will be some difference between the two, such as when consumers are unwilling to pay for all the medical services physicians think are needed or when they want services that physicians feel are unnecessary or inappropriate. The latter case is exemplified by the demand by seemingly healthy young adults for annual physical examinations. Figure 27 shows the effects of economic barriers by indicating that total demand is substantially greater than effective demand. Furthermore, much of the increase in the "total demand" circle overlaps the "need" circle, suggesting that many of the people who would demand health services but are prevented from doing so by financial barriers are regarded by professionals as those most in need of care. Total demand may be only an academic concept, with little relevance to the planner's day-to-day activities, unless the planner hopes to change the nation's economic system by removing most of the financial barriers to health care.

Institutional planners in particular will focus on effective demand since the development of service capacity that is underutilized could lead to economic losses, perhaps even to bankruptcy. In fact, the

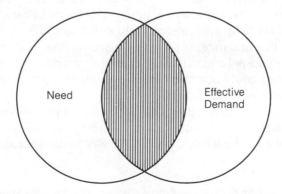

Figure 26   Need and effective demand.

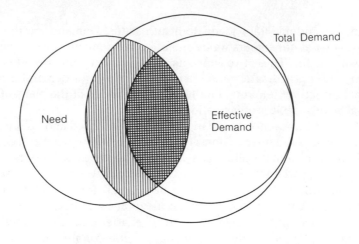

Figure 27   Need, effective demand, and total demand.

institutional planners will need specific policy guidance on whether capacity should be limited to the amount of service for which reimbursement can be expected.

Although health services utilization data reflect effective demand, they can be used as a basis for estimating need and uncovering latent demand that could become the focus of a growth strategy. The data should be collected from a sample survey within the target community by well-qualified professionals. This was done in the late 1960s in Rochester, New York, where a team of professionals visited a sample of community residents to assess their actual health status and to determine whether they were receiving appropriate levels of care.[5] Planners can use the data from such a sample to construct ratios for an entire community. For instance, if planners discover that within a certain population only 75 percent of those needing a particular type of care are receiving it, they could determine need by multiplying the current utilization by a factor of 1.33 (i.e., 100 ÷ 75).

Holloway and his colleagues have proposed an improved, 10-step method for carrying out such a study.[6] Their proposal is intended to deal with some of the weaknesses in the Rochester approach. At this

[5]Walter Wenkert, John G. Hill, and Robert L. Berg. "Concepts and Methodology in Planning Patient Care Services." *Medical Care, 7*(4):327, July–August 1969.
[6]Don C. Holloway et al. "Determining Appropriate Levels of Care." In: *The Priorities of Section 1502,* pp. 92–101.

writing, however, they have published no reports on the application of their method.

In general, requirements can be estimated as follows:

1. Multiply the population at risk by the appropriate requirement factor[7] to obtain the service requirement.
2. Divide the service requirement by the unit productivity measure for the resource involved to determine the resource requirement.
3. Multiply the resource requirement by acquisition and operating costs to determine financial requirements.

Service Requirements

Ambulatory service requirements usually are defined in terms of an encounter or visit. Ancillary services, such as laboratory and x-ray, are computed on the basis of a ratio, usually historical, between the basic unit of service and the use of the ancillary service. The "visit requirement" can be based on either total population or subgroups. For subgroups, both the size and the service-usage rates of the subgroup must be known. Although this combination of data frequently is not available, every effort should be made to obtain it whenever possible, because it can reflect significant variations. For instance, in the case of office visits to physicians, the national rate in 1975 was 2.7 visits per person per year, but, for people 65 and older, the rate was 4.3 visits per person per year. There were equally important differences based on such factors as sex and race.[8] An interesting variation on the ratio approach has been proposed by Pollack.[9] Rather than relying only on population size, he proposes the construction of a set of indicators for ranking various communities. For instance, in estimating requirements for mental health services, some of the factors considered are the percentage of households with only one person, those headed by women, the percentage of divorced or separated men, and so forth.

---

[7]The requirement factor should take into account the possibility of future changes in service delivery (e.g., when ambulatory surgery is substituted for inpatient surgery). An illustration of this can be found in John R. Griffith and Robert A. Chernow, "Cost Effective Acute Care Facilities Planning in Michigan," *Inquiry,* *14*(3):235–238, September 1977.

[8]U.S. Department of Health, Education, and Welfare, National Center for Health Statistics. *Ambulatory Medical Care Rendered in Physician's Office in the United States, 1975.* Advance Data from NCHS Vital and Health Statistics No. 12. Washington, D.C., 1977, p.7.

[9]Earl S. Pollack. *Mental Health Demographic Profile for Health Services Planning.* Statistical Notes for Health Planners No. 4. Washington, D.C., U.S. Department of Health, Education, and Welfare, 1977.

This allows a ranking of communities based on need for service. Next, some measure of service availability is obtained, and the same communities are ranked on that basis. An analysis of the relation between the measures of need and service availability should provide a basis for ranking areas according to unmet needs for health services.

Pollack states that there are many ways to conduct such an analysis and proposes one based on a regression equation designed to predict expected resource availability given the index of need previously computed. This expected rate is then compared to the actual resource rate to produce a ratio. When the ratio is greater than 1.0, the community has fewer resources than it needs, given the probability of health problems that can be inferred from its population characteristics.

Inpatient services also are measured in terms of encounters, which are called *admissions*. Since these encounters are of relatively long and widely variable duration, units of service usually are expressed as patient days. A typical approach to estimating inpatient service requirements is to multiply the population by the rate of admissions per 1,000 by the average length of stay. An alternative method is to multiply the population by the number of patient days per 1,000. For the community population as a whole, the end result of these calculations should be the same. Working with total population data is seldom desirable, however, because the rate and length of hospitalization vary considerably among age and sex groups. It is better to deal with small groups within a population and to consider the types of service they are likely to require. For instance, women of ages 15–44 have a relatively high rate of hospitalization and a very low average length of stay; this can be attributed to the number of admissions for obstetrical reasons.[10]

The difference between types of services is so great that it is undesirable to consider all hospital admissions as a homogeneous group. This is illustrated by comparing the average hospital stay for patients with complications related to pregnancy, childbirth, and the puerperium (3.7 days) with the average stay for all conditions (7.7 days). Not only is the 3.7-day stay lower than the average stay, it is lower than that for virtually every disease category. Furthermore, this set of conditions accounts for the highest rate of discharge in the U.S. population (373 per 10,000 compared with the next highest rate of 222.4 per 10,000 for diseases of the female genito-urinary system), or 12 percent of all

---

[10]U.S. Department of Health, Education, and Welfare, National Center for Health Statistics. *Persons Hospitalized by Number, Episode, and Days Hospitalized in a Year, United States—1972.* NCHS Vital and Health Statistics Series 10, No. 116. Washington, D.C., 1977, pp. 12, 27.

discharges.[11] The third largest group (5.4 percent of all discharges) is for heart disease victims, who have an average stay of 11.3 days.

When relating service requirements to a population, the planners need not restrict their consideration of that group to a single dimension. With other methods of analysis, they can consider many factors; specifically, they can use regression analysis, with independent variables such as age and sex, to obtain the expected number of bed days for each age/sex cohort and can sum these estimates to obtain the total bed days required.[12]

Crane[13] has described an unpublished report on the use of a ratio approach based on an unusually complex technique involving age and sex cohorts to which mortality rates are applied. Morbidity/service required ratios are then used to estimate service requirements.

VARIABILITY IN DEMAND

An approach that considers the number of admissions and the average length of stay, rather than simply the total number of bed days, is preferable for assessing service requirements. Length of stay has been declining rapidly since the advent of the medicare prospective price reimbursement system. Consequently, the effects of this variable should be considered explicitly in forecasts of patient day requirements. Furthermore, the length of stay is an important determinant of the variability in the daily level of service use. The following discussion of this variation is limited to inpatient service, since relatively small changes in demands for those services will produce a large percentage change in total demand. (Note, however, that demand variability also can be a significant factor in the requirement for ambulatory services, especially those for medical emergencies.) The variability in inpatient demand leads to occupancy rates of considerably less than 100 percent. This apparent inefficiency in resource use raises serious policy questions on appropriate standards for occupancy.

---

[11]U.S. Department of Health, Education, and Welfare, National Center for Health Statistics. *Inpatient Utilization of Short Stay Hospitals by Diagnosis, United States—1974.* NCHS Vital and Health Statistics Series 13, No. 30. Washington, D.C., 1977, p. 16.

[12]Rachel Doyle et al. "Estimating Hospital Use in Arkansas." *Public Health Reports,* 92(3):211–216, May 1977.

[13]Robert M. Crane. "Methods Used in Determining Health Service and Facility Requirements." In: *Health Regulation: Certificate of Need & 1122.* Edited by Herbert H. Hyman. Germantown, Md., Aspen Systems Corp., 1977, pp. 105–134.

OCCUPANCY RATES AS MEASURES OF VARIABILITY

Issues

Efficiency. Does a high occupancy rate necessarily reflect efficient use of beds? In general, the answer is yes; however, there is some evidence that, in the short run, occupancy rates and lengths of stay increase together.[14] Since increased length of stay might also cause increased revenue in a hospital with otherwise low occupancy rates, the increases in length of stay may be attributable to nonmedical factors.[15] Thus, to assure that an occupancy standard achieves its intended purpose, there should be a related criterion requiring analysis of medical necessity of hospital utilization.

Need. Although the occupancy rate may reflect efficient use of beds for those who are hospitalized, if used alone it may still mask inefficiencies. In other words, a measure of the use of an available hospital does not take into consideration the aggregate level of need in the service area. Patient days per 1,000 population is a widely used indicator of whether services are overused, are being used to meet legitimate demand, or are insufficient to meet the community's needs. If the rate of hospitalization days per 1,000 deviates widely from the expected rate, the supply of beds may be influencing the use rate in an undesirable way. Thus, this measure also should be used as a criterion in conjunction with the occupancy rate standard.

A related concern is the use of historical data as the basis for planning decisions, since planning supposedly affects the future. If there are likely to be substantial changes in the characteristics of the service area's population or in the practice of medicine, historical data are irrelevant except as a baseline for making a judgmental forecast of future events.

Measurement. There are two concerns in this category: the basis of measurement and the computational method.

A primary consideration regarding the basis of measurement is the distinction between licensed beds and staffed beds. If the number of licensed beds exceeds the number of staffed beds, the result will be a lower occupancy rate if licensed beds are the basis of measurement. If the number of licensed beds is equal to the number of beds that could

---

[14]Roice D. Luke and Melissa D. Culverwell. "Hospital Bed Availability and Discharge Patterns in the Short Run." *Inquiry, 17*:54–61, Spring 1980.

[15]Under a prospective price system with fixed amounts of reimbursement for episodes of hospitalization, there is an incentive to maximize reimbursement by reducing length of stay per admission (episode) and increasing the number of admissions.

realistically become staffed beds, the occupancy rate will be valid. If, on the other hand, the number of licensed beds includes some beds that could never be staffed beds (e.g., because ancillary services have expanded to the space allocated for the "phantom" beds), then the resulting occupancy rate will be an invalid measure.

The computational methods differ in their approaches to dealing with a major and fundamental problem: the variability in the level of demand for hospital services. The demand for hospitalization arises from incidence of disease and injury, which are largely random events. Some demand for hospitalization can be scheduled, but a substantial portion must be met immediately to prevent death, disability, or needlessly prolonged suffering. Consequently, industrial models of productivity and efficiency are inappropriate. The health services models presently available fall into four categories: expert judgment, theoretical distribution, empirical distribution, and controlled demand.

The expert judgment model is usually some variant of the Hill-Burton model, in which the annual productivity of a hospital bed is estimated to be some percentage of the 365 days in a year (e.g., 85 percent). The percentage represents the best judgment of the average number of days a hospital bed will be filled during a year if the total number of beds is sufficient to meet peak demand whenever that occurs. Historically, an additional 10 beds were added to the results obtained from this formula to account for special circumstances when the hospital would have unusually high relative demand. Shonick[16] developed the concept of relative demand, which shows that one occupancy level for all hospitals, regardless of size, clearly is inappropriate.

The widely used theoretical distribution model is based on the normal approximation of the Poisson distribution.[17] It is frequently referred to as the Normile method or the average daily census (ADC) method. Its basis is the assumption that the levels of demand will be approximately normally distributed around the ADC and that the frequency of various levels of demand can be estimated by using the standard deviation (defined as the square root of the ADC). For instance, in a normal distribution, 90 percent of all events will be below the level $ADC + 1.28 \cdot \sqrt{ADC}$. Consequently, if $ADC = 100$ and $\sqrt{100} = 10$, the demand for hospitalization 90 percent of the days in the year (328 days) would be 113 beds $(100 + [1.28 \cdot 10] = 112.8 \approx 113)$ or less.

---

[16]William Shonick. "Understanding the Nature of the Random Fluctuations of the Hospital Daily Census." *Medical Care, 10*:123, March–April 1972.
[17]Public Health Service Region VIII. "The Square Root Formula: A Tool for Estimating the Number of Hospital Beds Needed." Denver, Colo., January 1980. Mimeographed.

The proponents of the empirical distribution methods correctly point out that the demand for hospitalization is not completely random and that some portion can be scheduled. Since this invalidates or at least seriously weakens the estimates made with theoretical distribution models, the use of historical data is suggested. (It can be inferred that proponents of empirical distribution would agree to an adjustment of historical data to reflect anticipated changes in use patterns.) A good example of this is the work of Phillip.[18] His model is particularly interesting because it incorporates measures of both efficiency (use of available beds) and effectiveness (ability to meet the community's demands for service). It can only be used, however, when there are data on the number of people who wanted to enter the facility each day, including those turned away and those who did not seek admission due to overcrowding. (The latter group probably gained their knowledge of the hospital's overcrowding from their physicians.)

The best known of the controlled demand models was developed by Griffith and Chernow[19] and by Hancock and his colleagues[20,21,22,23] at the University of Michigan. It is a simulation model that recognizes both immediate and controllable demand. The controllable demand is subdivided into scheduled and call-in categories. It operates on the premise that occupancy levels can be maximized by minimizing the prescheduling of controllable admissions and using last minute call-ins of waiting controllable admissions to fill the gap between the total available beds and the number of beds required to satisfy the scheduled and immediate demand. Use of the scheduling system on which the model is based could make it possible to achieve much higher occupancies than when relying on the other models.[24]

Facility or Area. Demand peaks usually will not occur at all facilities at the same time. Consequently, fewer beds will be needed to meet peak demands if patients can be diverted from an overcrowded facility

---

[18]P. J. Phillip. "Some Considerations Involved in Determining Optimum Size of Specialized Hospital Facilities." *Inquiry, 6*:44–48, December 1969.

[19]John R. Griffith and Robert A. Chernow. "Cost Effective Acute Care Facilities Planning in Michigan." *Inquiry, 14*:229–239, September 1977.

[20]Walton M. Hancock et al. "Maximum Average Occupancy for Hospital Units, NCHSR-81-214." Ann Arbor, Mich., University of Michigan Press, 1980, pp. 156–158.

[21]_____. "Parameters Affecting Hospital Occupancy and Implications for Facility Sizing." *Health Services Research, 13*:276–289, Fall 1978.

[22]_____. "Simulation-Based Occupancy Recommendations for Adult Medical/Surgical Units Using Admissions Scheduling Systems." *Inquiry, 15*:25–32, March 1978.

[23]Walton M. Hancock and Paul F. Walter. *The "ACSC" Inpatient Admission Scheduling and Control System.* Ann Arbor, Mich., AUPHA Press, 1983.

[24]Walton M. Hancock et al. "Parameters Affecting Hospital Occupancy and Implications for Facility Sizing," p. 276.

to one that is experiencing only normal levels of demand. MacStravic[25] has shown, however, that for clusters of hospitals, the Poisson model consistently underestimates peaks of demand and that the underestimation becomes increasingly severe as the size of the total demand increases. To remedy this problem, he proposes a measure called the *synthetic standard deviation* to estimate peak demand within an area as opposed to peak demand for an individual institution.

Facility Size. Shonick's[26] concept of relative variability is the clearest exposition of the notion that the size of a facility is a significant factor in estimating the resources required to cope with the variability in demand. For instance, if the average variability is 10, the relative variability of a 100-bed institution would be 10 percent and the relative variability of a 500-bed institution would be 2 percent. This can also be seen by applying the ADC formula to a population needing an average of 80 beds per day. To meet the demand 95 percent of the time, it would be necessary to have 95 beds; if the same need were to be met by two separate facilities, 102 beds would be required:

ADC	$\sqrt{ADC}$	$ADC + (1.65 \cdot \sqrt{ADC})$	=	*Beds Needed*	*Percent Occupancy*
		ONE FACILITY			
80	8.94	$80 + (1.65 \cdot 8.94)$	=	95	84
		TWO FACILITIES			
40	6.32	$40 + (1.65 \cdot 6.32)$	=	51	78
40	6.32	$40 + (1.65 \cdot 6.32)$	=	51	78
	TOTAL			102	

Also see Table 19.

Bed Uses. The problems of adequately dealing with variability in demand are compounded when the beds under consideration are used for different purposes. In other words, the demand for some services is much more volatile than the demand for others. A typical example is obstetrical services, in which there is little opportunity for scheduling and in which the demand cannot be postponed. This situation is gener-

---

[25]R. E. MacStravic. "Areawide Fluctuations in Hospital Daily Census." *Medical Care, 17*: 1229–1237, December 1979.
[26]William Shonick. "Understanding the Nature of the Random Fluctuations of the Hospital Daily Census," p. 123.

TABLE 19   Interaction of Occupancy and Size

| | Required Occupancy | | | | | | | | |
	91.5 percent			90 percent			85 percent		
Number of Beds	130	230	330	130	230	330	130	230	330
ADC at Required Occupancy	119	210	302	117	207	297	111	196	281
Standard Deviation = $\sqrt{ADC}$	10.9	14.5	17.4	10.8	14.4	17.2	10.5	14.0	16.8
Beds − ADC	11	20	28	13	23	33	19	34	49
Number of S.D. = (Beds−ADC) ÷ $\sqrt{ADC}$	1.00	1.38	1.61	1.20	1.60	1.92	1.81	2.43	2.92
Percent of Total Demand that Could Be Met	84.1	91.6	94.6	88.5	94.5	97.3	96.5	99.3	99.8
Days per Year on Which Demand Could Not Be Met	58	31	20	42	20	10	13	3	1

ally recognized by establishing lower occupancy rates for obstetrical beds. Unfortunately, medical/surgical (M/S) beds are often treated as though they provide a homogeneous set of services, but this is not so. Some services, such as detoxification, have relatively long lengths of stay, and the admissions are often not of critical urgency. On the other hand, coronary care units (CCU) deal with life-threatening situations and, thus, must be able to meet virtually all demand as it occurs. Since the CCU beds are not interchangeable with standard M/S beds, there must be enough CCU beds to meet the peak demand. Consequently, average occupancy of CCU beds is relatively low; this, in turn, lowers the total average occupancy of all M/S beds (see Table 20).

Stability of Occupancy. Even if the standard is applied only to a more-or-less homogeneous type of bed, there is still a substantial amount of seasonal variability in demand that makes it difficult to attain a high average occupancy level. The term seasonal simply means within different time periods. Variability within a day can affect the "official" count of the midnight census. For instance, if a decision to discharge a patient is made late in the day, it may not be possible to prepare the room and contact an elective (call-in) admission on that day; consequently, the midnight census will be reduced by one. The weekend decline in census due to the wishes of patients and physicians is a widely realized phenomenon. Less widely discussed, but equally important, are the monthly/quarterly variations in admissions that are attributable to numerous factors such as the seasonal incidence of certain diseases. All of this variability, some of which is beyond the control of either clinicians or managers, means that to attain a high level of average occu-

TABLE 20   Results of Separate Consideration of Critical Care Beds

Bed Type	Number of Beds	ADC	Occupancy, in percent
Critical Care	18*	9	50
Adult Medical/ Surgical	112	110†	98†
Total	130	119	91.5

*Assumes 18 critical care beds must meet 99+ percent of urgent demand for this type of treatment ($18 = $ ADC $+ 3\sqrt{\text{ADC}}$ or $18 = 9 + 3\sqrt{9}$).
†These values are implicitly required to meet the standard of 91.5 percent overall occupancy when 18 of the 130 beds are allocated to critical care.

pancy, a hospital must be able to obtain and sustain very high levels of use at some time to offset the lower levels that inevitably occur.

Facility Configuration.   All of the models in use assume that each unfilled bed is available for occupancy. This actually is true only in the case of a facility with private rooms only. In this situation, the initial capital cost of the facility is relatively high and one could argue that staffing costs also would be higher than for a facility with multibed rooms. If the facility does not have all single rooms, then there will be occasions when empty beds cannot be filled (e.g., when one person in the room must be isolated; when the first occupant is of a different sex than the available admittee; when smoking preferences are taken into account for patient comfort).

Feasibility

The issues just discussed all bear on the feasibility of attaining a stipulated level of occupancy. (A minimum level of 90 percent frequently has been suggested as a standard for efficient use of hospital beds.) It is possible to examine feasibility more directly from theoretical and empirical perspectives. The theoretical perspective will be based on the models already identified.

The widely used Poisson model is the basis for the first phase of theoretical analysis. If different occupancy level requirements are applied to facilities of different sizes, it becomes evident that the required occupancy level and the facility size interact to produce significant changes in an institution's ability to meet demand. This is illustrated in Table 19, which shows that a smaller unit with a high level of average occupancy (130 beds at 91.5 percent) will probably be unable to meet total demand on 58 days out of each year, whereas a larger unit with a lower level of average occupancy (330 beds at 85 percent) will seldom be unable to meet the needs of its community. In other words, the net effect is that smaller communities that cannot support large facilities are placed at greater risk of being unable to meet peak demand when high average occupancy rates are required. Of course, these communities are often distant from other facilities, with the result that the diversion of a patient to another, less-crowded, facility becomes much more problematic.

Difficulty in meeting total demand can be dealt with by setting aside beds to meet urgent needs. The data for a typical community hospital can be used in simplified form to demonstrate the results of this approach. If the hospital's 130 M/S beds are divided into two groups (18 critical care and 112 M/S) and if it is assumed that there is a sufficient number of critical care beds to meet all urgent demand, the critical care beds will have an ADC of 9 for an occupancy rate of 50 percent. These computations and the effects on occupancy of M/S beds are shown in Table 20. The most significant effect is the extraordinarily high occupancy rate (98 percent) for the M/S beds that must be maintained to achieve the desired average overall occupancy of 91.5 percent. Also, it must be noted that since the difference between 100-percent occupancy in M/S beds (112) and the implicitly required occupancy (110) is only two beds, there must be at least one day on which all beds are filled to compensate for each occasion when there is a decline of more than 2 percent in ADC. For instance, if the weekend census dropped from 110 to 108, then the hospital would have to be completely filled at least 104 weekdays (52 weekends × 2 days per weekend) throughout the year. In other words, on 40 percent of the weekdays the facility would be unable to accommodate peaks in demand for M/S admissions except by inappropriately placing the M/S patient in a vacant critical care bed, if one were available; canceling scheduled M/S admissions, if the urgent need were known before the scheduled patients had actually been admitted; prematurely discharging other M/S patients; or setting up extra beds "in the halls."

Obviously, none of these alternatives is desirable, and, therefore, efforts have been made to overcome the sort of difficulties illustrated by devising managerial methods to control the flow of patients. This requires a more complex model that takes into account the various categories of demand for hospital services and attempts to meet all urgent demand while maintaining high occupancy by managing the flow of nonurgent admissions. The most promising and best known of these models was developed by Hancock and his colleagues.[27,28] They assert that their scheduling procedure makes it possible to attain higher levels of occupancy than would be possible "with any other presently documented admissions system."[29] They support this assertion with impressive data from simulation runs and from several sites where the system has been implemented. They do, however, stress that these levels can be achieved only if certain assumptions are met. The implications[30] of

---

[27]Walton M. Hancock and Paul F. Walter. *The "ASCS" Inpatient Admission Scheduling and Control System.*

[28]John R. Griffith and Robert A. Chernow. "Cost Effective Acute Care Facilities Planning in Michigan," p. 237.

[29]Walton M. Hancock and Paul F. Walter. *The "ASCS" Inpatient Admission Scheduling and Control System,* p. V-64.

[30]Walton M. Hancock et al. "Maximum Average Occupancy for Hospital Units, NCHSR-81-214," pp. 156–158.

these assumptions are that the attainable maximum occupancy increases as

1. Unit bed size increases
2. Percentage of emergency admissions decreases
3. Percentage of scheduled (as opposed to call-in) admissions decreases
4. Acceptable level of turnaways increases
5. Acceptable level of cancellations increases

It is significant that the simulation runs which demonstrated these levels of occupancy apparently did not take into account seasonal variations in demand, except for holidays.

A final and extremely important factor affecting the feasibility of the scheduling system is acceptance. To fulfill the assumptions underlying Hancock's high levels of achievement, it is necessary to change radically the behavior and expectations of patients, physicians, and hospital staff. Student's[31] account of attempts to do this, however, is rather discouraging. Still, his report is now somewhat dated, and, consequently, it can only be suggested that, even in the best of circumstances, full implementation of this system is a long and difficult process. In today's environment, with its emphasis on competition between health services providers, it is also necessary to ask whether an institution or administrator implementing such an unpopular course of action could survive.

The last phase of the feasibility analysis presents a summary of empirical evidence gleaned from a survey of state and local health plans and several analyses of data from a typical community hospital.

The validity of results obtained from models is often suspect due to the simplified assumptions used, such as those enumerated for the Hancock model. Thus, it is useful to verify results by an examination of actual experience. Several representative studies and 46 plan documents developed by typical planning agencies were surveyed for this purpose.

One study was conducted by a state agency in Florida. Florida established its occupancy standards on the basis of a lengthy study process

---

[31]For example, see Kurt R. Student, "Understanding Changes in the Hospital," in: *Cost Control in Hospitals,* edited by John R. Griffith et al., Ann Arbor, Mich., Health Administration Press, 1976, pp. 372–384.

completed with the help of a nationally renowned consulting firm.[32,33] A standard average occupancy rate of 80 percent was adopted with the observation that "It is very likely that standards established for maximum access time or patient flow patterns will in some cases conflict with minimum service volume desired."[34] In this instance, Florida gave priority to accessibility and established a travel time standard for 90 percent of the population of 30 minutes in urban areas and 45 minutes in rural areas.[35] Georgia's approach exhibits even greater concern for flexibility to adapt standards to local situations. First, it uses several quantitative models and then a normative approach to adapt the results to local needs in such a way that there are explicit policy decisions concerning the appropriate use rate and its effects on other characteristics of the health services system.[36]

The plans included in this survey represent the current best judgment of health planning agencies in 12 northeastern states. No agency established a standard higher than 90 percent for M/S occupancy and only eight agencies (17 percent) used the 90-percent level. These eight were all located in New York or Massachusetts, and the documents show that in most cases the 90-percent standard was accompanied by provisions for adjustments (e.g., for nonurban or nonteaching hospitals or both). In several instances where data were provided, they indicated that a 90-percent occupancy rate frequently could not be sustained, even in large institutions.[37,38]

In summary, a survey of the products of a substantial number of planning agencies showed that

1. There is widespread agreement that an occupancy rate standard should be established only after its interactions with other factors are explicitly considered.

---

[32]Kathryn J. Brown et al. "Beyond Hill-Burton: The Development of an Improved Acute Care Need Methodology in Florida." Tallahassee, Fla., Department of Health, 1979. Mimeographed.

[33]Florida Bed Need Task Force. "Recommended Acute Care Facility Need Methodology: Final Report." Tallahassee, Fla., February 1978.

[34]Ibid., p. 55.

[35]Kathryn J. Brown et al. "Beyond Hill-Burton: The Development of an Improved Acute Care Need Methodology in Florida," p. 29.

[36]Paul R. Justison. "Bed Requirements Methods and Processes." Denver, Colo., PACT Health Planning Center, February 1979, p. 3.

[37]NY-Penn HSA. *HSP 1981–1986*. Appendix. December 1980, p. 217.

[38]"Report and Recommendations of the Finger Lakes Health Systems Agency, Part 709.2, Task Force on 1985 Bed Need in the Southern Tier, Appendix B." Rochester, N.Y., August 25, 1982, pp. 9–10. Mimeographed.

2. The highest level set is 90 percent, and this level has been adopted only by a small number of the agencies surveyed.

3. Even when the 90-percent level is used (with appropriate adjustments), it frequently has not been achieved.

Resource Requirements

Resource requirements are based on service requirements during a certain period of time, divided by resource productivity during a comparable period. For example, if a service requirement is expressed as the number of bed days during a year, this number would be divided by 365 days to determine the number of beds actually required. Thus, if 36,500 bed days were required during the year, then 100 beds would be needed. This assumes that the beds would be used every day of the year, and, as we know, this is not likely to be the case. Consequently, there must be some adjustment for resource productivity.

FACILITIES

In the case of facilities, particularly inpatient facilities, the preceding discussion on service requirements essentially describes the major steps in estimating the number of beds actually required, with one important exception: "Market share" is discussed in Chapter 9, on pp. 227–236.

It is important to consider the effects of the migration of patients between service areas, especially for tertiary services. The same effects apply, although in a smaller percentage of cases, to primary and secondary care activities. Planners, therefore, must consider the relevance of the service for the community and also must estimate the amount of demand from persons who live outside the service area. Following are the factors involved in computing resource requirements for a health services facility:

1. Population served.
2. Market share of that population.
3. The service use rate per period of time by that population.
4. Duration of service.
5. The portion of service duration during which the specific facility is used. For example, in the case of a hospital admission, the patient might spend part of a hospital stay in an intensive care unit and the remainder in a medical bed. The planner would need to know the distri-

bution of this activity to identify precisely the needs for different types of services.

6. A complex set of factors affecting the variability of resource use.

Frequently, all of these factors are subsumed in a single occupancy rate. As illustrated previously, however, this is generally a mistake, because a uniform occupancy rate leads to inappropriate estimates of facility use levels. Other factors that planners should consider explicitly include the distribution of arrivals or demands for the service, the duration of the service, the amount of waiting time that is acceptable, the risk of not meeting emergency demands for service, the portion of the demand that cannot be postponed, the size of the facility, the level of use required for satisfactory financial results (i.e., to exceed the break-even point of operation), and a facility's productivity for a year. This is measured by multiplying the number of days during the year that the facility would be in use by the number of services that could be produced during each day of use. For example, a clinic facility used five days per week, 52 weeks per year, with an average of 200 visits per day, would have a productivity of 52,000 visits. Such a facility would be adequate for a population of approximately 10,000 people who, on the average, needed or demanded 5.2 ambulatory care visits per person per year. The entire population could be served by this facility so long as there were no large variations in the daily level of demand for services.

PERSONNEL

For health manpower, seven specific planning approaches have been identified.[39] The first is the *resource-to-population ratio,* mentioned on p. 215. Although generally regarded as the least satisfactory approach, it is probably the one predominantly used, mainly because the data needed for the other methods are not available.

The second approach, called *service targets,* computes manpower requirements by multiplying the population size by the number of services per person required during a given period of time, then dividing the product by the productivity per unit of manpower during the same time period.

[39]U.S. Department of Health, Education, and Welfare, Bureau of Health Planning and Resources Development. *Methodological Approaches for Determining Health Manpower Supply and Requirements.* Vol. II. Health Planning Methods and Technology Series No. 2. Washington, D.C., U.S. Government Printing Office, 1976, pp. 36–93.

The *health needs approach,* a variant of the service targets method, assumes that the planner can identify all conditions requiring health services. The manpower requirement is computed by multiplying the population served by the number of conditions occurring per year. This product is multiplied by the number of services required for each person experiencing that condition, and that product is multiplied by the average time required to provide each service. The final product is divided by the time worked each year by the average member of the manpower pool being considered (e.g., the average physician).

The fourth approach, *budgeted vacancies,* assumes that most health manpower requirements exist within large organizations that prepare formal budgets and are willing to reveal them to decision makers. For personnel who are unlikely to be employed outside of institutions, this crude approach may be satisfactory, but, in general, it has several major weaknesses. First, institutions vary considerably in the content of their budgets, with some using budgets as rigorous control documents and others using them as "wish lists." Second, when providers are competing, they are unlikely to be willing to release budgetary data for public consumption. Finally, there are few occupations that are employed entirely within large institutions that prepare budgets.

The fifth method, *constant utilization rate with changing population,* estimates future personnel requirements by multiplying current manpower by a ratio of present to forecast utilization. In effect, this approach assumes that current utilization rates will prevail in the future. Thus, these rates are multiplied by both current and future population subgroups, with results summed for the two categories. The ratio between present and future population is multiplied by the present manpower supply to determine what future personnel requirements will be.

This method assumes that the present manpower supply is adequate and is being used efficiently. Also, if one assumes a uniform usage rate over all parts of the population, the ratio will simply become the size of the forecast population to the size of the present population. The hazards of making such an estimate have been discussed (see *Simple projection,* p. 159), and it is hoped that population forecasts will at least indicate the size of the different age cohorts within that population.

The sixth personnel planning approach is similar to the fifth, except that it assumes changing income rates and then hypothesizes that those changes will affect usage rates. This approach requires a consideration of the income elasticity of demand, as well as changes in the size of the population subgroups. The necessary statistical analysis is complex and is probably infeasible for widespread use at present because of the lack of reasonable data for making estimates of the income elasticity of demand.

The seventh method is called the *industry occupational matrix*. It is useful only for total manpower requirements or for a few of the large categories identified by the Bureau of Labor Statistics (BLS). It requires the use of BLS data on total employment and ratio of categories of health manpower to total manpower. This method might be useful for checking the feasibility of large expansions of manpower requirements in the following way:

1. Determine the historical ratio between the health manpower category the planner is concerned with and the number of persons in the work force during the same period of time.
2. Multiply this ratio by the size of the work force projected for the planning horizon.
3. Compare the results of this process with the estimated requirements for the manpower category to determine whether the projected requirements will substantially exceed the number of persons in that occupation who would be in the work force if the historical relationships prevailed.

The seven methods just described generally assume a constant level of productivity for each type of health manpower. Since this is unlikely to be the case, the planner must consider the following factors that could affect the productivity of any health manpower category: substitution of other types of personnel, organizational changes, quality changes in the manpower itself, substitution of capital for personnel, greater patient involvement in the provision of health services, changes in reimbursement schemes, and changes in technology.[40]

DOLLAR REQUIREMENTS

Health facilities and personnel become available as community resources only to the extent that the community has the financial ability to acquire those resources. Consequently, the final step in the process of estimating resource requirements is to translate facilities and manpower requirements into dollar requirements. Decision makers must understand that dollar requirements involve both capital outlays and operating costs. Frequently, decisions are based on only one of these factors. For instance, decisions to build hospitals are often made on the basis of their initial or capital cost without regard for the need to provide

---

[40]Jack Hadley. "Research on Health Manpower Productivity: A General Overview." In: *Health Manpower and Productivity*. Edited by John Rafferty. Lexington, Mass., D. C. Heath, 1974, pp. 143–203.

funds for their operation after the construction process has been completed. Similarly, in the case of personnel, decision makers frequently overlook the capital cost involved in training and consider only the operating costs represented by wages or salaries. The incidence of these costs may be shifted from the group represented by the decision maker, but, nevertheless, a valid analysis of the resource requirements should take into account total cost.

The method for doing this is called *life-cycle costing*. It has only recently been adapted to the needs of the health services industry.[41] The concept is particularly important because it allows decision makers to make significant trade-offs between capital and operating costs and to choose the alternative that, in the long term, will result in the lowest total cost for the community. For instance, although building a more expensive structure (e.g., one with interstitial space for utility maintenance and modification) might represent a larger investment at the outset of a project, it could, over the life of the facility, result in savings in operating costs because the savings resulting from the ease with which utilities can be maintained and/or modified would exceed the added capital cost. On the other hand, it is equally likely that some expensive aspects of a construction project may turn out to be unjustified in terms of savings in operating costs over the useful life of the facility.

The five steps in life-cycle costing follow:

1. Describe the project in sufficient detail to allow the analyst to determine the productive life of the resource and to make reasonably sound estimates of both capital and operating costs.

2. Determine the capital cost.

3. Learn operating costs and service volumes. Including service volumes in the analysis is important, but, at this point, planners should remember that the relationship between service volumes and operating costs may not be linear. In other words, there may be economies or diseconomies of scale.

4. Compute the project's life-cycle costs. This involves summing the capital and operating costs for the total life span of the project, discounted at an appropriate rate.

5. Analyze the life-cycle cost with particular reference to the cost per unit of output. This is especially important when one is comparing alternatives that may be of very different scales, since the basic issue as far as the decision maker is concerned is not how many dollars are spent but rather what the cost will be for each unit of service provided.

---

[41]Abt Associates, Inc. "L.C.C.: A Manual on Life Cycle Costs Analysis for Health Planners." Cambridge, Mass., December 1976. Mimeographed.

Life-cycle cost analysis does not include a study of the financial feasibility of any project. Although such an analysis would be a logical first step toward determining financial feasibility, the life-cycle costing process does not provide the essential revenue data.[42]

SELECTING ALTERNATIVES AND ESTABLISHING PRIORITIES

Why Choices Must Be Made

The main reason for making choices is simply that there are not enough resources to do everything one wishes. For a time, however, this constraint did not seem to exist within the health industry. With minor exceptions, it was generally agreed that improvement of health services toward the end of improvement of health status was a crucial undertaking not to be challenged on crass economic grounds. This attitude was reflected at the organizational level by a process of reimbursement for all "reasonable" costs incurred.

Because of this attitude, and for a number of other reasons, health care expenditures within the United States have been rising rapidly. The *absolute* amount of health care expenditures for the entire country nearly doubled between 1955 and 1965 and tripled between 1965 and 1975. Health expenditures as a *percentage* of gross national product (GNP) increased from 4.6 percent in 1955 to 5.9 percent in 1965, 8.3 percent in 1975, and 10.0 percent in 1983. Since the percentage of GNP spent on health care has increased, outlays in other spending categories must be reduced.

An examination of personal consumption expenditures from 1950 to 1975 reveals that medical care increased from 4.6 percent to 8.7 percent of total personal spending, whereas food, alcohol, and tobacco outlays decreased from approximately 30 percent to 23 percent and clothing expenditures declined from 12 percent to 8.4 percent. Expenditures for other items, such as housing, rose during this period, but their rate of increase was far lower than that experienced for medical care. Indeed, it is with good reason that the residents of the United States are becoming increasingly concerned about rising health costs.

---

[42]Those interested in aspects of analysis of financial feasibility, see Lester Gorsline Associates, *Guide to Financial Analysis and Introduction to Economic Impact Analysis for Health Planning,* Health Planning Methods and Technology Series No. 3, Rockville, Md., Bureau of Health Planning and Resources Development, U.S. Department of Health, Education, and Welfare, 1976. (HRA 76-14513)

This problem is not unique to the United States; in fact, it seems to be common to most industrial nations. A study of five Western European countries[43]—West Germany, England (and Wales), France, the Netherlands, and Sweden—points out that cost containment has been a driving force in the health planning programs of all these nations. Some—for example, England—have set a limit on total expenditures and have compelled service providers to operate below that ceiling. Other countries have followed the United States and are attempting to limit additions to the system. (It should be noted, however, that within the United States experiments are now being conducted on the basis of the principle of *budgetary* limitation.)

The concern of the private sector is illustrated by an insightful article written in 1976 by the physician Howard H. Hiatt.[44] He points out that "Nobody would deny that there is a limit to the resources any society can devote to medical care. . . .We risk reaching a point where marginal gains to individuals threaten the welfare of the whole. . .and priorities have been set at best by well-intentioned policymakers with information of limited quantity and quality and at worst in anarchic fashion."

Within the public sector, both legislative history and the language of P.L. 93-641 clearly indicate concern among legislators and the executive branch about costs. Section 1513(a)(3) of P.L. 93-641 states that one of the purposes of the health system agency is to restrain "increases in the cost of providing health care services." Section 1532(a)(4) requires consideration of the availability of less costly alternatives when agencies are reviewing uses of federal funds, proposals for new institutional health services, and the appropriateness of existing institutional health services. Finally, federal guidelines implementing the portion of the law on plan development state that "attention to cost of health care is an immediate national priority."

This shift of emphasis from improving the availability, accessibility, and quality of health services to containing costs has put planners in a difficult situation, since many members of the public do not yet understand the points made by Hiatt. Thus, it is essential that planners be in a position to show that their decisions are based on a thorough consideration of all aspects of the issue. In the private sector, traditional measures such as return on investment (ROI) and return on equity (ROE)

---

[43]Jan Blanpain et al. "International Approaches to Health Resources Development for National Health Programs." Leuven, Belgium, Institute for European Health Research, Leuven University, 1976. Mimeographed.
[44]Howard H. Hiatt. "Protecting the Medical Commons: Who Is Responsible?" *Trustee*, 29(10):14–17, October 1976.

are available as guides for decision making. Cost-benefit analysis serves the same purpose in the public sector.

In its broadest application, cost-benefit analysis is a technique that allows the planners to assess the relative value of alternative courses of action. The list of plan development activities in Table 4 includes those activities that involve the types of choices discussed here. Specifically, choices must occur in step 3, where decision makers strive for a balance between the levels of such attributes as quality, accessibility, and cost; in steps 16 and 17, in which issues are placed in priority sequence; and in steps 9, 14, and 19, where decision makers must select a preferred course of action from among several possibilities.

Cost-Benefit Analysis

From a theoretical point of view, the objective sought in a cost-benefit analysis is the attainment of Pareto Optimality, a condition in which changes occur only if they make someone better off and no one else worse off. This formulation does not consider the relative status of individuals who might be affected; in other words, no attempt is made to consider the individual's wealth or poverty. Pareto Optimality simply focuses on the determination of whether it is possible to increase the general welfare in the aggregate. There are few circumstances in which this criterion can be applied; therefore, other economists have devised supplementary considerations.

The best known of these is the Kaldor-Hicks criterion, which states that a change is desirable if it makes someone so much better off that he or she could compensate those who are made worse off and still have something left. This statement indicates only that the gainer can compensate the loser; it does not guarantee that compensation will in fact occur. Nevertheless, the Kaldor-Hicks criterion has become the basis for cost-benefit analyses that try to identify situations wherein the benefits to one person will exceed the costs regardless of who pays.

History

Cost-benefit analysis is not really new. In 1844, the Frenchman Dupuit wrote on the utility of public works. In the United States, the River and Harbor Act of 1902 required the U.S. Army Corps of Engineers to select projects on the basis of benefits to commerce and the cost of these benefits.[45] Cost-benefit analysis is more widely used now because of the

---

[45]A. R. Prest and R. Turvey. "Cost-Benefit Analysis: A Survey." *The Economic Journal,* *73*(4):683, December 1965.

development of operations research methods during and since World War II. The methods developed provide the necessary techniques for cost-benefit analysis, and the increased availability of computers has made the necessary computations feasible in everyday situations.

At first, the use of cost-benefit analysis outside the defense establishment received little publicity. Congress, however, began to take some interest in the possibility of applying cost analysis, both in its own decision-making processes and as a requirement for receiving grants-in-aid to ensure that federal funds would be spent wisely by nonfederal recipients.[46] In addition, the use of the Planning-Programming-Budgeting System (PPBS), a process that relies heavily on cost-benefit analysis, has been endorsed by such state and local government organizations as the Council of State Governments, the International City Managers' Association, the National Governors' Conference, and the U.S. Conference of Mayors.[47] Individual institutions also are beginning to use cost-benefit analysis in the selection of such devices as computers and automated laboratory systems.

Purpose

Cost-benefit analysis, usually regarded as a technique for making societal decisions, is analogous to capital budgeting in business and industry. Both techniques deal with the same problems, such as measuring benefits, establishing priorities, measuring the costs of capital and of intangible factors, and, ultimately, choosing the best of several competing proposals. In a more definitive vein, cost-benefit analysis is the systematic examination of alternative courses of action for a complex and uncertain future.

A systematic examination of alternatives is a radical departure from the requirements approach to budgeting. With the latter, an agency decided what it wanted to do and then adjusted its program to include whatever activities could be supported with available funds. This approach, which focused on activities, often led to selection of a program that offered very little improvement in relation to its cost. By contrast,

---

[46]U.S. Congress, Joint Economic Committee, Subcommittee on Economy in Government. *Economic Analysis of Public Investment Decisions: Interest Rate Policy and Discount Analysis.* 90th Congress, 1st Session. Washington, D.C., U.S. Government Printing Office, 1967, p. 17.

[47]Harry P. Hatry. "Criteria for Evaluation in Planning State and Local Programs." In: U.S. Congress, Senate, Subcommittee on Intergovernmental Relations. *Planning-Programming-Budgeting: Selected Comments.* 90th Congress, 1st Session. Washington, D.C., U.S. Government Printing Office, 1967, p. 12.

the objective of cost-benefit analysis—or a systematic examination of alternatives—is to focus the analysis on a final output, which can be produced in several ways. Although this focus can be difficult to develop (because the connection between inputs and outputs is not always well known), it can prevent the building of hospitals merely for the sake of having hospitals. The results of the Hill-Burton program might have been considerably different if this cost-benefit method had been applied in 1948.

Because of complexities and uncertainties, cost-benefit analysis must involve a large element of qualitative analysis, as well as the quantitative methods stressed in the literature. One of the dangers of using the cost-benefit method is that analysts and decision makers may become so enthralled with the apparently neat answers derived that they disregard the simplifying assumptions necessary to arrive at those quantitative solutions.

All analytic techniques require simplification, but the cost-benefit approach has virtues that the others lack. First, it offers a way to derive numerical values that are logically consistent with one another and with the objective. Second, it accomplishes this goal by explicit processes that are open to critical evaluation or replication by others. Enthoven,[48] a leading proponent of the technique, stresses the second point by saying that cost-benefit analysis is neither occult nor synonymous with computers. A good analyst, he says, must be able to give the responsible decision makers a clear, nontechnical explanation of his methods and results.

As Fisher[49] says, cost-benefit analysis has a modest but significant role in decision making. Most major long-range decisions must be made on the basis of judgment, and the main purpose of analysis is to sharpen this judgment.

Categories

Cost-benefit analysis depends on the scope of the comparison, which can be intrasystem, intersystem, intraprogram, and interprogram. *Intrasystem analysis* compares alternative methods for a given system, (e.g., movement of patients by helicopters compared to movement by con-

[48]U.S. Congress, Senate, Subcommittee on National Security and International Operations. *Planning-Programming-Budgeting: Selected Comments.* 90th Congress, 1st Session. Washington, D.C., U.S. Government Printing Office, 1967, p. 2.
[49]G. H. Fisher. "The Role of Cost-Utility Analysis in Program Budgeting." In: *Program Budgeting.* Edited by David Novick. Cambridge, Mass., Harvard University Press, 1965, p. 67.

ventional ambulances). *Intersystem analysis* compares alternative systems within a program (e.g., a preventive medicine system compared to a curative medicine system). *Intraprogram analysis* compares alternative combinations of systems that are aimed at the same general objective, such as maximizing health during an entire life span. This is sometimes called *force structure analysis*. *Interprogram analysis* deals with programs that have different goals, such as health and education.

The significance of this categorization is that a move from intrasystem to interprogram analysis is accompanied by a gradual shift from very precise quantitative formulations to a much more qualitative mode of analysis. To some extent, this shift results from the increasing complexity of the problem, but primarily it is due to the greater difficulty encountered in developing equivalent measures of the outputs. For example, it is not too difficult to compare time lags in getting a patient to the hospital by various modes of transportation, but it is extremely difficult to determine the relative values of eradicating lung cancer and of ensuring that every citizen completes high school.

Other Types of Analysis

Although some of the original workers in the health care field see no difference between cost-benefit and cost-effectiveness,[50] most practitioners find it useful to make a distinction.[51] Essentially, in cost-benefit studies, both inputs and outputs are variable, whereas in cost-effectiveness studies, one of the two is held constant.

COST-EFFECTIVENESS ANALYSIS

Cost-effectiveness is used to avoid problems of measurement. In analyzing health services for the poor, for example, DHEW found that the many alternatives available were not mutually exclusive and, thus, could have been combined in an infinite number of ways. Consequently, DHEW established a fixed budget for inputs and presented a limited set of output combinations to decision makers.

The department's approach is an unusual one. In most cases, an attempt is made to determine the least-cost method of reaching a fixed level of output (e.g., reducing the incidence of lung cancer by 10 percent). Because of the difficulty in assigning values to outputs, this

---

[50]Roland N. McKean. *Public Spending*. New York, McGraw-Hill, 1968, p. 135.
[51]Royal A. Crystal and Agnes W. Brewster. "Cost-Benefit and Cost-Effective Analysis in the Health Field: An Introduction." *Inquiry, 3*(4):4, December 1966.

approach is favored by practitioners, although it has two disadvantages. First, it limits quantitative comparisons to the intrasystem level (i.e., to the level where outputs are identical). Second, as Ackoff [52] points out, the approach simply shows which is the better of two alternatives, with no guarantee that either one is optimal or even adequate. By holding constant either input or output, however, cost-effectiveness analysis keeps the user from falling into the trap of striving to maximize outputs and minimize inputs simultaneously. The cost-benefit method allows both to vary, but both cannot go to their opposite extreme values at the same time.

Benefit-Cost Ratio Analysis

Benefit-cost ratio analysis must be used with caution, since it can be misleading. Maximization of the ratio is considered the ideal, but actually the ratio is irrelevant. The real question is whether the extra output is worth the added cost or whether the program is operating at the proper scale. For example, a ratio of 20/10 is numerically equivalent to 200/100, but it does not mean the same to a person concerned with the absolute level of accomplishment. Interestingly, although many studies have used ratios as criteria, in the final analysis, decisions also were based on judgment regarding scale of programs and estimates of need.

Steps in Analysis

A full systems analysis involves the following phases:

Phase 1

    Establish the objectives
    Define the environment in which these objectives will be sought
    Develop alternative methods

Phase 2

    Determine the interrelationships among variables within the system
    Construct models of the system

---

[52]Russell L. Ackoff. "Toward Quantitative Evaluation of Urban Services." In: *Conference on Public Expenditure Decisions in the Urban Community.* Edited by Howard G. Schaller. Washington, D.C., Resources for the Future, 1963, p. 95.

Phase 3

Measure costs

Phase 4

Measure benefits

Phase 5

Document the analysis so that it can be reevaluated if necessary and present the results in terms suitable for the decision maker

Each of the first four steps will be discussed separately. Two approaches to Phase 5, documenting the results of the analysis, are discussed later in this chapter on pp. 300–301.

PHASE 1: ESTABLISH OBJECTIVES, ENVIRONMENT, AND ALTERNATIVES

Establishing the Objectives

During this phase, analysts must have the opportunity to work closely with decision makers, or they may produce a superb analysis that is utterly useless. The analysts must be sure that they are working toward the proper objective on the basis of acceptable assumptions, with methods that are politically feasible. For example, despite the doctrine of sunk cost, decision makers are bound to some degree by what has happened in the past; thus, in many areas, prior substantial investments may limit the courses of action that are practically available.

The most important characteristic of objectives is that they must be oriented to ends and not to means. This orientation is not necessarily easy to achieve, because the end results often are far less measurable than the means. For example, a study on ambulance services, in which the criterion was speed in transporting emergency patients to the hospital, failed to show that there was any demonstrable relationship between speed and patient welfare.

Also, the criteria used to measure attainment of objectives must be broad enough so that any unwelcome side effects of the proposal will be detected. For instance, costs can be reduced by failing to provide services (such as diagnosis and treatment), but the indirect costs (such as loss of productivity because of illness, disability, and debility) will continue. A side effect that often is overlooked in analysis but that is tremendously important to public decision makers is the redistribution of income. (In a hospital setting, the analogous effect is a shift of charges from one group of patients to another.)

Defining the Environment

A number of the assumptions about the system's environment are political in nature, which leads to much criticism of the cost-benefit method. Many critics of cost-benefit analysis either do not understand or do not believe that analysis is used as a supplement to judgment in the decision-making process. They allege that the analyses overemphasize efficiency without considering the consequences. In the words of one United States senator,[53] "the analysts emphasize crass materialism rather than American ideological values."

More rational critics insist that analysis depends on a prior political framework, within which analysis can be very useful. This view is certainly supported by other writers, one of whom[54] suggests that the practitioner may well find Banfield's *Political Influence* to be just as important a book as Hitch's *Decision Making for Defense.* The effect of political judgment on the dental care program analysis will illustrate this point. Fluoridation was shown to have a very high benefit-cost ratio, but, in the Johnson administration legislative proposal, it was replaced by a costlier, less-effective treatment program because of dread expressed by the very vocal "antifluoridites."[55]

Actually, analysts who ignore the political aspects of a program do so at their own risk. Few programs of any consequence can be initiated unilaterally, and the interests of other influential parties who were ignored in the analysis will very likely cause modification of the pure proposal to such an extent that achieving expected goals is most unlikely.

Developing Alternative Methods

This phase can be mutually beneficial to both analysts and decision makers. Often, decision makers do not have time to develop alternatives on their own, and this leads to rigidities—the hallmark of bad planning. There is no single right way; alternatives must be considered at every level of decision making, and cost-benefit analysis provides a more-or-less systematic method for defining and considering useful alternatives. For analysts, effort at this stage helps them to avoid the expenditure of effort required to develop a full study of alternatives that will never be discussed seriously.

---

[53]U.S. Congress, Senate, Subcommittee on National Security and International Operations. *Planning-Programming-Budgeting.* Hearings. 90th Congress, 2nd Session. Washington, D.C., U.S. Government Printing Office, 1968, p. 145.
[54]William L. Kissick. "Planning, Programming and Budgeting in Health." *Medical Care,* 5(4):201–220, July–August 1967.
[55]Elizabeth B. Drew. "HEW Grapples with PPBS." *Public Interest,* 7(2):27, Summer 1967.

PHASE 2: DETERMINE INTERRELATIONSHIPS IN THE SYSTEM AND CONSTRUCT MODELS OF ALTERNATIVES

Characteristics of Models

Once a set of alternatives has been selected, models of these alternatives must be constructed to determine the possible outcomes of each alternative. A model is an explicit representation of some system or object. It includes the components of the system, interrelationships among the components, and the boundaries within which the system operates. Models have three important characteristics:

1. *Abstraction.* Because it is developed at a higher level of generality than the specific object or system, the model represents the entire class or set of objects with which analysts are concerned.
2. *Simplification.* Closely related to abstraction, simplification deals with elimination of certain complexities that have very little influence over operation of the model-subject. For example, in modeling a multiphasic screening process, one might not necessarily include in the model details of how the patient moved from one part of the unit to another. The kind and degree of simplification must depend on the purpose for which the model is to be used.
3. *Substitution.* A model uses words, mathematical symbols, analog circuits, and the like, to represent the objects in which analysts are interested.

Reasons for Using Models

The reasons for using models rather than the actual object are based on the three characteristics just described. Following are five of those reasons:

1. *Cost saving.* Generally, it is much cheaper to use representations of the object than the object itself. Obviously, one cannot afford to build each of the alternative designs that might be considered for a health facility to choose the best facility.
2. *Time saving.* The actual object of system analysis often operates at a relatively slow pace, so the impact of changes cannot be seen for a long time. Models, however, can speed up the process by scaling down time. For example, if a model of a hospital admission system were constructed, a computer simulation could easily produce the results of a year's experience in less than one hour.

3. *Safety.* In the health field, attention often focuses on objectives involving people. Since models use representations in lieu of people, they allow analysts to make preliminary estimates of what the effects of alternative courses of action might be, without the risk of adverse effects on human beings.

4. *Understanding.* Because building a model requires that designers have a thorough understanding of all the components and their interrelationships, it forces them to obtain a clear conception of what goes on within the real system.

5. *Reproducibility.* The economies in time, money, and risk make it possible for analysts to reproduce their models, enabling them to examine a great many alternatives and, consequently, giving them a much wider range of choices in their analyses. Furthermore, this reproducibility allows those who enter the decision-making process at a later stage to use different inputs based on their respective judgments and to test the outcomes.

Model Types

The many types of models range from replicas, which look and function exactly like the real thing, to symbolic models, which use abstract symbols (e.g., diagrams or mathematical equations) to represent the real object. This discussion focuses primarily on symbolic models, in which statistical or engineering models are developed to represent some component of a health care delivery system. These types of models typically involve mathematical equations and take one of two possible forms: deterministic or probabilistic.

The deterministic model considers the relationship among components to be fixed. For example, such a model might state that one pediatrician can care for 15 patients during a four-hour shift in an outpatient clinic. The probabilistic model, on the other hand, might show that the relationship among components will vary in accordance with some sort of statistical distribution. For instance, a simulation of the same flow of patients might use a probability distribution and random numbers to determine which patients would require ancillary diagnostic services.

In practice, it is possible to combine both probabilistic and deterministic components in a single model; when this is done, however, the outcome must necessarily be treated as that of a probabilistic model. In such cases, each run of the model is considered an individual experiment. Therefore, it is necessary to take the mean value of the outcome of many experiments to determine the expected value for the real system.

Model Design

Two approaches to model design will be considered. The first of these deals with the statistical model, and the second deals with the engineering model. The former takes data from a large number of similar cases and then applies these data to estimate how the planned alternative would work. The data can be collected longitudinally—that is, for a few institutions over a long period of time—or on a cross-section basis—that is, from many similar institutions at a single point in time. On the basis of the longitudinal technique, one would have to assume that health institutions had not changed their methods of operation over many years; yet, this is not the case.

The difficulty with the cross-section technique in the health field is that it is virtually impossible to find a sufficient number of similar institutions from which to gather adequate data. There are differences in service offered among hospitals that, on the surface, appear to be quite similar. For example, among three large teaching hospitals in Washington, D.C., which appear to be very much alike, it is entirely possible that the management of a particular type of surgery varies substantially. Consequently, the resulting differences in resources used and in the assignment of costs would be significant.

The engineering method of model building assumes that the basic components of the object or system can be identified and that the relationships among them can be determined in order to build a total structure from these individual parts. One of the first problems encountered is the level of detail to which these components should be broken down. For example, in a model for a neighborhood health center, should the laboratory be treated as a single entity or should it be divided into parts, such as "chemistry" and "hematology"?

Frequently, the components and/or functions within a unit are irrelevant or unknown and are treated as black boxes. Specifically, they are considered only in terms of their input and output. For example, planners might know that the assignment of 3 cooks, 2 bakers, and 12 dietary aides will allow them to produce all the meals required for 300 patients during a seven-day week; they are not concerned with any details regarding the production of those meals.

If satisfactory data on the operation of the black box are not available, test results can substitute. Experimental operation is closest to reality and involves decision makers as actors in a real environment.

Demonstration projects are useful for getting data of this kind. Unfortunately, although demonstration projects are quite common in health care institutions, they seldom collect information on anything except direct clinical aspects of the program.

PHASE 3: MEASURE COSTS

Some of the most important economic concepts in cost-benefit analysis are the various types of costs and economies of scale. Decision makers must consider the proper costs, or they will almost certainly make the wrong choices. Because cost-benefit analysis is oriented toward selecting future programs, most alternatives probably will involve long-run costs based on nearly complete variability of inputs. Thus, possibilities of increasing or decreasing returns to scale become highly significant.

Types of Costs

Following are several types of costs that the health care practitioner is likely to encounter and must take into consideration when selecting future programs.

1. *Opportunity costs.* This type of cost, which usually is not very well understood, should be used when the supply of some input is strictly limited. Essentially, opportunity cost is the potential value of some action that cannot be taken because all of the available limited resource is being used in other activities. If the value gained from one of the other activities is less than the opportunity cost of any alternative, then the rational decision maker will feel obligated to discontinue that other activity and substitute for it the most valuable available alternative. For example, periodic physical examinations require many man-hours of physician effort, but no evidence exists that systematic screening detects a significant number of asymptomatic illnesses. Therefore, so long as the number of physicians is insufficient to provide all of the needed treatment, a program of widespread, complete physical examinations probably will not pass the test of opportunity cost.

2. *Sunk costs.* Those costs that will not be altered as a result of the decision making are known as sunk costs and are considered irrelevant. To determine whether a particular cost is a sunk cost will depend on the scope of a decision. For instance, ownership costs of a truck would be irrelevant in a decision relating to alternative uses for that truck but very relevant in a decision involving alternative types of vehicles.

3. *Incremental costs.* These are additional costs resulting from a change in activity. They arise from a decision and appear to be more relevant for decision making than those average costs that include sunk costs. For example, a share of depreciation should not be included in the cost of initiating a seven-day schedule in the operating room, since no additional facilities are required for the change in activity. In this situation, probably the only significant relevant costs would be salaries.

4. *Average costs.* Average costs are obtained by dividing total costs by total units of output, and they frequently mask important variations in unit costs. This masking effect is illustrated by the following finding in a study by Ingbar and Lee.[56] Health care data typically are presented in terms of cost per patient per day, but Ingbar and Lee's study of a domiciliary care program used special cost-collection techniques to avoid the usual aggregation and allocation that occurs in a hospital accounting system. They found that occupational therapist and physician visits cost an average of $0.14 and $0.44 a day, respectively, for all patients. But when they shifted focus to cost per day for patients using the service, the average cost for therapist visits was $0.52 and the cost for physician visits remained the same.

5. *Marginal costs.* These costs occur when one more unit is added. As the data from the previous example show, the average cost of a physician visit in terms of cost per day to users was less than the average cost of a visit by a social worker—in this case, an occupational therapist. Logically, the program director should substitute physicians for social workers, since the physician could presumably perform most, if not all, of the social worker's functions. Because the actual cost of an additional physician is greater than the actual cost of an additional occupational therapist (greater marginal cost), a decision based on average costs per day for both physician and therapist visits, rather than on the marginal costs of the additional manpower, would increase, not decrease, the total cost of the program. In many instances, marginal costs and incremental costs are synonymous.

Problems of Cost Measurement

A good technique for determining costs is to plot total cost as a function of the cumulative number of units produced. When this is possible, it

---

[56]Mary Ingbar and Sidney S. Lee. "Economic Analysis as a Tool of Program Evaluation: Costs in a Home Care Program." In: *The Economics of Health and Medical Care.* Ann Arbor, Mich., University of Michigan Press, 1964, pp. 173–210.

will provide total fixed cost, total variable cost, and marginal cost. To extrapolate beyond the observed data would be unwise, however, because these functions may not be linear. The use of this so-called accounting method of cost estimating is severely limited, because virtually all available health cost data are collected in accounting systems that do not separate relevant costs from irrelevant costs. As mentioned in the discussion on model design, the problems of incommensurability generally rule out the use of the statistical approach to these problems. Consequently, it appears that the engineering method of cost estimating will be the way to go at least for the foreseeable future. The engineering method involves identifying all of the components of a system, assigning a cost to each, and then aggregating these costs to arrive at the total costs for the system.

Long-Run Costs

The foregoing discussion was related primarily to the measurement of short-run costs—that is, costs of varying rates of output with a fixed level of plant or technology. In the planning process, the focus is on the long-run costs that arise when all factors are variable. The long-run cost function can be visualized as an envelope curve enclosing short-run cost curves, each of which represents one of the feasible plant sizes (for example, number of beds in a hospital) or production techniques. The long-run cost function is especially useful in determining the optimum plant size and/or measuring the costs of using other than optimum plant size to achieve a desired distribution of locations.

The data problems are particularly acute in the development of a long-run cost function, because the estimate must be based on comparable inputs and outputs for plants of many sizes. This is nearly impossible in the health field at the present time; however, the example of centralized or decentralized obstetrical service units on p. 271 illustrates the importance of this point.

Direct and Indirect Costs

When identifying relevant costs, it is important to distinguish between direct and indirect costs. Direct costs are out-of-pocket or private expenditures associated with the provision of some service; they should include both the actual cost of providing that service and the overhead cost associated with the activity. (Overhead costs include spending for functions such as agency management, research, and education.) Indirect costs include the expenses incurred by those seeking the service—

for example, travel time or time off the job. Indirect costs also should include social costs such as might be experienced when a new facility effectively destroys a neighborhood's cohesiveness.

PHASE 4: MEASURE BENEFITS

Many studies avoid the problem of benefit measurement by holding output at a constant level, but, by doing this, they drastically lower the level at which quantitative comparisons can be made. Frequently, benefits are expressed as costs or other undesirable events that have been (or will be) avoided. For example, if the cost of a disease or illness were expressed in years of life lost, the benefit would be the avoidance of these losses.[57]

The quantitative value of human life and health has been studied since the time of Sir William Petty in the seventeenth century, but there still is no widely accepted method for assessing it.[58] One analyst[59] set the value of an airplane accident victim at $373,000, and another[60] suggested that the appropriate value should be measured by the value that the target population places on avoiding risks. Most studies that use dollar values, however, tend to follow the concepts outlined in Mushkin's[61] landmark article, "Health as an Investment," which focuses on losses in productivity. This study was followed by two analyses[62] by the Federal Government on the cost of illness. In addition to actual cost estimates, these papers present excellent discussions of the pragmatic solutions to some very complex issues that arise in the

---

[57]Discussion of quality-adjusted life years is included in William B. Stason and Milton C. Weinstein, "Foundations of Cost-Effectiveness Analysis for Health and Medical Practices," *The New England Journal of Medicine, 296*(13):716–721, March 31, 1977. For an excellent guide to measuring years of life lost, see Joel C. Kleinman, "Age Adjusted Mortality Indexes for Small Areas: Applications to Health Planning," *American Journal of Public Health, 67*(9):834–840, 1977.

[58]A. W. Mitchell. *Cost/Benefit Analysis in Health.* Santa Monica, Calif., Rand Corp., 1965, p. 2.

[59]Gary Fromm. "Civil Aviation Expenditures." In: *Measuring Benefits of Government Investments.* Edited by Robert Dorfman. Washington, D.C., The Brookings Institution, 1965, p. 196.

[60]T. C. Schilling. "The Life You Save May Be Your Own." In: *Problems in Public Expenditure Analysis.* Edited by Samuel B. Chase, Jr. Washington, D.C., The Brookings Institution, 1968, pp. 127–176.

[61]Thelma J. Mushkin. "Health as an Investment." *The Journal of Political Economy, 70*(5):129–157, October 1962.

[62]Dorothy P. Rice, *Estimating the Cost of Illness,* Health Economics Series No. 6, Washington, D.C., U.S. Public Health Service, 1966; Barbara S. Cooper and Dorothy P. Rice, "The Economic Cost of Illness Revisited," *Social Security Bulletin, 39*(2):21–36, February 1976.

process of making estimates of costs and benefits. The following is a brief description of some of the more significant issues that the health planner might encounter.

Problems in the Measurement of Benefits

None of the methods for measuring benefits are free from measurement problems. These include how to handle taxes and transfer payments to avoid double counting; how to adjust earnings for possible future increases in productivity; whether it can be assumed that all those who avoid illness will be employed continuously in the future (e.g., should the possibility of another illness or a decline in the national employment level be considered?); whether that which is consumed by a person whose life has been saved should be deducted from how much the person will produce during the remainder of his or her life (*gross* benefit to society) to yield the person's net benefit to society; and what earnings should be imputed to homemakers or to children whose entrance into the labor force is delayed by illness.

Furthermore, there is the problem of quantifying unmeasurables. For example, Klarman[63] asserts that people will spend more to avoid a disease than the value of direct and indirect costs of cure. He proposes the "analogous disease" technique to estimate how much this indirect cost will be. In Klarman's example, psoriasis is used as an analog to syphilis because, although psoriasis is not disabling, it does have symptoms that people want to get rid of. If the cost of ridding oneself of the symptoms of psoriasis is $50, then this component of the cost of an episode of syphilis will be approximately the same. Weisbrod[64] argues that the distribution of nonmonetary costs (e.g., sorrow over death) is approximately that of total economic costs (i.e., both costs are highest at middle life and least in infancy and old age). Hatry suggests that a panel of experts could be used to rank alternatives subjectively when unquantifiable factors, such as amount of discomfort, are involved.[65] Another unmeasurable, which is frequently overlooked, is the benefit to the patient of having alternatives from which to choose. Too often, health care professionals are overly paternalistic, but how can the benefit of having choices be valued?

---

[63]Herbert E. Klarman. "Syphilis Control Programs." In: *Measuring Benefits of Government Investments.* Edited by Robert Dorfman. Washington, D.C., The Brookings Institution, 1965, p. 400.

[64]Burton A. Weisbrod. *Economics of Public Health.* Philadelphia, University of Pennsylvania Press, 1961, p. 96.

[65]Harry P. Hatry. (State-Local Finance Project, The George Washington University, Washington, D.C.) Personal interview. November 26, 1968.

After thoroughly analyzing four techniques to value benefits, Eastaugh[66] has concluded that although these are indeed difficult problems, they should not become an excuse for accepting "analytical nihilism." Although none of the various approaches are perfect, they can contribute to informed decision making. In particular, his analysis suggests that a "willingness to pay" approach generally will yield the most satisfactory results.

Finally, health programs are very likely to affect the distribution of incomes (e.g., from a reduction in unemployment); therefore, it is important to show which regions or population groups will benefit, and, in the overall picture, how much society will gain—both crucial issues in the political decision-making process. A vocational rehabilitation study[67] that attempted to show benefits and gains ultimately demonstrated that reductions in welfare payments plus taxes on income earned by rehabilitated persons were two to four times greater than the tax cost of the program.

INCLUDING QUALITATIVE CONSIDERATIONS

Consideration of those factors that can be quantified, and particularly those that can be translated into dollar terms, is generally insufficient for public decision-making processes. In the public sector, decision makers must consider the multiple effects implied by any decision. At the very least, they must consider the second- and third-order effects, which can be identified with an analytic matrix such as the one suggested in Chapter 3. In most cases, however, the decision maker must look further and consider effects outside the system (e.g., impact on unemployment rate).

Since the analyst will be dealing with considerations expressed in dissimilar terms, he must give attention to means by which the information can be presented to the decision maker. Two well-known techniques for such presentations are the Lichfield balance sheet and Hill's goal-achievement matrix.[68]

The Lichfield balance sheet shows the benefits and costs to many categories of people affected by a decision. It describes these costs in a

---

[66]Steven R. Eastaugh. "Placing a Value on Life and Limb: The Role of the Informed Consumer." *Health Matrix,* *1*(1):5–21, Winter 1983.

[67]U.S. Department of Health, Education, and Welfare. *Vocational Rehabilitation: Program Analysis 1967—13.* Washington, D.C., 1967, p. 37.

[68]Nathaniel Lichfield, "Cost-Benefit Analysis in Urban Expansion: A Case Study—Peterborough," *Regional Studies,* *3*(2):123–155, 1969; Morris Hill, "A Goal Achievement Matrix for Evaluating Alternative Plans," *Journal of the American Institute of Planners,* *34*(1):19–28, January 1968.

variety of ways—monetary, numeric, and qualitative—giving the analyst an opportunity to select an appropriate level of measurement. It also distinguishes between operating and capital costs. (Insofar as quantitative data are concerned, the distinction between capital and operating costs is unnecessary if the analyst adopts the life-cycle costing approach, which, in effect, combines the two kinds of costs in an effort to represent to decision makers the total impact of the choice to be made.)

Hill's goal-achievement matrix was designed specifically to improve on the Lichfield balance sheet. Unlike the balance sheet, the goal-achievement matrix does not lump together all effects; instead, it separates objectives or effects and assigns each a relative weight. It also differentiates groups, as does the balance sheet, but it goes one step further and assigns a relative weight to each group for each goal.

With the balance sheet, the decision maker is simply left with a display of what is usually a large amount of data relating to different facets of a choice. With the matrix, the decision maker is presented with weighted indexes of goal achievement. The indexes are based on measurement on the least rigorous of all the scales used—probably a nominal scale. Weights are applied to the scale values and aggregated for each of the options; a nominal scale might be positive effect, no effect, and negative effect, with corresponding ratings of $+1$, 0, or -1, respectively. If, for example, an alternative has a positive effect for an objective with a weight of 4 in relation to a group that has a weight of 2, the net score will be $+8$ $(+1 \cdot 4 \cdot 2)$.

The difficulty with this approach is that, from both theoretical and practical points of view, one should not aggregate values on nominal and ordinal scales, since there is absolutely no assurance that the values being combined are in any way homogeneous. For instance, an investment in a piece of new equipment might have a positive effect for both physicians and a hospital; however, the extent of such an effect on individual physician prestige might be far less than on the reputation of the hospital. Yet, both effects would be rated as $+1$ on the nominal scale. A more systematic approach to dealing with the values of multiple attributes is described on pp. 306–311.

ADJUSTING COST AND BENEFIT
QUANTITATIVE MEASUREMENTS

In most cases, both cost and benefit data must be adjusted for three factors: time value of money, price changes, and risk and uncertainty. Adjusting for time value of money makes it possible to compare projects with different life cycles and different patterns of cost outlay and receipt of benefits. Adjusting for price changes is necessary to compare the monetary data collected during different periods. Since cost-benefit analyses are designed for making decisions that will take effect in the future, there is inevitably a large amount of uncertainty. This can be dealt with in several ways; the most useful is sensitivity analysis, which allows the decision maker to change key factors in the analysis to determine the impact of such variations.

Time Value of Money

Many health goals are attainable by several means. Frequently, these means have significantly different time frames (e.g., the time required for research versus the time required for expanded application of existing knowledge). Thus, it is necessary to make intertemporal comparisons, usually through the time value of money, which is computed as a flow of funds discounted at an appropriate interest rate. Once again, this sounds simple, but it presents the difficult problem of selecting the proper discount rate.

A comparison of the costs of two programs for the prevention of the same disease, one having benefits with a present value of $46 million at a discount rate of 10 percent and one having benefits with a present value of $71 million at a discount rate of 4 percent, shows that this is not a trivial problem. Also, it must be remembered that the pattern of cash flow in both programs will bear on the importance of the rate of discount. For instance, if, in one program, most costs occur in the immediate future and benefits are not realized for many years, but, in another program, the costs and benefits tend to run concurrently, then the higher the discount rate, the less favorable the first program will appear.

There are three popular interest rates: cost of government borrowing; rate of return on private investments (not a unique value); and the weighted-average market interest rate that individuals receive on the money used to pay taxes.[69] Even among economists, however, there is little agreement on an appropriate rate (consider, for example, that the interest rates used in various studies range from 0 to 9 percent). Generally, a low rate of return is used when evaluating public projects, since people tend to undervalue the needs of future generations. The low interest rate encourages the acceptance of many government proposals and thus forces saving for the benefit of future generations.

---

[69]Martin S. Feldstein. "Opportunity Cost Calculations in Cost-Benefit Analysis." *Public Finance, 19*(2):120, 1964.

Baumol[70] suggests that the interest rate should be kept high to discourage excessive government investment projects and that the money saved should be diverted to consumption projects for those in need. Machlup[71] also urges higher rates for government projects. His contention is that, given the trend toward greater government involvement in everyday life, the use of a low discount rate could lead to the government undertaking a great variety of commercially unprofitable projects while the private sector was deprived of funds. This is a restatement of the opportunity cost argument.

The government has long struggled with setting a standard interest rate for use by all federal agencies. It is difficult to be sanguine about the outcome of this endeavor because of the political factors involved. To illustrate this point, it was noted in congressional hearings that every water project would be dropped if even the low rate of government borrowing were used as a criterion but that such an action would never be tolerated by either the legislative or executive branches because of political implications.[72] Similarly, the proponents of highway construction succeeded in getting legislation passed that required the Department of Transportation to use very low interest rates.[73]

Even when discount rates are established, they must be adjusted to compensate for changes that can reasonably be expected to occur during the life of the project. For example, in a study on chronic kidney disease, the discount rate was adjusted to show a change in productivity because of technological changes in dialysis. Interestingly, a different discount rate was used for hospital dialysis than for home dialysis,[74] implying that home methods would charge less than hospital techniques or that the labor of family members in performing home dialysis would be free.

Klarman,[75] whose method was followed consistently in DHEW studies, also makes an adjustment for increases in medical costs. His

---

[70]William J. Baumol. "On the Social Rate of Discount." *American Economic Review,* 58(4):799, September 1968.

[71]Fritz Machlup. "Comments on 'Preventing High School Dropouts.' " In: *Measuring Benefits of Government Investments,* Edited by Robert Dorfman. Washington, D.C., The Brookings Institution, 1965, p. 156.

[72]U.S. Congress, Joint Economic Committee, Subcommittee on Economy in Government. *The Planning-Programming-Budgeting-System: Progress and Potentials.* Hearings. 90th Congress, 1st Session. September 14, 19, 20, 21, 1967. Washington, D.C., U.S. Government Printing Office, 1967, p. 160.

[73]Robert L. Banks and Arnold Kotz. "The Program Budget and the Interest Rate for Public Investment." *Public Administration Review,* 26(6):283–296, December 1966.

[74]U.S. Bureau of the Budget. "Report of the Committee on Chronic Kidney Disease." Washington, D.C., September 14, 1967. Mimeographed.

[75]Herbert E. Klarman. "Syphilis Control Programs," p. 403.

study of syphilis showed a zero-percent rate of interest; apparently, he started with a positive discount rate and arrived at zero percent as a result of adjustments for cost increases.

Price Changes

Any historical monetary data used to estimate costs or benefits must be adjusted to a common value, preferably current dollars. Generally, such an adjustment is made with the consumer price index (CPI), but this is inappropriate for the health care delivery system. For example, in recent years, physicians' fees have risen faster than the CPI, and the cost of hospitalization has risen even more rapidly.

Because of uncorrected deficiencies in its original construction and differences in the quality of care, the price index for medical care is more vulnerable to criticism than the price index for nearly any other class of commodity. Scitovsky[76] argues that much of the difficulty arising from changes in methods of pricing medical care could be eliminated by shifting from pricing inputs (e.g., drugs, x-rays) to pricing outputs (e.g., appendectomy, cure of a streptococcal infection). Prospective pricing based on diagnosis-related groups (DRGs) is an important step in this direction. At present, there are no satisfactory techniques for making the necessary price adjustments; therefore, each analyst will have to choose a method. It is important that decision makers understand this so that they can insist that consistent methods be used in analysis of competing projects.

Uncertainty

Even in simple cases where a single-outcome deterministic model is an adequate representation of reality, the estimate developed will be affected by such things as the choice of methods, the assumptions made in establishing the ground rules for study, and the uncertainties about the parameter estimates used in determining models of alternatives. The primary concern of the analyst is to clearly indicate that uncertainties do exist and what the effects of these uncertainties might be. There are at least four ways to do this.

The first—probably the easiest but also the least satisfactory—is to include a qualitative discussion of the uncertainties.

---

[76]A. A. Scitovsky. "Changes in the Costs of Treatment of Selected Illnesses, 1951–65." *American Economic Review, 57*(5):1182–1195, December 1967.

The second allows the analyst to make a likelihood estimate—that is, to indicate the probability that certain conditions will prevail. Again, this tends to be rather subjective.

The third way permits a range of possibilities to be presented. For example, a kidney disease program analysis[77] used high and low cost assumptions for each treatment modality. The high data were based on an assumption of no change from today's methods, and the low data assumed technological advances. The low cost and high cost assumptions at the end of the fifth year were $1.0 billion and $1.5 billion, respectively, and, after 15 years, $1.8 billion and $2.8 billion, respectively. Similarly, in analyzing programs for delivery of health services to the poor, DHEW[78] used high and low estimates, because it had no assurance that the target population would utilize fully the services made available to it. Often, these estimates reflect three levels of outcome: optimistic, most probable, and pessimistic.

The fourth approach is a variant of the third. It is called *sensitivity analysis* and is designed to show the extent to which the outcome is affected by a change in some factor.[79] If, for example, a 20-percent change in a parameter caused only a 1-percent change in the outcome, the analyst and the decision maker could conclude that the system was relatively insensitive to that parameter; thus, even a large degree of uncertainty in estimating its value would not be especially dangerous. This approach is more satisfactory than the other three for displaying the degree of certainty. Moreover, the degree of sensitivity will indicate the level of accuracy and precision that should be sought in gathering parameter data.

In cases requiring more complex analyses producing more than a single estimated outcome, it is customary to distinguish between uncertainty and risk. When the decision maker can assign relative probabilities to the various outcomes, this is a situation involving risk. If probabilities cannot be assigned to the outcomes, then the decision maker is dealing with uncertainty. In both cases, the decision maker should be aware of the various techniques that have been developed as

---

[77]Kidney Disease Program Analysis Group. "Kidney Disease Program Analysis: A Report to the Surgeon General." Washington D.C., U.S. Public Health Service, 1967, p. 31. Mimeographed.
[78]U.S. Department of Health, Education, and Welfare. *Delivery of Health Services for the Poor: Program Analysis 1967—12.* Washington, D.C., 1967, p. 56.
[79]Technically, sensitivity analysis studies only the effect of changes in key parameters. Changes in assumptions are assessed by contingency analysis, but the concept is the same for both.

decision aids, including maximum and minimum regret rules and estimates of expected values.[80]

SETTING PRIORITIES

The discussion to this point has indicated that cost-benefit analysis is useful for making single choices. As a practical matter, however, the planner often will face situations in which the choice will be the construction of a subset of preferred actions from among a larger set of possible alternatives. This is the function of priority setting, which involves listing feasible alternatives according to their relative standing in a list of preferences. It is assumed that adoption of the entire list of alternatives would require more resources than are available. Consequently, the sequential ordering of alternatives is a first step in allocating scarce resources among desirable and feasible activities.

Many methods are available for setting priorities to guide decision makers in determining which choice is most suitable for their purposes. The following criteria are suggested:

1. The method should be objective to ensure consistency among decisions.
2. The method should emphasize analysis and explicitness, so that decision makers can explain and discuss the bases for their choices.
3. The method must be understandable; that is, it must have face validity to the persons to whom decision makers are accountable. The general public, for instance, will not be persuaded by an arcane mathematical process that has no apparent relationship to the relevant factors.
4. The method must be efficient. The time decision makers can commit to a process is scarce and must be used as wisely as possible. Consequently, the method chosen must be selected on a cost-benefit basis. The gain in information or the persuasiveness of the priority-setting method must exceed (or at least equal) the cost of the decision makers' time together with the time their staffs must invest in preparing data for consideration.

---

[80]See, for example, B. E. Fries, *Applications of Operations Research to Health Care Delivery Systems,* New York, Springer-Verlag, 1981; J. P. Kirschner, "An Annotated Bibliography of Decision Analytic Applications to Health Care," *Operations Research, 28*(1): 97, January–February 1980; Joel S. Greenberg, *Investment Decisions—The Influence of Risk and Other Factors,* New York, American Management Assn., 1982.

These methods fall into nine generic categories, which arise as a result of combining three scoring processes and three levels of analysis, as displayed in Figure 28.

Scoring Processes

The first scoring process, *ranking,* involves placing all available alternatives in a sequence from most preferred to least preferred. Ranks frequently are identified by numbers, so if the choice were to be from among 10 alternatives, number 10 would be assigned to the most preferred and number 1 to the least preferred alternative.

Paired comparisons can be used when the number of alternatives is so large that it is not feasible for the decision maker to consider each alternative in relation to all the others at a single moment. Rather, the decision maker examines each alternative in relation to every other alternative, indicating a preference within each pair. He then counts the number of times each alternative was preferred, and the decisions are placed in sequence from the highest number of choices to the lowest number of choices. This is illustrated in Table 21, where a hypothetical individual is making a choice among a variety of entrees for dinner. The preferred alternative is circled as each comparison is made. Then the number of times each alternative has been circled is added, giving the score for that alternative. In this instance, chicken is the least preferred entree, while lobster is the most preferred.

Unlike ranking and paired comparisons, which do not distinguish the relative level of preference assigned to each alternative, *rating* is based

LEVELS OF ANALYSIS

SCORING PROCESSES	Aggregate	Factor	Weighted Factor
Ranking			
Paired Comparison			
Rating			

Figure 28   Priority-setting methods.

TABLE 21   Example of Paired Comparisons

Alternatives	Paired Comparisons with Preferred Alternative Circled				Preference — Alternative	Preference — Score
1. Chicken	1 ⟨2⟩	1 ⟨3⟩	1 ⟨4⟩	1 ⟨5⟩	1	0
2. Steak		⟨2⟩ 3	2 ⟨4⟩	⟨2⟩ 5	2	3
3. Crab			3 ⟨4⟩	⟨3⟩ 5	3	2
4. Lobster				⟨4⟩ 5	4	4
5. Lamb Chops					5	1

on a ratio scale. Hence, it is possible to perform arithmetic operations on the results. A typical rating scale might range from 0 to 10, with 10 being the highest level of preference. Thus, one would know that if alternative A were rated as 10 and alternative B as 5, the decision maker meant that alternative A was twice as desirable as alternative B.

The rating process can be carried a step further by allocating a limited number of points and requiring the decision maker to indicate how many of these points are assigned to each of the alternatives. For instance, the decision maker might be allocated 100 points, which he would then assign in appropriate proportions to a set of five alternatives. This arrangement allows decision makers to express clearly the strength of their preferences and also provides a set of scores that can be aggregated, averaged, or whatever.

The decision alternative rational evaluation (DARE) method of rating, developed by Klee,[81] combines paired comparisons, relative scoring, and allocation of limited points, as shown in Table 22. The first step in the DARE process is to compare each alternative on a list with the one after it. In this instance, emergency medical services are rated as being half as important as establishing a trauma unit, which is consid-

---

[81] A. J. Klee. "DARE Makes Your Solid Waste Decision." *American City, 85*(2):100–103, February 1970.

TABLE 22   Example of DARE Method

Alternative	Paired Comparison	Relative Score	Allocation of Limited Points*
Improve Emergency Medical Services	0.5	1.5	21
Establish Trauma Unit	2.0	3.0	43
Develop Rehabilitation Services	1.5	1.5	21
Community Education	1.0	1.0	15
Total		7.0	100

*Normalized scores that are equivalent to percentages.

ered twice as important as developing rehabilitation services, which is deemed one and one-half times as important as community education. Because it is the last item in this list, community education cannot be compared with anything else. Consequently, it is assigned a basic value of 1.0.

To develop relative scores, computations begin with the base value of 1.0, assigned to community education. Because it was determined that rehabilitation services are one and one-half times as important as community education, rehabilitation services are assigned a score of 1.5 (1.0 × 1.5). Since it was determined that a trauma unit is twice as important as the rehabilitation services, the score for rehabilitation services (1.5) is multiplied by 2.0, resulting in a score of 3.0 for the trauma unit. The last score is multiplied by 0.5 to rate emergency medical services, which are considered only half as important as the trauma unit. The set of relative scores established by this process shows that community education is the least important activity and that establishing the trauma unit is the most important—in fact, three times more important than community education and twice as important as improving emergency medical services and developing rehabilitation services.

The process can be carried a step further through a technique sometimes called *normalizing,* which is, in effect, conversion of relative scores to amounts equivalent to percentages. This is done by adding the relative scores and using the sum as the base for establishing percentages. Consequently, in Table 22, the sum is 7.0 points and the score for the trauma unit is 43 percent of the total points allocated (3.0 ÷ 7.0). This technique is recommended because it facilitates understanding by stakeholders, since percentages are very common and widely accepted measures.

Levels of Analysis

The next step in describing methods of priority setting is to examine the level of analysis, the horizontal axis of the matrix in Figure 28. The first level is *aggregate,* which means that alternatives are examined and ranked, compared, or rated, with no explicit consideration of the issues that the decision maker took into account when assigning that rank or rating. In this situation, it is possible for two decision makers to assign similar ranks or ratings for totally different and perhaps conflicting reasons. It is also possible for them to assign divergent values to alternatives because they each are considering different aspects of those alternatives. Consequently, many believe that decision makers should make explicit the factors they are considering when making their choices (e.g., capital cost, research value, contribution to patient care, operating cost, contribution to the education of physicians).

If three alternatives were under scrutiny, each would be considered in relation to each factor and would be assigned a rank or weighting relative to that factor. For example, if one were discussing ranking on the factor of capital cost, alternative 1 might be ranked second, alternative 2 third, and alternative 3 first. The three alternatives would then be ranked on each of the remaining factors.

Because ranking does not distinguish the relative level of preference assigned to each alternative, it would not be possible to combine the ranks to obtain an aggregate standing. If, on the other hand, a rating method were used, the assigned values for each factor could be added to give a sum of ratings for each alternative. That sum would be the basis for placing the alternatives in priority order.

Decision makers generally are dissatisfied with a simple factor process, because it implies that all factors are of equal consequence, which is seldom the case. This difficulty can be overcome by assigning a relative weight to each factor. Once the weight for each factor has been determined, it is multiplied by an assigned rating to get a weighted factor score. These scores can then be summed and their aggregate used as the basis for assigning priorities among the alternatives. Table 22 illustrates this process, where alternative 1 is given precedence over alternative 2 on the basis of their total weighted scores (0.346 versus 0.293).

Factor weights can be determined by arbitrary allocation of points. Frequently, such a process is best accomplished by allocating 100 points among the factors, thereby reflecting the percentage of importance attached to each factor. Alternatively, a process such as the one described in the example of scoring can be used. The development of factor scores by this method is shown in Table 23.

TABLE 23   Example of DARE Method Using Weighted Factors

A. Set Factor Weights

Factors	Paired Comparison (R)	Relative Score (K)	Weight (Standardized Relative Score)
Capital Cost	0.20	0.64	0.10
Patient Care	9.90	3.22	0.50
Research Value	0.25	0.33	0.05
Operating Cost	1.30	1.30	0.20
Medical Education	1.00	1.00	0.15
Total		6.49	1.00

B. Set Relative Scores for Each Factor

Alternatives	R	K	Capital Cost Factor Score
Health Education	2.5	1.25	0.46
Preventive Screening	0.5	0.50	0.18
New Therapy	1.0	1.00	0.36
Total		2.75	1.00

C. Compute Weighted Scores for All Factors

Factor	Weight	Alternative 1 Score	Alternative 1 Weighted Score	Alternative 2 Score	Alternative 2 Weighted Score	Alternative 3 Score	Alternative 3 Weighted Score
Capital Cost	.10	.46	.046	.18	.018	.36	.036
Patient Care	.50	.20	.100	.40	.200	.40	.200
Research Value	.05	.40	.020	.20	.010	.40	.020
Operating Cost	.20	.60	.120	.15	.030	.25	.050
Medical Education	.15	.40	.060	.23	.035	.32	.056
Total			.346		.293		.362

Using Priorities to Allocate Resources

Once priorities have been established, decision makers must decide how to apply them in allocating resources. If it is assumed that resources are insufficient to implement all of the alternatives, decision makers must answer a number of questions: Should the first alternative on the list be funded to the maximum amount, even though its marginal productivity might decline rapidly at a higher level of input? Should available resources be divided among the top three or four alternatives, even though this will not produce "threshold" funding for one of the projects? As the second question implies, some projects require a substantial quantity of resources to be invested before even one unit of service can be produced. It is therefore possible that a simple process of allocating the funds on a proportional basis may result in some money being assigned to an alternative but not an amount sufficient for the minimum essential investment.

The number of alternative combinations for allocating resources can be extremely large, and, frequently, the results of different allocations are not intuitively obvious. In these circumstances, an operations research technique known as *mathematical programming* can be of great assistance to decision makers. In many cases, more sophisticated approaches, such as integer programming and goal programming, might be the method of choice, but often simple linear programming, as suggested by Pollack,[82] will do much to clarify the opportunities available to decision makers.

The use of linear programming is illustrated by the example in Table 24, in which a total budget of $1 million is to be allocated among five mental health projects. The projects have been assigned priority scores used essentially as benefit measurements, with the intent of maximizing the benefit derived from the allocation of funds. Other known data are the cost per case (part A of Table 24) and certain limitations on the number of cases that can be handled during the budget period (part B). These limitations are expressed as a set of constraints.

In addition to the case limitation, constraints arise due to problems of manpower availability. For instance, both drug abuse and alcoholism programs use the same types of manpower, and the supply within the community is so limited that only 200 cases can be handled (see part D of Table 24).

---

[82]See R. I. Pollack, "Allocation of Resources for Neighborhood Improvement," *Journal of Environmental Systems, 1*(3):269–281, September 1971; S. M. Lee, *Goal Programming for Decision Analysis*, Philadelphia, Pa., Auerbach Publishing, 1972.

TABLE 24   Linear Programming Solution to Resource Allocation Problem (Total Budget $1 Million; Five Mental Health Projects)

A.

Project	Weights	Cost per Case
Drug Abuse (DA)	.444	$ 3,000
Alcoholism (AL)	.254	1,500
Mental Retardation (MR)	.350	30,000
Suicide Prevention (SP)	.202	500
Family Counseling (FC)	.147	1,000

B. Limits on cases that can be handled during budget period

	Number of Cases
DA	100
AL	200
MR	30
SP	1,000
FC	150

C. Objective Function

$Z = 444 \text{ DA} + 254 \text{ AL} + 350 \text{ MR} + 202 \text{ SP} + 147 \text{ FC}$

D. Constraints

Total		$1,000,000
DA	≤	100
AL	≤	200
MR	≤	30
SP	≤	1,000
FC	≤	130
DA and AL	≤	200 (Both use same type of manpower)
SP and FC	≤	1,000 (Both use same type of manpower)

TABLE 24   (Continued)

E.

Project	Project Size (Number of Persons Served)	Project Cost	Priority Points
DA	100.00	$300,000	44,400
AL	100.00	150,000	25,400
MR	1.66	19,800	581
SP	1000.00	500,000	202,000
FC	0.00	—	—
Total		$969,800	272,381

With a simple linear programming model, decision makers can determine the size and cost of each project and the benefits or priority points that can be realized from establishing projects of those sizes. Table 24, part *E,* shows that, given the established constraints, the maximum amount of money that can be allocated is $969,800, which will yield a total of 272,381 priority points. In this case, because a simple linear programming model was used, the results include an impossible allocation—one that would establish a mental retardation program serving 1.66 persons. Had more sophisticated integer programming been used, this result would not have occurred, since the project sizes would be expressed only in whole numbers. Nevertheless, decision makers can readily see that no more than two mental retardation cases should be handled during the course of a year. Because this is such a small number, the program may be of insufficient size to be economically viable, in which case the decision maker could place another constraint on the allocation of resources—one that would establish a minimum size for the mental retardation program. The linear program model might then yield a different result. As in all other cases, however, the decision maker must continually bear in mind that the results obtained by applying these various methods are simply an aid to judgment. They do not produce incontrovertible answers to difficult problems.

SUMMARY

Objectives—steps toward achievement of goals—are reached by carrying out programs or projects. Since there are many ways to accomplish objectives, planners must identify the feasible alternatives and analyze them so that the preferred alternative can be chosen for implementation.

This choice is based on a cost-benefit analysis, in which the amount of service to be provided and the resources required to create these services are estimated. The estimation of service requirements must proceed on the basis of need or demand. Policymakers should determine which concept is appropriate for their organization or system. Because health services frequently are needed urgently and because the level of need or demand fluctuates markedly, service capacity decisions must take into account the trade-offs between efficiency and effectiveness. The tension between the two concerns can be reduced by managerial actions that will tend to smooth out the level of demand experienced by the service production components of the systems.

Resource requirements encompass personnel, technology, facilities, and funds. The requirement estimates should reflect resource productivity in relation to the planned service capacity. All resource requirements can be expressed in financial terms, since money is required to obtain the other types of resources. Cost estimates should be made for the entire life cycle of the program so that comparisons with other programs will be valid and so that decision makers will understand fully the effects of their choices.

Cost-benefit analysis provides a useful framework for developing the information needed by decision makers. Cost-effectiveness analysis is an alternate approach to be used in circumstances where either the benefits sought or the amount spent will be the same for all alternatives considered. Cost-benefit analysis provides a means for excluding infeasible alternatives from further consideration and tentatively ranking the feasible alternatives.

Usually, the cost-benefit analysis process will be used to select a preferred alternative for each program or project. Then, choices must be made concerning which projects will receive any share of the limited resources available and how the resources will be distributed among the chosen programs. Priority-setting methods provide guidance for making these decisions.

REFERENCES

Ackoff, Russell L. "Toward Quantitative Evaluation of Urban Services." In: *Conference on Public Expenditure Decisions in the Urban Community.* Edited by Howard G. Schaller. Washington, D.C., Resources for the Future, 1963, p. 95.

Alpha Center for Health Planning. "A Planning Framework for Reducing Excess Hospital Capacity, Volume I." Bethesda, Md., July 1981.
———. "A Planning Framework for Reducing Excess Hospital Capacity, Volume III." Bethesda, Md., July 1981.

Banks, Robert L., and Arnold Kotz. "The Program Budget and the Interest Rate for Public Investment." *Public Administration Review,* 26(6):283–296, December 1966.

Barzel, Yoram. "Costs of Medical Treatment: Comment." *American Economic Review,* 58(4):936–940, September 1968.

Baumol, William J. "On the Social Rate of Discount." *American Economic Review,* 58(4):799, September 1968.

Blanpain, Jan, et al. "International Approaches to Health Resources Development for National Health Programs." Leuven, Belgium, Institute for European Health Research, Leuven University, 1976. Mimeographed.

Brown, Kathryn J., et al. "Beyond Hill-Burton: The Development of an Improved Acute Care Need Methodology in Florida." Tallahassee, Fla., Department of Health, 1979. Mimeographed.

Cooper, Barbara S., and Dorothy P. Rice. "The Economic Cost of Illness Revisited." *Social Security Bulletin,* 39(2):21–36, February 1976.

Crystal, Royal A., and Agnes W. Brewster. "Cost-Benefit and Cost-Effectiveness Analyses in the Health Field: An Introduction." *Inquiry,* 3(4):4, December 1966.

Drew, Elizabeth B. "HEW Grapples with PPBS." *Public Interest,* 7(2):27, Summer 1967.

Eastaugh, Steven R. "Placing a Value on Life and Limb: The Role of the Informed Consumer." *Health Matrix,* 1(1):5–21, Winter 1983.

Falk, Shoshana. "Average Length of Stay in Long-Term Institutions." *Health Services Research,* 6(3):251–255, Fall 1971.

Feldstein, Martin S. "Opportunity Cost Calculations in Cost-Benefit Analysis." *Public Finance,* 19(2):120,1964.

Finch, Larry E., and Jon B. Christianson. "Rural Hospital Costs: An Analysis with Policy Implications." *Public Health Reports,* 96:423–433, September–October 1981.

Fisher, G. H. "The Role of Cost-Utility Analysis in Program Budgeting." In: *Program Budgeting.* Edited by David Novick. Cambridge, Mass., Harvard University Press, 1965, p. 67.

Florida Bed Need Task Force. "Recommended Acute Care Facility Need Methodology: Final Report." Tallahassee, Fla., February 1978.

Fries, B. E. *Applications of Operations Research to Health Care Delivery Systems.* New York, Springer-Verlag, 1981.

Fromm, Gary. "Civil Aviation Expenditures." In: *Measuring Benefits of Government Investments.* Edited by Robert Dorfman. Washington, D.C., The Brookings Institution, 1965, p. 196.

Gardner, Elmer A. "The Use of a Psychiatric Case Register in the Planning and Evaluation of a Mental Health Program." In: *Program Evaluation in the Health Fields.* Compiled by Herbert C. Schulberg and Alan Sheldon. New York, Behavioral Publications, 1969, pp. 538–561.

Greenberg, Joel S. *Investment Decisions—The Influence of Risk and Other Factors.* New York, American Management Assn., 1982.

Griffith, John R., and Robert A. Chernow. "Cost Effective Acute Care Facilities Planning in Michigan." *Inquiry, 14*(3):229-239, September 1977.

Gross, P. F. "Urban Health Disorders, Spatial Analysis and the Economics of Health Facility Location." *International Journal of Health Services, 2*(1):63-83, February 1971.

Hancock, Walton M., et al. "Maximum Average Occupancy for Hospital Units, NCHSR-81-214." Ann Arbor, Mich., University of Michigan Press, 1980, pp. 156-158.

_____. "Parameters Affecting Hospital Occupancy and Implications for Facility Sizing." *Health Services Research, 13*:276-289, Fall 1978.

_____. "Simulation-Based Occupancy Recommendatio \]s for Adult Medical/ Surgical Units Using Admissions Scheduling Systems." *Inquiry, 15*:25-32, March 1978.

Hancock, Walton M., and Paul F. Walter. *The "ACSC" Inpatient Admission Scheduling and Control System.* Ann Arbor, Mich., AUPHA Press, 1983.

Hatry, Harry P. "Criteria for Evaluation in Planning State and Local Programs." In: U.S. Congress, Senate, Subcommittee on Intergovernmental Relations. *Planning-Programming-Budgeting: Selected Comments.* 90th Congress, 1st Session. Washington, D.C., U.S. Government Printing Office, 1967, p. 12.

_____. (State-Local Finance Project, The George Washington University, Washington, D.C.) Personal interview. November 26, 1968.

Hiatt, Howard H. "Protecting the Medical Commons: Who Is Responsible?" *Trustee, 29*(10):14-17, October 1976.

Hill, David R. "Hill-Burton Program Planning Model Found Faulty" *Hospitals, 45*(24):46-50, December 16, 1971.

Hill, Morris. "A Goal Achievement Matrix for Evaluating Alternative Plans." *Journal of the American Institute of Planners, 34*(1):19-28, January 1968.

Ingbar, Mary, and Sidney S. Lee. "Economic Analysis as a Tool of Program Evaluation: Costs in a Home Care Program." In: *The Economics of Health and Medical Care.* Ann Arbor, Mich., University of Michigan Press, 1964, pp. 173-210.

Justison, Paul R. "Bed Requirements Methods and Processes." Denver, Colo., PACT Health Planning Center, February 1979. Mimeographed.

Karniewicz, Alfred J., Jr. "Estimating Coronary Care Bed Needs." *Hospitals, 44*(18):51-53, September 16, 1970.

Kidney Disease Program Analysis Group. "Kidney Disease Program Analysis: A Report to the Surgeon General." Washington, D.C., U.S. Public Health Service, 1967, p. 31. Mimeographed.

Kirschner, J. P. "An Annotated Bibliography of Decision Analytic Applications to Health Care." *Operations Research, 28*(1):97, January-February 1980.

Kissick, William L. "Planning, Programming and Budgeting in Health." *Medical Care, 5*(4):201-220, July-August 1967.

Klarman, Herbert E. "Syphilis Control Programs." In: *Measuring Benefits of Government Investments.* Edited by Robert Dorfman. Washington, D.C., The Brookings Institution, 1965, pp. 400-403.

Klee, A. J. "DARE Makes Your Solid Waste Decision." *American City,* *85*(2):100–103, February 1970.

Lee, S. M. *Goal Programming for Decision Analysis.* Philadelphia, Pa., Auerbach Publishing, 1972.

Lichfield, Nathaniel. "Cost-Benefit Analysis in Urban Expansion: A Case Study—Peterborough." *Regional Studies, 3*(2):123–155, 1969.

Luke, Roice D., and Melissa D. Culverwell. "Hospital Bed Availability and Discharge Patterns in the Short Run." *Inquiry, 17*:54–61, Spring 1980.

Machlup, Fritz. "Comments on 'Preventing High School Dropouts.' " In: *Measuring Benefits of Government Investments.* Edited by Robert Dorfman. Washington, D.C., The Brookings Institution, 1965, p. 156.

MacStravic, R. E. "A Case for a Hospital Census Variation and Bed Needs Formula." *American Journal of Health Planning, 3*:51–60, April 1978.

———. "Areawide Fluctuations in Hospital Daily Census." *Medical Care, 17*:1229–1237, December 1979.

———. "Admissions Scheduling and Capacity Pooling: Minimizing Hospital Bed Requirements." *Inquiry, 18*:345–350, Winter 1981.

———. "Average Life-cycle Occupancy: A Radical New Approach to Bed Needs and Appropriateness Review Decisions." *Health Care Planning and Marketing, 1*:25–33, April 1981.

———. "What Are Appropriate Occupancy Levels?" *Hospitals, 56*:93–98, September 16, 1982.

Mandel, Mark D. "Planning Report Series Generated by Acute Care Bed Need Model Based on Statewide Uniform Hospital Discharge Abstracts." Boston, University Center for Health Planning, November 1978. Mimeographed.

Marshall, A. W. *Cost/Benefit Analysis in Health.* Santa Monica, Calif., Rand Corp., 1965, p. 2.

McKean, Roland N. *Public Spending.* New York, McGraw-Hill, 1968, p. 135.

Mushkin, Thelma J. "Health as an Investment." *The Journal of Political Economy, 70*(5):129–157, October 1972.

Normile, F. R., and H. A. Ziel. "Too Many OB Beds?" *Hospitals, 44*(14):61, July 16, 1970.

Phillip, P. J. "Some Considerations Involved in Determining Optimum Size of Specialized Hospital Facilities." *Inquiry, 6*:45–48, December 1969.

Pollack, R. I. "Allocation of Resources for Neighborhood Improvement." *Journal of Environmental Systems, 1*(3):269–281, September 1971.

Prest, A. R., and R. Turvey. "Cost-Benefit Analysis: A Survey." *The Economic Journal, 73*(4):683, December 1965.

Public Health Service Region VIII. "The Square Root Formula: A Tool for Estimating the Number of Hospital Beds Needed." Denver, Colo., January 1980. Mimeographed.

"Report and Recommendations of the Finger Lakes Health Systems Agency Part 709.2, Task Force on 1985 Bed Need in the Southern Tier, Appendix B." Rochester, N.Y., August 25, 1982, pp. 9–10. Mimeographed.

Rice, Dorothy P. *Estimating the Cost of Illness.* Health Economics Series No. 6. Washington, D.C., U.S. Public Health Service, 1966.

Schilling, T. C. "The Life You Save May Be Your Own." In: *Problems in Public Expenditure Analysis.* Edited by Samuel B. Chase, Jr. Washington, D.C., The Brookings Institution, 1968, pp. 127–176.

Scitovsky, A. A. "Changes in the Costs of Treatment of Selected Illnesses, 1951–65." *American Economic Review, 57*(5):1182–1195, December 1967.

_____ . "Costs of Medical Treatment: Reply." *American Economic Review, 58*(4):936–940, September 1968.

Shonick, William. "Understanding the Nature of the Random Fluctuations of the Hospital Daily Census." *Medical Care, 10*:118–142, March–April 1972.

Siegel, Earl D. M., et al. "Measurement of Need and Utilization Rates for a Public Family Planning Program." *American Journal of Public Health, 59*(8):1322–1330, August 1969.

Student, Kurt R. "Understanding Changes in the Hospital." In: *Cost Control in Hospitals.* Edited by John R. Griffith et al. Ann Arbor, Mich., Health Administration Press, 1976, pp. 372–384.

U.S. Bureau of the Budget. "Report of the Committee on Chronic Kidney Disease." Washington, D.C., September 14, 1967. Mimeographed.

U.S. Congress, Joint Economic Committee, Subcommittee on Economy in Government. *Economic Analysis of Public Investment Decisions: Interest Rate Policy and Discount Analysis.* 90th Congress, 1st Session. Washington, D.C., U.S. Government Printing Office, 1967, p. 17.

_____ . *Planning-Programming-Budgeting: Selected Comments.* 90th Congress, 1st Session. Washington, D.C., U.S. Government Printing Office, 1967, p. 2.

_____ . *The Planning-Programming-Budgeting-System: Progress and Potentials.* Hearings. 90th Congress, 1st Session. September 14, 19, 20, 21, 1967. Washington, D.C., U.S. Government Printing Office, 1967, p. 160.

U.S. Congress, Senate, Subcommittee on National Security and International Operations. *Planning-Programming-Budgeting.* Hearings. 90th Congress, 2nd Session. Washington, D.C., U.S. Government Printing Office, 1968, p. 145.

Wenkert, Walter; John G. Hill; and Robert L. Berg. "Concepts and Methodology in Planning Patient Care Services." *Medical Care, 7*(4):327–331, July–August 1969.

HEALTH PLANS

Western Massachussetts HSA. *HSP,* January 1983, pp. 5.10–5.11.

Central New York HSA. *HSP,* August 1982, p. 451.

Northeastern New York HSA. *HSP,* December 1981, pp. 909–910.

NY-Penn HSA. *HSP 1981-1986,* Appendix, December 1980, pp. 97–113.

Hudson Valley HSA. *HSP,* October 1979, p. 143.

New York State. *Health Plan Volume I,* 1982, p. 217.

AUTHOR INDEX

SUBJECT INDEX

325